MALNUTRITION,
BEHAVIOR,
AND SOCIAL
ORGANIZATION

MALNUTRITION, BEHAVIOR, AND SOCIAL ORGANIZATION

Edited by
LAWRENCE S. GREENE

Department of Anthropology
University of Massachusetts/Boston
Boston, Massachusetts

ACADEMIC PRESS   New York   San Francisco   London   1977

A Subsidiary of Harcourt Brace Jovanovich, Publishers

ACADEMIC PRESS, INC.
111 Fifth Avenue, New York, New York 10003

United Kingdom Edition published by
ACADEMIC PRESS, INC. (LONDON) LTD.
24/28 Oval Road, London NW1

Library of Congress Cataloging in Publication Data

Main entry under title:

Malnutrition, behavior, and social organization.

    Includes bibliographies and index.
    1.   Malnutrition—Social aspects.   2.   Malnutrition in
children—Complications and sequelae.   3.   Social
structure.   4.   Developmental psychobiology.   I.   Greene,
Lawrence S.
RA645.N87M35   362.5   76-55975
ISBN 0-12-298050-6

PRINTED IN THE UNITED STATES OF AMERICA

Contents

List of Contributors

Numbers in parentheses indicate the pages on which the authors' contributions begin.

GEORGEDA BUCHBINDER (109), Department of Anthropology, Queens College, CUNY, Flushing, New York

EUGENE G. D'AQUILI (233), Departments of Psychiatry and Anthropology, University of Pennsylvania, Philadelphia, Pennsylvania

EDWARD FOULKS (219), Departments of Psychiatry and Anthropology, University of Pennsylvania, Philadelphia, Pennsylvania

LAWRENCE S. GREENE (55, 267), Department of Anthropology, University of Massachusetts/Boston, Boston, Massachusetts

SOLOMON H. KATZ (219, 253). University of Pennsylvania and the W. M. Krogman Center, Children's Hospital of Philadelphia, and the Eastern Pennsylvania Psychiatric Institute, Philadelphia, Pennsylvania

MARGARET MEAD (259), The American Museum of Natural History, New York, New York

GARY J. MIHALIK (233), Departments of Pediatrics and Psychiatry, University of Pennsylvania, Philadelphia, Pennsylvania

EDWARD MONTGOMERY (143), Department of Anthropology, Washington University—St. Louis, St. Louis, Missouri

ERNESTO POLLITT (19), Department of Nutrition and Food Science, Massachusetts Institute of Technology, Cambridge, Massachusetts

MERRILL S. READ* (95), National Institute of Child Health and Human Development, Bethesda, Maryland

B. ABBOTT SEGRAVES (173), Museum of Anthropology, The University of Michigan, Ann Arbor, Michigan

JOHN B. STANBURY (39), Department of Nutrition and Food Science, Massachusetts Institute of Technology, Cambridge, Massachusetts

ROBERT M. SUSKIND (1), Clinical Research Center, Massachusetts Institute of Technology, Cambridge, Massachusetts

CAROL A. THOMSON (19), Department of Nutrition and Food Science, Massachusetts Institute of Technology, Cambridge, Massachusetts

* Present address: Division of Family Health/Nutrition, Pan American Health Organization, Washington, D. C.

Preface

This book describes the widespread and significant effect of mal-nutrition and environmental impoverishment on the behavioral characteristics of members of many human populations. It also indi-cates how this behavioral variation then influences the sociocultural characteristics of these communities. The work argues that there is an environmentally produced biological basis for some portion of the behavioral variation that we see both within and among human popu-lations. Most previous writings have stressed genetic or sociocultural factors as the main determinants of behavioral variation. We feel that there is evidence indicating that malnutrition and experiential depri-vation have significant and enduring effects on neurological develop-ment and behavioral capacity, and that this evidence is now strong enough to require some modification of these earlier concepts so as to include environmental components.

These chapters suggest that many communities contain significant numbers of individuals with discrete behavioral limitations as a con-sequence of the interaction between early moderate to severe malnu-trition, intermittent diarrheal and respiratory disease, and physical–social experiential deprivation. We have developed a model that shows how the uneven distribution of essential resources within and among societies is the major cause of these high rates of behavioral retardation in the less-developed world and among the lower socioeconomic strata of some industrialized societies. We thus suggest that future analyses of sociocultural dynamics and change must in-clude a more systematic consideration of the effect of the differential division of environmental resources on the biologically based be-havioral characteristics of human subpopulations.

This book raises questions that are of great theoretical and practical concern to all disciplines interested in human biological and sociocultural variability. Our major focus is anthropological, which is reflected in a strong orientation toward a consideration of nutritional, disease, and experiential variation within a population or community context. We are thus less concerned with the single clinical entity than with the prevalence of environmentally induced behavioral limitation within a population and the effect of this phenomenon on the organization of human social units. In addition to its interest to anthropologists, this volume should be particularly useful to sociologists, psychologists, epidemiologists, nutritionists, regional planners, and community development specialists who are concerned with the interrelationships between the environment, behavior, and sociocultural processes.

The first five chapters outline the problem of malnutrition and its effect on behavioral development. In the first chapter Suskind discusses the characteristics and causation of protein–calorie malnutrition, with special emphasis on the interrelationship between nutrition and disease. The synergistic effect of malnutrition and disease experience in affecting behavioral development is an important point that is emphasized in most of the succeeding discussion.

Thomson and Pollitt then follow with a careful review of the influence of various types and degrees of protein–calorie malnutrition on behavioral capacity. This is an extremely common deficiency disease estimated to afflict more than 100 million children in its moderate and severe forms. The importance of age of onset and covarying experiential factors are considered in detail.

Stanbury reviews the effect of iodine malnutrition and hypothyroidism on nervous system development and behavior in human populations. Although uncommon in most of the industrialized world, iodine malnutrition, endemic goiter, and cretinism are still quite prevalent in many parts of the less-developed world—and were much more widespread in the recent past.

Building upon the previous chapters, Greene then describes the extremely high percentage of individuals with neurologically based behavioral limitations in a community in highland Ecuador where iodine, and to a lesser extent protein–calorie, malnutrition are common. The impact of these individuals on the sociocultural characteristics of the community is discussed and a model is presented that outlines the interrelationships among environmental, biological, and sociocultural systems.

In the fifth chapter, Read comments on the previous contributions and expands our considerations to include more moderate forms of protein–calorie malnutrition and their effect on human performance.

Chapters 6 and 7 consider different aspects of nutritional stress in two human populations. In Chapter 6, Buchbinder presents an exhaustive evaluation of the relationships among malnutrition, disease experience, and postcontact population decline among the Maring of highland New Guinea. She then proceeds to develop a general model that relates overpopulation, environmental degradation, and nutritional and disease stress to population decline.

Montgomery deals with the social structuring of nutrition in southern India. His chapter is primarily concerned with an attempt to isolate those social factors that are the best predictors of nutritional status in the community under study. The complexity of the problem is emphasized and tentative answers are presented.

The next three chapters by Segraves, Foulks and Katz, and d'Aquili and Mihalik discuss the broader question of the general relationships among malnutrition, behavior, and social organization. Segraves begins with a careful consideration of the effect of overpopulation on the biological and sociocultural characteristics of human populations. She stresses the point that excessive numbers is perhaps the major strain placed on all biological populations, and suggests that malnutrition and increased mortality are the inevitable outcome of population expansion, and its necessary regulator. She also takes the position that the implications of malnutrition are different for biological and sociocultural systems.

Foulks and Katz emphasize the relationships among nutrition, behavior, and culture by drawing upon their own extensive work among the North Alaskan Eskimo and a number of other ethnographic studies. They emphasize the responsiveness of the sociocultural system to environmental stresses and to the behavioral variation produced within a human population as a consequence of environmental factors.

D'Aquili and Mihalik use a biogenetic structuralist model to discuss the effect of malnutrition on the cognitive capacity of the individual. They conclude that in areas of severe endemic malnutrition it is likely that many affected individuals have rigid cognitive structures that do not easily undergo transformation. They suggest that populations containing significant numbers of such individuals are less capable of generating new social structures, and, owing to this inflexibility, are at a selective disadvantage when faced with the problem of dealing with environmental change.

The final three chapters are synthetic. Katz emphasizes the point that good parental nutrition is important if the parent is to supply adequate social stimulation to the developing child. He also points out the problem of cross-cultural behavioral comparisons, which has been raised by several of the papers. An interesting suggestion, which should be seriously considered, is the possible utility of a "nutritional protection agency" which would be empowered to mandate nutritional impact statements for various foods or programs.

In her commentary Mead suggests that the "population" and "food" problems are not beyond human influence. She stresses that the degree to which we actively or passively affect these questions will essentially be a function of our beliefs. Mead also raises a number of important moral questions concerning societal attitudes toward individuals who may have behavioral limitations. Perhaps her most salient point has to do with the uncertainties concerning the reversibility or irreversibility of neurological deficits and the danger in labeling people as such.

In the final chapter Greene picks up on Mead's comments and discusses the profound influence of experiential factors on brain growth and behavior in animal models. He also comments at some length on a number of points that have been raised throughout the volume.

This volume takes an ambitious first step toward evaluating the relationship between malnutrition and other environmental stresses, behavior, and social organization. We strongly believe that our data and arguments are convincing enough to require a reformulation of the current social scientific conceptualization of sociocultural organization and change so as to include a much broader biological perspective.

Acknowledgments

This volume is an outgrowth of a symposium held at the Annual Meeting of the American Association for the Advancement of Science in February 1976. A grant from the Hershey Food Corporation helped to organize that session. The cooperation of Mr. Arthur Herschman and the AAAS Meetings Office was also greatly appreciated. Dr. John B. Stanbury, at M.I.T., helped in many aspects of the organization of the symposium and was instrumental in facilitating my fieldwork in Ecuador as was Dr. Rodrigo Fierro-Benítez, at the Escuela Politecnica Nacional in Quito. Dr. Solomon Katz, Director of the Krogman Growth Center at the Children's Hospital of Philadelphia, also provided institutional support for this effort.

The staff from Academic Press provided excellent support, and a number of different typists and students helped in many ways. As always, my wife Sylvie and my children Jennifer, Dicken, and Jeremy sustained me.

1

Characteristics and Causation of Protein–Calorie Malnutrition in the Infant and Preschool Child

ROBERT M. SUSKIND

Massachusetts Institute of Technology

SIGNIFICANCE OF MALNUTRITION AS A HEALTH PROBLEM

A recent study of the mortality of children living in Latin American countries revealed that malnutrition was either directly or indirectly responsible for over one-third of the deaths of children under 5 years of age (Pan American Health Organization, 1971). A nutritional survey of over 190,000 children in 46 communities in Asia, Africa, and South America between 1963 and 1972 demonstrated a prevalence of moderate and severe forms of protein–calorie malnutrition (PCM) of up to 80% (Bengoa, 1974) (Table 1.1). From the above figures, it is estimated at the present time that roughly 100 million children under 5 years of age are severely or moderately malnourished. Malnutrition is a problem of the developed as well as the developing world. Although primary PCM is not commonly seen in hospitals in the United States, physicians are becoming increasingly aware that malnutrition secondary to other disease states such as renal, liver, or cardiopulmonary disease does exist. Secondary nutritional deficits must also be considered when looking at the nutritional status of children throughout the world.

1

TABLE 1.1

Worldwide Prevalence of Protein–Calorie Malnutrition (PCM)[a]

Region	Number of communities surveyed	Number of surveys	Number of children examined in each survey (range)	Percentage prevalence of PCM (range)		
				Severe forms	Moderate forms	Severe and moderate forms
Africa	16	32	34–184	0–9.8	5.6–66.0	7.3–73.0
Asia	10	16	43–326	0–20.0	13.0–73.8	14.8–80.3
Latin America	20	29	116–179	0–12.0	3.5–32.0	4.6–37.0
Total	46	77	34–326	0–20.0	3.5–73.8	4.6–80.3

[a]Adapted from Bengoa (1974).

CLASSIFICATION OF PCM

Gomez, Galavan, Cravioto, and Frenks (1955) were among the first to define malnutrition in terms of deficits in weight for age. Using local standards, they defined first-, second-, and third-degree malnutrition in terms of 75-90% of weight for age, 60-75% of weight for age, and less than 60% of weight for age, respectively. Today, Gomez's classification has been modified. Instead of using local standards, we use, as a basis of comparison, internationally accepted standards that have been derived from the mean weights and heights of healthy children from North America of Europe (Waterlow, 1974). Inasmuch as there is little or no evidence that genetic differences affect growth potential during the early years of life (Habicht, 1974), the norms of developed countries are applicable to communities where malnutrition is common.

Height for age and weight for height are often more useful tools for defining an individual's nutritional status than is weight for age, which does not take into consideration the height deficit caused by chronic malnutrition. The child who has a decreased weight for height is wasted or acutely malnourished, while the child who has a decreased height for age is stunted or chronically malnourished. In many cases, the malnourished child has evidence of both wasting and stunting. Waterlow (1974) has constructed a table by which a child can be classified according to his degree of malnutrition and retardation

TABLE 1.2

Classification According to Degree of Malnutrition and Retardation[a]

Grade	Retardation	Malnutrition
	Expected height for age (%)	Expected weight for height (%)
0	>95	>90
1	90–95	80–90
2	85–90	70–80
3	<85	<70

[a]Adapted from Waterlow, J. C. Some aspects of childhood malnutrition as a public health problem. *British Medical Journal*, 1974, 4, 88.

(Table 1.2). Studies from several developing countries have shown that both wasting and stunting are commonly seen in children between the ages of 1 and 2. By 3 or 4 years of age, children who may still be underweight for age are largely stunted rather than wasted (Waterlow, 1974). In other words, they have stopped growing linearly but are of normal weight for height. The purpose of the above classification of wasting and stunting is to serve as a guide for the development of intervention programs at a public-health and community level. Those children who have evidence of wasting need nutritional rehabilitation either as inpatients or outpatients. For those who are stunted but not wasted, the question becomes one of public-health intervention.

SEVERE MALNUTRITION: MARASMUS AND KWASHIORKOR

Children develop marasmus secondary to severe deprivation of both protein and calories with resultant growth retardation, weight loss, muscular atrophy, and severe decrease of subcutaneous tissue (Figure 1.1). Children with kwashiorkor, on the other hand, show signs and symptoms resulting from acute protein loss or deprivation. Children with "classic kwashiorkor" have a picture characterized by edema, skin lesions, hair changes, apathy, anorexia, an enlarged fatty liver and decreased serum total protein and albumin (Figure 1.2). These children have abundant subcutaneous fat and recover rapidly on a high protein diet (Behar, Viteri, Bressani, Arroyave, Squibb, & Schrimshaw, 1958). Obviously, there is a continuum between normality, marasmus, and kwashiorkor, each of which may be superimposed

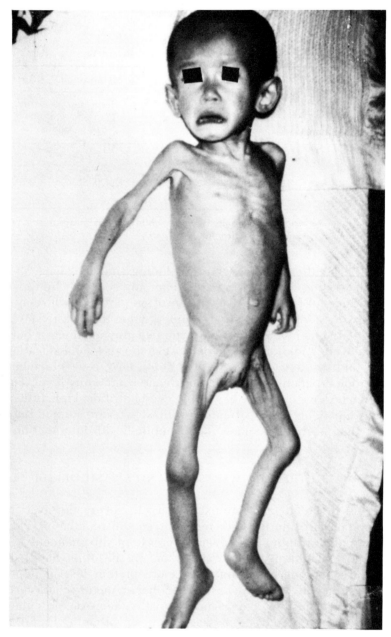

Figure 1.1. Marasmic child with evidence of growth retardation, weight loss, muscular atrophy, and severe loss of subcutaneous tissue. Reprinted with permission from Suskind (1975). (Courtesy of Medical Staff, Anemia and Malnutrition Research Center, Chiang Mai, Thailand.)

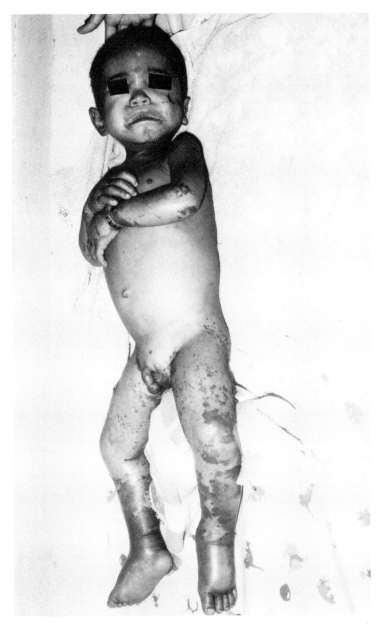

Figure 1.2. Child with kwashiorkor with evidence of edema, skin lesions, hair changes, apathy, anorexia, an enlarged fatty liver, and decreased serum total protein and albumin. Reprinted with permission from Suskind (1975). (Courtesy of Medical Staff, Anemia and Malnutrition Research Center, Chiang Mai, Thailand.)

5

on the other at any stage. The child with marasmus-kwashiorkor who combines the characteristics of both marasmus and kwashiorkor has a reduction in statural growth, weight, marked diminution of sub-cutaneous fat, a much greater degree of muscular wasting than do children with kwashiorkor, and a liver that has evidence of mild to moderate fatty infiltration. These children may have mild to moderate amounts of edema that disappear within a few days of the initiation of nutritional therapy, leaving only evidence of marasmus. The child with marasmus–kwashiorkor has total serum protein and serum albu-min values considerably lower than a child with marasmus in whom the values are usually only slightly below normal.

Because of variations in feeding practices and host requirements, the various states of malnutrition have characteristic age distributions. Marasmus usually occurs in children under 1 year of age when the quantity of mother's breast milk is not sufficient to provide adequate protein and calories for the growing child and when the supplemen-tary feeding is inadequate (Waterlow, Cravioto, & Stephen, 1960). Kwashiorkor, on the other hand, most commonly occurs after the age of 1 when a borderline diet becomes deficient in protein relative to calories as a result of superimposed infection (Scrimshaw & Behar, 1964).

Gopalan has outlined the differences between children with

TABLE 1.3

Kwashiorkor and Marasmus: Salient Features[a]

	Marasmus	Kwashiorkor
Age of maximal incidence	6–18 months	12–48 months
Emaciation	3+	1–2+
Edema	None	1–3+
Fatty infiltration of liver	None to 1+	3+
Skin changes	Infrequent	Frequent
Serum albumin	Almost normal	Markedly decreased
Serum enzymes		
Lipase	Normal	Markedly decreased
Amylase	Normal	Decreased
Esterase	Slightly decreased	Decreased
Serum lipids		
Triglycerides	Normal	Normal
Cholesterol	Normal	Lowered
Nonesterified fatty acids	Increased	Increased

[a]Adapted from Gopalan, C. Kwashiorkor and Marasmus: Evolution and distinguish-ing features. In R. A. McCance and E. M. Widdowson (Eds.), *Calorie deficiencies and protein deficiencies.* Boston: Little, Brown, 1968.

marasmus and kwashiorkor (Gopalan, 1968) (Table 1.3). His observations are similar to others who have described these syndromes from various parts of the world. Children with marasmus are generally younger than those with kwashiorkor. Serum proteins, including transferrin, albumin, lipase, amylase, esterase, and others, are relatively normal in children with marasmus, while they are significantly depressed in those children with kwashiorkor. There is fatty infiiltration of the liver in the children with kwashiorkor, while relatively normal liver histology is found in those with marasmus (Gopalan, 1968).

INFECTION AND MALNUTRITION

The role played by infection in the development of primary PCM has been outlined by Scrimshaw (1975), who noted that infection alters the nutritional status of the individual. The mechanisms by which the infection worsens nutritional status include reduction of appetite; a tendency for solid foods to be withdrawn, especially those of animal origin; increased metabolic losses of nitrogen, and decreased nitrogen absorption when infection involves the gastrointestinal tract. The use of purgatives and various home remedies may also have an adverse effect on absorption (Scrimshaw, 1975). The prevalence rates for infectious disease range from 50 to 60% during the 6–24-month age period.

The child's weight gain during the first 4–6 months is more or less normal, but thereafter the child develops recurrent infectious diseases leading to a leveling off of his weight and height gain. During the period when there is no significant weight gain, there is usually no increase in height, and the child's weight for height remains unchanged. However, should an intercurrent infection develop, a resultant decrease in weight for height would occur simultaneously, with a worsening of the child's nutritional status. The frequency of infectious diseases for the population of an Indian village in the Guatemalan highlands has been evaluated by Reyna-Barrios, Habicht, and Guzman (1971). Upper respiratory infections and acute diarrheal diseases were major problems for some children up to 7 years of age, with the peak incidence of both diseases occurring between 6 and 24 months of age.

Similar observations with regard to the frequency of infectious diseases in developing countries have been reported elsewhere. In the 1968 World Health Organization (WHO) monograph "Interactions of Nutrition and Infection," Scrimshaw (1968) outlined very clearly the consequences of infection on the nutritional status of man. It is now realized that even the mildest infectious diseases lead to increased urinary nitrogen excretion (Beisel, 1976a). The increased nitrogen excretion results mainly from increased mobilization of amino acids from peripheral muscle for gluconeogenesis in the liver with deamination and the excretion of nitrogen in the form of urea. Unless the loss of nitrogen is compensated for through increased dietary intake, depletion will occur with precipitation of a kwashiorkor-like syndrome.

Metabolic losses include not only nitrogen but potassium, magnesium, zinc, phosphorus, sulphur, and such vitamins as A, C, and B_2 (Beisel, 1976b). In addition to negative nitrogen balance, increased utilization, sequestration, or diversion from normal metabolic pathways of several nutrients occurs. In spite of the mobilization of amino acids from the peripheral muscle, there is a decrease in whole-blood amino acids after exposure to an infectious agent (Feigin, Klainer, Beisel, & Hornick, 1968).In addition to increased gluconeogenesis, there is increased diversion of amino acids for the synthesis of acute-phase proteins such as haptoglobin, C-reactive protein, alpha-I-antitrypsin, and alpha-II-macroglobulin in response to infection (Beisel, Cockerell, & Janssen, 1976).

MALNUTRITION AND THE IMMUNE RESPONSE

Cell-Mediated Immune Response

Several investigators have demonstrated that malnutrition affects all parameters of the host's immune response (Chandra, 1977; Douglas & Schopfer, 1977; Edelman, Suskind, Sirisinha, & Olson, 1973). Several host defenses have been implicated, including the cell-mediated immune response (Edelman et al., 1973), antibody production (Chandra, 1977), phagocytic and killing function of leukocytes (Douglas & Schopfer, 1977), and the complement system (Sirisinha, Suskind, Edelman, & Kulapongs, 1977).

The cell-mediated immune response, which is mediated through the thymus-dependent lymphocyte, plays a major role in the host's defense against viruses, mycobacteria, and fungi (Edelman, 1977). Malnutrition has been observed to have an adverse effect on the host's response to tuberculosis (Rich, 1951). The cell-mediated immune response is evaluated *in vivo* by intradermal skin testing and *in vitro* by the enumeration of T lymphocytes and by antigen and mitogen stimulation of isolated lymphocytes. Thymus-dependent lymphocytes are present in the peripheral blood, thymus, spleen, and peripheral lymph nodes.

Jackson was the first to call attention to lymphoid atrophy associated with severe PCM (Jackson, 1925). He noted at autopsy that children with kwashiorkor had atrophied thymus glands that were represented by only a few strands of tissue. In addition to atrophy of the thymus, lymph nodes, and tonsils, the spleen appears to be smaller in malnourished children (Mugerwa, 1971; Work, Ikekwunigwe, Jelliffee, Jelliffee, & Neumann, 1973; Smythe *et al.*, 1971). Several investigators have noted decreased numbers of positive tuberculin skin tests in children with PCM (Edelman, 1977). They have also found that with the nutritional rehabilitation, there was repair of the defective skin-test response (Edelman, 1977).

In vitro evaluation of lymphocytes from malnourished children reveals a decreased rate of DNA synthesis as determined by the uptake of tritiated thymidine by mitogenically stimulated peripheral lymphocyte (Edelman, 1977). With nutritional recovery *in vitro*, lymphocyte transformation becomes normal (Edelman, 1977). There is also a decreased number of circulating T cells in malnourished children (Chandra, 1974; Kulapongs, 1977). The thymus-dependent lymphopenia improves with nutritional recovery (Kulapongs, 1977). In the malnourished child, the depressed reaction to skin-test antigens correlates well with depressed *in vitro* lymphocyte function.

Recovery of both the *in vivo* and *in vitro* deficits occurs with improvement of nutritional status. The depressed cell-mediated immune response in malnourished children may be secondary to deficiencies of protein, calories, vitamins, or minerals, or to the suppressive effect of superimposed infection. These nutritional factors interact with the cell-mediated immune system, leading to its depression and the subsequent increase in susceptibility to those infections that are handled by it.

Humoral Immune Response

A secondary population of circulating lymphocytes, the B cell (bursa cell) or thymus-independent lymphocytes, is responsible for immunoglobulin production. Although the majority of malnourished children have elevated circulating immunoglobulins secondary to intercurrent infection, many of the children are unable to respond to various antigenic stimuli at the time of admission to the hospital (Chandra, 1977). In addition to the depressed antibody response to foreign antigens, the malnourished host is found to have depressed secretory IgA in nasopharyngeal and salivary secretions (Sirisinha, Suskind, Edelman, Asvapaka, & Olson, 1975). Chandra (1975) demonstrated that the secretory IgA antibody response to polio vaccine is reduced in malnourished children. Other changes that accompany the decreased secretory immunoglobulins are reduced digestive enzymes, atrophied gut wall, and an impaired hepatic reticuloendothelial system, all of which play an important role in the host's susceptibility to gram-negative organisms, especially from the gastrointestinal tract (Chandra, 1975)

Polymorphonuclear Leukocyte Response

Polymorphonuclear (PMN) leukocyte activity has also been studied in children with PCM using the Rebuck skin window. These studies have demonstrated normal PMN leukocyte mobilization and decreased mononuclear cell migration (Freyre, Chabes, Poenape, & Chabes, 1973). *In vitro* evaluation of the PMN leukocyte includes (1) chemotaxis or its ability to be attracted to a foreign subject; (2) phagocytosis or engulfment of the particle; and (3) the ability to form a phagocytic vacuole in order to digest and kill the microbe. The *in vitro* chemotactic response, although exhibiting some initial delay, appears to be normal at the end of a 3-hour *in vitro* assay (Douglas & Schopfer, 1977).

Phagocytosis of various particles by the PMN leukocyte is not affected by the child's nutritional state (Rosen, Geefhuysen, Anderson, Joffe, & Rabson, 1975; Seth & Chandra, 1972). In addition, the opsonic activity of the plasma in PCM does not appear to be depressed (Seth & Chandra, 1972). Electron microscopic studies of the PMN leukocyte from children with kwashiorkor using *Staphylococcus aurea, Escherichia coli*, and *Candida albicans* reveal no apparent abnormality in vacuole formation or degranulation (Douglas & Schopfer, 1977). The results of *in vitro* killing assays of PMN leukocytes from children with PCM have not been consistent. Some investigators have found defects in the ability of PMN leukocytes to kill the above organisms (Douglas & Schopfer, 1977), while others found no significant defect in bactericidal killing (Leitzmann, Vithayasai, Windecker, Suskind, & Olson, 1977).

The Complement System

The complement system, which is made up of several protein fractions, is important in chemotaxis of PMN leukocytes, monocytes, and eosinophils, opsonization of fungi, endotoxin inactivation, lysis of virus-infected cells, and bacteriolysis (Johnston, 1977). Sirisinha *et al.* (1977) found that most of the complement components were depressed in children with PCM. Hemolytic activity was also depressed. In addition, it was found that children with PCM had evidence of anticomplementary activity in their serum. It is well known that several substances, including endotoxin and immune complexes, activate complement or have anticomplementary activity. Klein, Suskind, Kulapongs, Mertz, and Olson (1977) have found that up to 50% of children with PCM have evidence of circulating endotoxin on admission. This may be one of the sources of anticomplementary activity found in many of these children.

In summary, the malnourished child is susceptible to infections that occur secondary to a depression of several host defenses. Once infected, the nutritional status further deteriorates, and he becomes even more susceptible to secondary infection. With either food supplementation or medical care, the continuous synergetic interaction of infection, nutrition, and immune status can be broken with subsequent improvement in the child's well-being.

INTRAUTERINE MALNUTRITION

Severe nutritional deficits during pregnancy affect intrauterine growth. Intrauterine growth deficits may be considered an indicator of maternal well-being as well as socioeconomic status (Gruenwald, 1968). The effects on fetal growth depend on the timing, severity, and duration of the nutritional insult. Subacute fetal distress occurs when the fetus is overdue and deprived of appropriate supplementation for days prior to birth, leading to a long, thin infant who is wasted but of normal length. In chronic fetal distress, deprivation extends over weeks and results in cessation of growth at an earlier period. Inasmuch as the fetus has not acquired any excess body fat, deficits in weight proportional to that of length occur. The external body proportions do not differ from those of the preterm infant of similar weight. The postterm sequelae of chronic fetal intrauterine malnutrition include height and weight retardation, in which the neonate tends to remain small for his age, in addition to defects in immunocompetency similar to those found in the postnatally malnourished child.

Several etiologic factors are involved in the development of intrauterine malnutrition, including maternal nutrition. The role of maternal nutrition in determining ultimate fetal weight has been pointed out by Lechtig, Yarbrough, Delgado, Habicht, Martorell, and Klein (1975), who found that caloric supplementation during pregnancy produced a significant increase in neonatal birth weight in short women from the lower socioeconomic group.

ETIOLOGY OF MALNUTRITION

The development of malnutrition depends on a complex interaction among nutrient, host, and environment (Scrimshaw & Behar, 1964). In nutritional deficiency states, nutrient quantities at the cellular level seem insufficient to satisfy metabolic needs (Scrimshaw & Behar, 1964). When considering protein intake, it is important to determine whether the protein contains adequate essential amino acids for body requirements. If there is, in fact, a lack of specific essential amino acid in the dietary protein of an individual, the consequences are the same with respect to protein synthesis by the body as if all essential amino acids were deficient in the food being considered. The body requires a supply of essential amino acids in proportion to those found in good-quality protein (Scrimshaw & Behar, 1964). The biological value of a food depends not only on its amino acid composition but on the degree to which amino acids are liberated during the process of digestion. Unless all of the essential amino acids are available at approximately the same time, complete utilization cannot occur (Scrimshaw & Behar, 1964). In addition, the caloric value of the diet has an effect on the biological value of the protein. If the diet is lacking in calories, dietary protein will be used for energy, with the same result as if the diet were inadequate in protein to that degree. Conversely, excess calories will spare the utilization of protein for energy. In many parts of the world, as a source of calories children consume foods that are grossly deficient in essential nutrients. In some underdeveloped countries, the high consumption of starchy vegetables such as sweet potato or cassava contributes to protein deficiency (Behar et al., 1958; Jelliffe, 1955).

Host factors affecting nutritional status include age, sex, activity, growth, pregnancy, lactation, and various pathological states. The nutrient requirements of a growing child are much different from those of an adult. During pregnancy and lactation, there are increased nutrient requirements. Activity and genetic variability must also be considered with regard to nutrient requirements. Environmental factors that affect the availability of nutrients include food production, food cost, food processing, food distribution, and population density (Scrimshaw, 1964). Temperature, humidity, and sunlight are other environmental factors that affect nutrient requirements of the host. Cultural influences, however, are among the most important environmental factors that determine what foods an individual eats (Scrimshaw & Behar, 1964). As an example, from the time of birth, northern Thai children are started on supplemental rice and bananas. These are often given prior to breast-feeding and lead to a decreased consumption of breast milk. As a result, children from northern Thailand often have protein deficits from early infancy from which they never recover. Prejudices such as the belief that cow's milk should not be fed to young infants because it causes diarrhea leads to decreased utilization of this important source of protein in certain parts of the world. Religious taboos such as the Hindu prohibition of beef consumption in India have greatly affected efforts to improve the nutritional status of the population. When a child has an acute case of diarrhea or another infection, kwashiorkor often develops as a result of the withdrawal of food and the metabolic loss of nitrogen. The nutritional status of the child is further stressed when he receives strong purgatives to eliminate parasites that the mother believes cause the diarrhea. These are only a few of the cultural factors that lead to a deficient nutritional status.

GENERAL PREVENTIVE MEASURES

Before initiating preventive measures, one must define the objectives of such a program. Some of the objectives that one might consider include: (1) detection of early signs of malnutrition in order to take remedial action; (2) reduction of the frequency and severity of infectious disease; (3) improvement of the nutritional status of women of childbearing age particularly through adolescence, pregnancy, and lactation; (4) reduction of the number of low-birth-weight infants and perinatal mortality and morbidity; (5) spacing of pregnancies at reasonable intervals (Bengoa, 1974).

Ignorance of nutritional requirements and the nutritive value of foods often plays an important role in the etiology of malnutrition (Scrimshaw & Behar, 1964). Nutrition education should be an integral part of all educational activities. However, educational measures must take into account the background of the population, including existing food habits and prejudices. If these factors are not taken into consideration, proposed nutritional changes are likely to be unrealistic and unacceptable (Scrimshaw & Behar, 1964). Relatively small alterations in established food habits are easier to put into effect than improving nutrition through radical changes. Nutrition education programs should recommend locally available foods.

The prevention of malnutrition requires that the basic principles of nutrition be included in the curriculum of teachers, nurses, social workers, agricultural extension workers, home economists, and other professionals who participate in community activities (Scrimshaw & Behar, 1964). In addition, political authorities and professionals at the university level in fields of medicine, public health, biological sciences, agriculture, economics, and other subjects directly or indirectly related to health and nutrition should be included.

Education and intervention programs should be aimed at those factors that will affect the nutritional status of the child. Early weaning practices are a problem with far-reaching consequences in developing countries (Bengoa, 1975). The risks of early weaning arise in large part from infection associated with poor hygiene, especially with respect to bottle preparation, and from the lack of knowledge and money to prepare a nutritious substitute. Mothers should be encouraged to breast-feed for as long as possible.

Supplementary feeding programs have been used on a wide scale for improving the nutritional state of the population. Pregnant and lactating women are frequently the recipients of such distribution. School lunch programs also play an important role in improving the nutritional status of children. Nutritional rehabilitation centers are another way in which supplementary feeding programs can be carried out (Bengoa, 1975). Nutritional and educational benefits of such a program are significant. These low-cost day-care-center programs are particularly intended for mild to moderately malnourished children who can be rehabilitated without the expense of full hospitalization. In addition to these rehabilitation centers, day-care centers have been set up in different parts of the world for children over 2 years of age. Children receive supplementation in these centers as well as in home visits. In terms of mother and family—child interaction, the supplemented child often receives more stimulation, rewards, and deferences than the unsupplemented child. The picture of the supplemented child is that of an active, independent, playful youngster who frequently verbalizes and demands. This behavior appears to stimulate the parent, resulting in more frequent and varied two-way interaction between child and parent and child and environment.

A relatively small addition of animal products to the diet of populations living on predominantly vegetable products can be beneficial (Scrimshaw, Taylor, & Gordon, 1961). The lysine deficiency of wheat and the tryptophan and lysine deficiency in corn are readily corrected by supplementation with animal products. Institute of Nutrition of Central America and Panama (INCAP) studies have demonstrated that adequate combinations of vegetable products result in food and diets with protein values comparable to those containing protein of animal origin.

Control of infectious disease should be given the highest priority because of the adverse effects of infection on the nutritional status of the child. Two programs with the highest priority for preventing the consequences of infection are immunization and the rehydration of children with diarrhea. Both of these steps are important in minimizing the metabolic response of children who are exposed to an infectious agent. Family planning is of paramount importance in most developing countries (Bengoa, 1975). It appears that a close relationship exists between malnutrition on the one hand and timing and spacing of the number of pregnancies on the other (Bisweswara, Rao, & Gopalan, 1969). The cumulative effect of pregnancies starting very early in life often leads to nutritional depletion of the mother. Therefore, family planning should be given its proper role in the prevention of PCM (Bengoa, 1974).

Successful implementation of the above programs should lead to a decreased prevalence of PCM throughout the world.

REFERENCES

Behar, M., Viteri, F., Bressani, R., Arroyave, G., Squibb, R., & Scrimshaw, N.S. Principles and treatment and prevention of severe protein malnutrition in children (kwashiorkor). *Annals of the New York Academy of Sciences*, 1958, 69, 954.

Beisel, W. R. Malnutrition as a consequence of stress. In R. M. Suskind (Ed.), *Malnutrition and the immune response*. New York: Raven Press, 1977. (a)

Beisel, W. R. Non specific host defense factors. In R. M. Suskind (Ed.), *Malnutrition and the immune response*. New York: Raven Press, 1977. (b)

Beisel, W. R., Cockerell, G. L., & Janssen, W. A. Nutritional effects on the responsiveness of plasma acute phase reactant glycoproteins. In R.M. Suskind (Ed.), *Malnutrition and the immune response*. New York: Raven Press, 1977.

Bengoa, J. M. The problem of malnutrition. *WHO Chronicle*, 1974, *28*, 3.
Bengoa, J. M. Prevention of protein calorie malnutrition. In R. E. Olson (Ed.), *Protein calorie malnutrition*. New York: Academic Press, 1975.
Bisweswara, R., Rao, K. N., & Gopalan, C. Nutrition and family size. *Journal of Nutrition and Diet*, 1969, *6*, 258.
Chandra, R. K. Rosette-forming T lymphocytes and cell-mediated immunity in malnutrition. *British Medical Journal*, 1974, *3*, 608.
Chandra, R. K. Reduced secretory antibody response to live attenuated measles and polio virus vaccines in malnourished children. *British Medical Journal*, 1975, *2*, 583.
Chandra, R. K. Immunoglobulins and antibody response in malnutrition. In R. M. Suskind (Ed.), *Malnutrition and the immune response*. New York: Raven Press, 1977.
Douglas, S., & Schopfer, K. Peripheral blood phagocytic disorders in children with protein energy malnutrition. In R. M. Suskind (Ed.), *Malnutrition and the immune response*. New York: Raven Press, 1977.
Edelman, R. Cell-mediated immune function in malnutrition. In R. M. Suskind (Ed.), *Malnutrition and the immune response*. New York: Raven Press, 1977.
Edelman, R., Suskind, R., Sirisinha, S., & Olson, R. E. Mechanisms of defective cutaneous hypersensitivity in children with protein–calorie malnutrition. *Lancet*, 1973, *1*, 506.
Feigin, R. D., Klainer, A. S., Beisel, W. R., & Hornick, R. B. Whole blood amino acids in experimentally induced typhoid fever in man. *New England Journal of Medicine*, 1968, *278*, 293.
Freyre, E. A., Chabes, A., Poenape, O., & Chabes, A. Abnormal rebuck skin window response in kwashiorkor. *Journal of Pediatrics*, 1973, *82*, 523.
Gomez, F., Galavan, R. P., Cravioto, J., & Frenks, S. Malnutrition in infancy and childhood with special reference to kwashiorkor. *Advances in Pediatrics*, 1955, *7*, 131.
Gopalan, C. Kwashiorkor and marasmus: Evolution and distinguishing features. In R. A. McCance & E. M. Widdowson (Eds.), *Calorie deficiencies and protein deficiencies*. Boston: Little Brown, 1968.
Gruenwald, P. Fetal growth as an indicator of socio-economic change. *Public Health Report*, 1968, *83*, 867.
Habicht, J. P. Height and weight standards for preschool children. How relevant are ethnic differences in growth potential? *Lancet*, 1974, *1*, 611.
Jackson, C. M. *The effects of inanition and malnutrition upon growth and structure*. New York: McGraw-Hill, 1925.
Jelliffe, D. B. Infant nutrition in the subtropics and tropics. *World Health Organization Monograph Series*, 1955, No. 25.
Johnston, R. B. The biology of the complement system. In R. M. Suskind (Ed.), *Malnutrition and the immune response*. New York: Raven Press, 1977.
Klein, K., Suskind, R. M., Kulapongs, P., Mertz, G., & Olson, R. E. Endotoxemia, a possible cause of decreased complement activity in malnourished Thai children with protein–calorie malnutrition. In R. M. Suskind (Ed.), *Malnutrition and the immune response*. New York: Raven Press, 1977.
Kulapongs, P. *In vitro* cellular immune response in Thai children with protein–calorie malnutrition. In R. M. Suskind (Ed.), *Malnutrition and the immune response*. New York: Raven Press, 1977.

Lechtig, A., Yarbrough, C., Delgado, H., Habicht, J. P., Martorell, R., & Klein, R.E. Influence of maternal nutrition on birth weight. *American Journal of Clinical Nutrition*, 1975, 28, 1223.

Leitzmann, C., Vithayasi, V., Windecker, P., Suskind, R., & Olson, R. E. Phagocytosis and killing function of polymorphonuclear leukocytes in Thai children with protein–calorie malnutrition. In R. M. Suskind (Ed.), *Malnutrition and the immune response*. New York: Raven Press, 1977.

Mugerwa, J. W. Lymphoreticular system in Kwashiorkor. *Journal of Pathology*, 1971, 105, 105.

Pan American Health Organization. Inter-American investigation of mortality in childhood, first year of investigation, provisional report. Pan American Health Organization, Washington. D.C., 1971.

Reyna-Barrios, J. M., Habicht, J. P., & Guzman, G. Method to increase coverage and improve the quality of ambulatory patient care in rural areas of Guatemala, using medical auxiliaries. Condresco Nacional de Salud, Documentos de trabajo, Tena II-6, pp. 1–16. *Revista del Colegio Medico de Guatemala*, 1971, 22, 134.

Rich, A. E. *The pathogenesis of tuberculosis.* (2nd ed.) Springfield, Illinois: Charles C. Thomas, 1951.

Rosen, E. U., Geefhuysen, J., Anderson, R., Joffe, M., & Rabson, A. R. Leukocyte function in children with kwashiorkor. *Archives of Diseases of Child*, 1975, 50, 220.

Scrimshaw, N. S. Interactions of nutrition and infection. *World Health Organization Monograph Series*, 1968, No. 57.

Scrimshaw, N. S. Interactions of malnutrition and infection: Advances in understanding In R. E. Olson (Ed.), *Protein–calorie malnutrition*. New York: Academic Press, 1975.

Scrimshaw, N. S., & Behar, M. Causes and prevention of malnutrition. In G. H. Beaton (Ed.), *Nutrition a comprehensive treatise*. New York: Academic Press, 1964.

Scrimshaw, N. S., Taylor, C. E., & Gordon, J. E. All-vegetable protein mixture for human feeding V clinical trials with INCAP mixtures 8 & 9 and with corn and beans. *American Journal of Clinical Nutrition*, 1961, 9, 196.

Seth, A., & Chandra, R.K. Opsonic activity of phagocytosis and bactericidal capacity of polymorphs in undernutrition. *Archives of Diseases of Children*, 1972, 47, 282.

Sirisinha, S., Suskind, R., Edelman, R., Asvapaka, C., & Olson, R. E. Secretory and serum IgA in children with protein–calorie malnutrition. *Pediatrics*, 1975, 55, 166.

Sirisinha, S., Suskind, R., Edelman, R., & Kulapongs, K. The complement system in protein–calorie malnutrition. In R. M. Suskind (Ed.), *Malnutrition and the immune response*. New York: Raven Press, 1977.

Smythe, P. M., Schonland, M., Breton-Stiles, K. K., Coovadia, H. M., Grace, H. J., Leoning, W. E. K., Mafoyane, A., Parent, M. A., & Vos, G. H. Thymic lymphatic deficiency and depression of cell–mediated immunity in protein calorie malnutrition *Lancet*, 1971, II, 939.

Suskind, R. M. Gastrointestinal changes in protein–calorie malnutrition. *Pediatric Clinics of North America*, 1975, 22, 873–883.

Waterlow, J. C. Some aspects of childhood malnutrition as a public health problem. *British Medical Journal*, 1974, 4, 88.

Waterlow, J. C., Cravioto, J., & Stephen, J. M. L. Protein malnutrition in man. *Advances in Protein Chemistry*, 1960, 15, 138.

Work, T. H., Ikekwunigwe, A., Jelliffe, D. B., Jelliffe, P., & Neumann, C. G. Tropical problems in nutrition. *Annals of Internal Medicine*, 1973, 79, 701.

2

Effects of Severe Protein–Calorie Malnutrition on Behavior in Human Populations[1]

CAROL A. THOMSON AND
ERNESTO POLLITT

Massachusetts Institute of Technology

INTRODUCTION

In the early 1900s, Correa (1908) described a pathological condition, *culebrilla*, in which young children appeared to be suffering from deficient intakes of animal foodstuffs. Later reports from South and Central America, India, Africa, China, Southeast Asia, the Middle East, and the Philippines helped to identify the disease, now called protein–calorie malnutrition (PCM). PCM refers to a deficiency disease caused by inadequate intake of proteins and/or calories.

Table 2.1 illustrates the point prevalence of severe and moderate forms of malnutrition in Latin America, Africa, and Asia. According to estimates from the World Health Organization (WHO, 1974) PCM among young children is "the most important urgent nutritional problem that must be faced by the developing countries." The point prevalence of severe PCM in those countries is approximately 0.5–

[1]Supported in part by funds from the Grant Foundation and Research Grant No. 1R22 HDO9228–01 from the National Institute of Child Health and Human Development.

19

TABLE 2.1

Ranges of Percentage Point Prevalence of Protein–Calorie Malnutrition in Community Studies Made between 1963 and 1972 in Three Regions the World[a]

Region	Number of communities	Number of surveys	Number of children examined	Percentage prevalence of PCM		
				Severe forms	Moderate forms	Severe and moderate forms
Latin America	20	29	116,179	0–12.0	3.5–32.0	4.6–37.0
Africa	16	32	34,184	0– 9.8	5.6–66.0	7.3–73.0
Asia	10	16	43,326	0–20.0	13.0–73.8	14.8–80.3
Total	46	77	193,689	0–20.0	3.5–73.8	4.6–80.3

[a] From Bengoa (1974, p. 5).

20.0% (median, 2.6%) of the population, whereas the point prevalence of more moderate forms of the same disease is 3.5–46.4% (median, 18.9%; Bengoa, 1974).

The focus of this paper is on the behavioral consequences of PCM in its severe forms: marasmus, kwashiorkor,[2] and marasmus-kwashiorkor. Our intentions are to review the data on severe PCM both during and after a severe episode, to identify problems in the design and method of studies used to gather these data, and to draw specific conclusions from the data within the context of the experimental errors identified.

Kwashiorkor is generally thought to result from an inadequate intake of proteins relative to calories, whereas marasmus arises from an inadequate intake of both calories and proteins. The marasmic individual is often in a state of starvation or near starvation. Cases of pure kwashiorkor or marasmus are rare. Rather, most severely malnourished individuals show signs and symptoms of both conditions or, at times, alternate between marasmus and kwashiorkor (Scrimshaw & Behar, 1961). This alternating or combined condition is sometimes referred to as marasmus–kwashiorkor (Waterlow & Alleyne, 1971).

Scrimshaw and Behar (1961) have advanced the idea that kwashiorkor and marasmus represent the extremes of a continuum of nutritional deficiency diseases. The base of the obtuse triangle in Figure 2.1 illustrates this continuum. Sides N–K and N–M indicate the paths taken by those children who develop kwashiorkor and marasmus, respectively. Lines b, c, and d illustrate various paths in the development of marasmus-kwashiorkor, and line a shows a child who initially showed signs of marasmus but eventually developed full-blown kwashiorkor.

In contrast to the idea of a kwashiorkor-marasmus continuum, Waterlow and Rutishauser (1974) maintain that the two deficiency conditions have different developmental histories. According to their data, distinct growth patterns emerge soon after birth in children with marasmus or kwashiorkor. As shown in Figure 2.2, the child with kwashiorkor grows normally for approximately the first 6 to 8 months of life. The growth rate then begins to decline, and by 14–18 months of age the child's weight for age has fallen to 60–80% of the standard (Boston Growth Norms; Nelson, Vaughn, & McKay, 1969). The child with marasmus shows poor growth from birth. Even in the first few

[2]Kwashiorkor, a word from the African Ga language meaning "displaced child," was associated with protein deficiency by Cicely Williams in 1935.

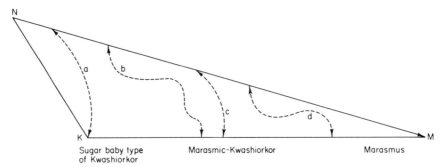

Figure 2.1.   Schematic representation of the development of the different types of protein malnutrition in children. (From N. S. Scrimshaw and M. Behar, Protein malnutrition in young children. *Science*, *133:* 2039–2047, 1961, p. 2045, with permission of the publisher. Copyright 1961 by the American Association for the Advancement of Science.)

months of life, the marasmic child has a large weight-for-age deficit (<60% of standard) and at no time shows normal weight gain.

The different natural histories of kwashiorkor and marasmus have also been documented by McLaren (1966) in Lebanon. His identification of the events that precede each deficiency disease appears in Figure 2.3. Marasmus is precipitated by an early abrupt weaning followed by ingestion of formula that has become contaminated by dirty water or unclean preparation. The child then suffers repeated gastrointestinal infections during which the mother withholds all foods in order to cure him. The combined effect of little or no food intake and repeated infections eventually results in marasmus. The history associated with a kwashiorkor child begins when he/she is weaned (at approximately 6 to 8 months) from breast milk and placed on the high-carbohydrate, low-protein family diet. Weaning often occurs when the mother finds she is again pregnant—hence, the term *displaced child*. The rapidly growing 6-month-old infant is severely weakened by this inadequate diet and succumbs to acute infections. Shortly, the child is in a state of acute kwashiorkor.

Validation of factors identified as diagnostic of kwashiorkor or marasmus is difficult because few data exist on the premorbid condition of these children and because etiologic factors vary with sociocultural (including dietary) practices, incidence of infection, and geographical area. Nevertheless, evaluation of existing data on postmorbidity allows several conclusions to be drawn that are pertinent to a discussion of the effects of PCM on behavior: (1) Marasmus usually develops shortly after birth and, by definition, is chronic; (2)

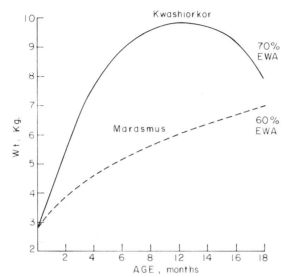

Figure 2.2. Hypothetical diagram of natural histories of kwashiorkor and marasmus, showing percentage of expected weight-for-age (EWA) for each syndrome. (From
Waterlow, J. C., and Rutishauser, I. H., Malnutrition in man. In J. Cravioto, L. Hambraeus, and B. Vahlquist (Eds.), *Symposia of the Swedish Nutrition Foundation* [*Vol.
XII*]: *Early malnutrition and mental development.* Stockholm: Almquist & Wiksell,
1974, p. 15.)

kwashiorkor usually occurs in the second year of life and is most likely
to be an acute, rather than a chronic, condition; (3) marasmus appears
to have multiple etiologic factors, whereas kwashiorkor is likely to be
the result of a dietary deficiency.

Clinical descriptions documenting the behavior of children with
acute kwashiorkor have been available since the 1950s (Autret &
Behar, 1954; Geber & Dean, 1956; Jelliffe, 1965). Apathy, irritability,
anorexia, and withdrawal are the most commonly observed symptoms,
with immobility present in the most severe cases. Neurological
examinations have frequently shown hypotonia, poorly developed
motor skills, and, occasionally, cortical and subcortical atrophy (Marcondes *et al.*, 1973). Some researchers found they could not obtain
measurable responses on mental-development scales from children
severely affected with kwashiorkor (Geber & Dean, 1956).

Fewer behavioral and neurological data exist for the marasmic condition. However, reduced activity, hypotonia, cortical atrophy, and
reduced brain weight have been reported in children with marasmus
(Marcondes *et al.*, 1973; Winick & Rosso, 1969). Also, the marasmic

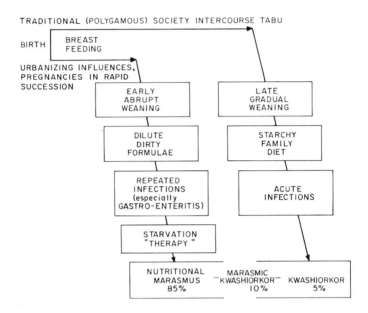

Figure 2.3. Paths leading from early weaning to nutritional marasmus and from protracted breast feeding to kwashiorkor. Percentages of types of malnutrition are based on figures for Jordan but are typical for many other countries. (From D. S. McLaren, A fresh look at protein–calorie malnutrition. *Lancet*, 1966, 2:485–488, p. 485.)

child, unlike the anorexic kwashiorkor child, is often reported to be hungry (McCance & Widdowson, 1966).

Two recent studies have provided new data on the behavioral signs of children suffering from PCM. One of these studies, by Lester and colleagues in Guatemala (Lester, 1975; Lester, Klein, & Martinez, 1975), examined the attentional processes of malnourished children. The other, conducted in India by Graves (1976), focused on the social interaction of children with PCM.

Lester and co-workers conducted two experiments in which they tested 12-month-old infants diagnosed as having second- and third-degree malnutrition according to the classification devised by Gomez *et al.* (1956). In the second and more rigorous of the two experiments, these infants and a control group of normal-weight infants listened to an intermittent 90-dB tone, which was alternated between sets of trials at 750 or 400 Hz. During the trails, the infants' heart rates were monitored to record cardiac deceleration, a reaction previously shown to correlate with the orienting reflex to a novel stimulus. While the normal infants showed the cardiac-orienting response to both the onset and change of the tones, the malnourished group showed no cardiac-orienting response to either condition. In addition, the normal group became habituated to repeated tones, whereas the malnourished infants evidenced inconsistent and minimal responses.

The results of this experiment indicate that malnourished infants are less responsive to environmental stimuli than infants of normal weight and, as a result, process less information from the environment. These researchers (Lester et al., 1975) point out that reduced responsivity or attention to impinging environmental stimulation may be the source of the poor performance of these children on psychological tests. There is some evidence, as will become clear later, that rehabilitation from malnutrition does not attenuate this attentional defect.

The mother–child interaction and exploratory behavior of 23 children afflicted with second-degree PCM were investigated by Graves (1976) in West Bengal, India. She found that age was an important determinant of the amount of exploratory behavior and the quality of mother–child interaction for the malnourished children but not for the well-nourished controls. Older malnourished children (13–18 months) received less attention from their mothers and in their exploratory behavior were less vigorous than controls of comparable age. There were no differences between malnourished children and controls in the younger group (7–12 months) on either of these measures. It was noted that the older malnourished children maintained close physical contact with their mothers despite the lack of attention given to them.

Although neither Graves (1976) nor Lester and colleagues (1975) identified the type of malnutrition (kwashiorkor, marasmus, or marasmus–kwashiorkor) suffered by their index groups, both studies have contributed excellent quantitative data that have furthered our knowledge of the behavior of children afflicted with PCM.

Let us now turn to studies that focus on the behavioral sequelae of severe malnutrition. Because almost all of these studies employed retrospective research designs, many of them lack diagnostic information and, therefore, make comparisons between and within samples difficult. For this reason, we have selected for discussion only those studies in which the index children were hospitalized for their nutritional condition. Studies of children with marasmus, kwashiorkor, marasmus–kwashiorkor, or unspecified severe malnutrition will be dealt with in order.

MARASMUS

Research on children rehabilitated from nutritional marasmus has been conducted by Brockman and Ricciuti (1971) and Pollitt and Granoff (1967) in Peru; Monckeberg (1968) in Chile; Cabak and Najdanvic (1965) in Yugoslavia, and Yaktin and McLaren (1970) and McLaren, Yaktin, Kanawati, Sabbagh, and Kadi (1973) in Lebanon. (See review by Pollitt, 1973.) These studies show that in almost all cases in which the anthropometric data indicated a state of marasmus, the children's performance on global intelligence or developmental tests, which were standardized in industrialized countries, was approximately 1–2 standard deviations below the average IQ of 100. In addition, one study (Yaktin & McLaren, 1970) showed that psychological stimulation increased the IQ scores of a group of severely malnourished children by about 28 points, but their scores were still below the level indicative of normal functioning.

These findings, however, must be evaluated in terms of the problems in study designs and the limitations of the methods used to measure intellectual functioning in severely malnourished children. With the *ex post facto* design, data seldom are found on developmental characteristics of the children before the onset of malnutrition. Their birth weights, attainment of developmental landmarks, or morbidity prior to the onset of PCM are usually unavailable. These unknown antecedent variables could well have been limiting factors in the children's mental development. In brief, because of insufficient premorbid data, the cause of the intellectual impairment observed in rehabilitated PCM children cannot unequivocally be established.

Socioeconomic factors, such as level of maternal education, per capita income of the family, and occupation of the father, are also known to correlate with the IQ score. A thorough investigation of these variables was not undertaken in any of the four studies. It is possible that one or several socioeconomic factors could have operated in favor of the control group. While the use of siblings or matched pairs for control subjects (as in the studies of Pollitt and Granoff [1967] and Brockman and Ricciuti [1971]) diminishes the effect of these nonnutritional factors, it does not eliminate the problem. More will be said on the use of siblings and matched pairs as controls later.

It is noteworthy that the average age at which the malnourished children were hospitalized in each of these 5 studies was less than 1 year (10.6 months). This finding is consistent with the observation of Waterlow and Rutishauser (1974) that marasmus occurs early in life—earlier, as we shall see shortly, than kwashiorkor.

KWASHIORKOR

Investigators studying the effects of kwashiorkor have also used the *ex post facto,* or retrospective, design and standardized global intelligence tests for IQ measurement. These studies, then, suffer from the same limitations in design and methodology as those dealing with marasmus. Premorbid development variables and socioeconomic factors that may affect the IQ score are for the most part unknown.

Kwashiorkor has been studied by Geber and Dean (1956) in Africa; Cravioto and Robles (1965) and Birch, Pineiro, Alcalde, Toca, and Cravioto (1971) in Mexico; Champakam, Srikantia, and Gopalan (1968) in India; Barrera-Moncada (1963) in Venezuela; and Evans, Moodie, and Hansen (1971) in South Africa. (See review by Pollitt, 1973.)

Examination of the data from these studies yields a picture somewhat different from that drawn from studies of marasmic children. Evidence shows that, although early kwashiorkor may, in some cases, depress intellectual functioning as measured by intelligence tests, the sequelae is not as severe as that observed in children with a history of early marasmus. It appears, in fact, that the detrimental effects of early kwashiorkor on intellectual functioning may ameliorate with time.

Notably, the mean age at which children were hospitalized for kwashiorkor was later than for marasmus. In all studies reviewed in which the age at hospitalization could be determined, admission occurred after 12 months of age; in four of the studies, the mean age of admission was greater than 15 months. The average ages at hospitalization for marasmus (10.6 months) and for kwashiorkor (> 15 months), then, correspond well to the developmental patterns for the two deficiencies illustrated in Figure 2.2.

These studies on kwashiorkor highlight a methodological problem in measuring intellectual function in severely malnourished children. The use in other cultures of intelligence tests developed and standardized in Great Britain or the United States precludes meaningful interpretation of the IQ scores obtained. In other words, cross-cultural application of these tests results in distorted data of questionable significance. For example, in the study by Birch *et al.* (1971), the mean score of the index group was a statistically significant 13 points below that of the control group. The means of both groups, however, were well below average by United States standards. Without an appropriate reference group, in this case, lower-class Mexican children ranging in age from 5 to 13 years, it is impossible to interpret the test scores accurately. In other words, without knowledge of the mean or standard deviation of the population from which the reference group is drawn, no meaningful statements can be made about the levels of functioning of these two groups. For example, if the mean score for this population were 80 with a standard deviation (SD) of 5, the index group with a mean score of 68 would indeed be subnormal. If, on the other hand, the SD were 16, the index group would be functioning within the normal range. Finally, if the normal mean were 90, with an SD of 10, both groups would be functioning at a subnormal level. Thus, cross-cultural transference of a test without restandardization can, at best, yield only a gross indication of relative IQ scores with little meaningful interpretation. Problems associated with cross-cultural transference of standardized tests will be explored further in the discussion section.

SEVERE UNDIFFERENTIATED, OR MIXED-TYPE PCM

The studies reviewed in this section also focus on severely malnourished children who were hospitalized for their condition, but the authors either did not specify the type of malnutrition or included several types within their target sample.

This section includes studies conducted by the following researchers: Fisher, Killcross, Simonsson, and Elgie (1972) in Zambia; Chase and Martin (1970) in the United States; Cravioto and DeLicardie (1972, 1973) and DeLicardie and Cravioto (1974) in Mexico; Klein, Lester, Yarbrough, and Habicht (1975) in Guatemala; and Hertzig, Birch, Richardson, and Tizard (1972), Richardson, Birch, and Hertzig (1973), Richardson (1974), and Richardson, Birch, and Ragbeer (1975) in Jamaica. (See review by Pollitt, 1973.)[3] Again, nearly all of the studies included in this broadly defined category utilized retrospective designs and intelligence tests standardized in the United States and Great Britain.

Data from studies reviewed in this section are difficult to summarize. The children's ages at admission and testing, the degree and type of malnutrition, as well as the type of test used to assess intellectual functioning vary widely from study to study. The longitudinal investigation of Richardson et al. (1973, 1975; Richardson, 1974),

---

[3]Two other studies that would usually fall in this category have been omitted because the subjects were not hospitalized, the index samples were too small, or the IQ data were highly variable. (See, Graham & Adrianzen, 1972; Winick, Meyer, & Harris, 1975.)

however, illustrates the necessity of making progressive modifications in hypotheses regarding the effects of malnutrition on intellectual functioning. Hertzig *et al.* (1972), in the first paper on the project in Jamaica, reported findings on IQ tests given to malnourished children, their siblings, and a comparison group. The results show that IQ test scores differed among the three groups: The healthy controls scored higher than the siblings of the index group, who, in turn, scored higher than the affected children. A second paper (Richardson *et al.*, 1973) dealt with school achievement, grades, and teacher evaluations of these same children. The between-group differences found on these measures led to an examination of the quality of home life (Richardson, 1974) and home behavior (Richardson *et al.*, 1975) of the malnourished sample.

The complexity of the factors affecting the relationship between malnutrition and IQ unfolded as this study progressed, causing continual modification of the original hypotheses. The emergent network of interrelated factors surrounding the malnourished child led the investigators to suggest that the entire ecology surrounding the malnourished child must be the target of investigation rather than simply measurement of IQ. Two other studies in this section lend substantial support to this suggestion. In a longitudinal study, Cravioto and De-Licardie (1973) and DeLicardie and Cravioto (1974) found significant differences in the quality of home life from 6 months of age between children who developed malnutrition and those who did not, but no differences on gross measures of socioeconomic status. Similarly, Chase and Martin (1970) found that analyses of socioeconomic environmental variables revealed few differences between malnourished and control groups; however, there appeared to be more environmental stress on the families of index children.

In summary of the section, while generalization on these mixed or undifferentiated studies is not feasible because of methodological variability, several of them have elucidated the importance of the ecology surrounding the malnourished child.

DISCUSSION

To date, the data on the behavioral effects of early severe malnutrition do not present a clear picture. The validity of the findings remains questionable because of (1) limitations inherent in the *ex post facto* design; and (2) methodological problems in the measurement of the dependent variable.

In an attempt to cope with the problems of *ex post facto* design and to control score variability due to nonnutritional factors, some investigators have matched index and control children for demographic, social, and economic correlates of intelligence (e.g., Champakam *et al.*, 1968). Despite such efforts, it is likely that the technique of matching only accounts for a few of the variables that actually differentiate malnourished from well-nourished children. An episode of severe malnutrition must be considered the "lawful product of numerous antecedents (Campbell & Stanley, 1972)." Thus, while matching achieves some measure of control over selected variables, large numbers of known and unknown factors continue to contribute considerable error to the study design. For example, different nutritional states may result from differences in child-care practices and maternal attitudes.

Another way of attempting to control for extraneous variability is to select siblings of the index children to act as controls (Pollitt & Granoff, 1967; Birch *et al.*, 1971). This method is based on the belief that environmental influences on mental development are constant for all siblings. To the contrary, however, use of this method may result in selective unmatching. Malnutrition in one child when his siblings are healthy signals the possibility that differential treatment is being applied, that the malnourished child himself is responding differently to the same treatment, or that both factors are operating conjointly. Thus, the apparent control is deceptive.

Social ecology data on severely malnourished children support the contention of nonequivalence between index and control children in the studies reviewed. Longitudinal studies on populations in which malnutrition is endemic show that low birth weight—an indication of prenatal malnutrition—often precedes the development of severe postnatal PCM (Stickney, Beghin, Urrutia, Mata, Arenales, Habicht, Lechtig, & Yarbrough, unpublished ms.). The probability of normal intellectual development among children with low birth weights is diminished (Babson & Henderson, 1974; Davies & Tizard, 1975; Fitzhardinge & Steven, 1972). Also, many studies in South America (Graham & Morales, 1963; Wray & Aguirre, 1969), Central America (Richardson, 1974), Asia (Levinson, 1974; Rao, Pralhad, & Swaminathan, 1969), and Africa (Kanawati, Darwish, & McLaren, 1974) have found that families of children with third-degree malnutrition are more disadvantaged than the typical or average family living in the same locale. Families of malnourished children are often more crowded, poorer, and more unstable than families in which the children are adequately nourished. Mothers of malnourished children were found to be less educated, more illiterate, and in poorer health than mothers of well-nourished children. Additionally, while some studies (DeLicardie & Cravioto, 1974) have reported no differences on broad indicators of socioeconomic status between control and index families, significant differences were found on measures of maternal care in favor of families having adequately nourished children. Therefore, those socioeconomic and behavioral factors that distinguish populations with prevalent malnutrition from those without also serve to distinguish families with and without malnutrition within a population.

In all fairness, then, it must be said that the available studies fall short of satisfying the criteria of internal validity in scientific research or "the basic minimum without which any experiment is uninterpretable (Campbell & Stanley, 1972, pp. 5–6)." There is no way of determining the contribution of nonnutritional factors in the observed effects. Consequently, the data thus far collected on the nutrition factor, independent from or in interaction with the other intervening variables, fulfill the role of hypotheses generating more than hypotheses testing.

The longitudinal research design used by Cravioto and DeLicardie (1972, 1973; DeLicardie & Cravioto, 1974) in Mexico is unique in that it includes extensive data on the children's postnatal development from the time of birth. Thus, it was possible to identify antecedent variables that were characteristic of children who developed malnutrition before the age of 5. This design allows one to determine the specific onset of the nutritional deprivation, its clinical nature, and final course. Such data are simply unavailable elsewhere. Apparently, however, the authors did not measure the duration of the index children's deficiencies. As data on duration and subsequent mental effects are sorely lacking in the literature, this was an unfortunate omission.

Limitations in the method of measuring the dependent variable also must be recognized. With few exceptions, the investigators used global intelligence tests, such as the Binet, Wechsler, or Bayley Scales, and compared average IQ or DQ scores between groups for the purpose of inferring statistical differences in levels of intellectual function. In other words, global standardized tests often are used as though the validity of their constructs is transferable from one culture to another.

The study by Hertzig et al. (1972) illustrates the erroneousness of this assumption. Although these investigators have stated that the test was used to obtain relative differences in IQ scores, the question of construct validity is pertinent. Using norms established in the United

States on the Wechsler IQ test, Hertzig *et al.* (1972) compared the
scores of severely malnourished Jamaican children (N = 71), their
siblings (N = 38), and a control group (N = 71). The mean full-scale
scores were: 57.72 (SD = 10.75) for the malnourished children, 61.84
(SD = 10.82) for their siblings, and 65.99 (SD = 13.59) for the controls.
These scores were all significantly different from one another at the
0.10 level or better. Even so, the highest mean IQ, that of the control
group, was approximately four points below the level used in the
United States to indicate mental retardation. Despite this fact,
teachers were reported rating only 28% of the controls as doing poor or
severely backward school work and 41% as having outstanding, good,
or above average work (Richardson, 1974). A chi square test between
the control children's full scale IQ scores and the overall evaluation of
their school performance was significant. Statistical evidence to the
contrary, it is apparent that the mean IQ of the control group is
conceptually discrepant with the reported school performance. If
these children were participants in special-education programs, the
discrepancy might be explainable. In this context, both IQ scores and
school evaluation would be valid. However, none of the reports on
this study suggest such a possibility. These data, therefore, must be
accepted *prima facie* and the assumption made that the discrepancy
arose from unidentified cultural and social idiosyncrasies of the population sampled, or the validity of the IQ scores must be questioned.
The second alternative is perhaps more reasonable, considering that
the numerical differences between groups are relatively small (although statistically significant at some arbitrary probability level) and
are of no specific behavioral significance.

CONCLUSIONS

The research problems described above notwithstanding, an
analysis of the studies to date does provide a basis for some inferences. First, only the marasmic studies report consistent findings of
detrimental effects. Studies on kwashiorkor, by contrast, yield inconsistent results. Second, victims of marasmus were observed to perform
about 1–2 standard deviations below control groups on mental
tests—a deficit greater in magnitude than victims of other types of
malnutrition. Third, marasmus, unlike other types of malnutrition,
does not appear to ameliorate with age. (The intervention study of
Yaktin and McLaren [1970] was the only study reporting evidence to
the contrary.) Conversely, when detrimental effects are reported with

kwashiorkor, they are of relatively small magnitude and often ameliorate with age.

Observed differences in the magnitude of cognitive deficits between marasmic and kwashiorkor children may stem from the different development patterns of the two deficiency diseases. Nutritional marasmus is a chronic condition with an onset in early postnatal or even in prenatal life. Kwashiorkor, on the other hand, is acute and generally occurs after the first year of life. These differences in timing—in onset and duration—may determine the severity of behavioral sequelae for two reasons: First, the onset of marasmus occurs during a period of accelerated brain growth; second, it results in a lengthy disruption of child–environment interaction that is damaging to intellectual development.

Research data have indicated that the severely malnourished child is characterized by apathy, withdrawal, low responsivity to environmental stimuli, and poor attention maintenance. This lethargic behavior ensures that the child fares poorly in competition for attention with others in the environment. As a result, learning experiences are curtailed because of reduced reciprocal mother–child interaction. Low-level functioning also limits the child's capacity to act on his own environment. According to the theories of Piaget, limitations in child-environment interactions interfere with intellectual development. In Piagetian terms, the child and the environment form an interlocking system whose interactions generate mental structures, which are the substrates of knowledge. The low level of interaction typical of the malnourished child thus leads to developmental retardation.

Under conditions in which the nutritional deprivation is severe but of short duration, with an onset during the second year of life, the vulnerability of the child appears to be largely reduced. In addition to the possibly decreased vulnerability of the brain during this time, the child is already working with signs and symbols. Contact with the environment and learning experiences is, therefore, only temporarily interrupted.

Regarding the issue of timing and vulnerability, it must be noted that some of the studies reviewed attempted to establish correlations between the onset of nutritional conditions, as defined by age at hospitalization, and magnitude of subsequent intellectual deficit (e.g., Cravioto & Robles, 1965; Chase & Martin, 1970). The rationale was that the younger the brain, the more vulnerable it was to subsequent damage. However, most studies have little, if any, data on the nutritional and developmental histories of the target children before they were hospitalized. Consequently, error in estimated time of onset produces inconsistent findings regarding periods of heightened or lessened vulnerability. At this time, no definitive statements can be made regarding brain vulnerability and age of onset within relatively small (± 6 months) time periods. Valid inferences on this relationship are possible for gross time periods only, such as comparing year one with year two.

Some conclusions on PCM and intellectual development can now be presented for populations in which malnutrition is endemic. First, a child who suffers severe, chronic protein–calorie deficiency in the first 12 months of life may show a severe intellectual impairment (DQ 1–2 standard deviations below average) when compared with standards from his population. Second, a child suffering severe, acute protein–calorie deficiency in the second year of life may, but generally does not, show intellectual impairment (as measured by developmental tests) when compared with standards from his population. Third and finally, the question of intellectual impairment resulting from either acute, severe PCM in the first 12 months of life or chronic, severe PCM occurring in the second year of life cannot yet be answered because of insufficient data.

REFERENCES

Autret, M., & Behar, M. *Sindrome policarencial infantil (kwashiorkor) and its preven-tion in Central America.* Rome: Food and Agricultural Organization of the United Nations, 1954.

Babson, S. G., & Henderson, N. B. Fetal undergrowth: Relation of head growth to later intellectual performance. *Pediatrics*, 1974, 53, 890–894.

Barrera-Moncada, G. *Estudios sobre alteraciones del crecimiento y del desarrollo psicologico del sindrome pluricarencial (kwashiorkor).* Caracas, Venezuela: Editora Grafas, 1963.

Bengoa, J. M. The problem of malnutrition. *WHO Chronicle*, 1974, 28, 3–7.

Birch, H. E., Pineiro, C., Alcalde, E., Toca, T., & Cravioto, J. Relation of kwashiorkor in early childhood and intelligence at school age. *Pediatric Research*, 1971, 5, 579–585.

Brockman, L., & Ricciuti, H. Severe protein-calorie malnutrition and cognitive development in infancy and early childhood. *Developmental Psychology*, 1971, 4, 312.

Cabak, V., & Najdanvic, R. Effect of undernutrition in early life on physical and mental development. *Archives of Disease in Childhood*, 1965, 40, 532–534.

Campbell, D. T., & Stanley, J. C. *Experimental and quasiexperimental designs for research.* (9th ed.) Chicago: Rand McNally, 1972.

Champakam, S., Srikantia, S., & Gopalan, C. Kwashiorkor and mental development. *American Journal of Clinical Nutrition*, 1968, 21, 844–852.

Chase, H. P., & Martin, H. P. Undernutrition and child development. *New England Journal of Medicine*, 1970, *232*, 933.

Correa, P. G. Que es la culebrilla? *Revista Medicina Yucatan*, 1908, 3(6).

Cravioto, J., & DeLicardie, E. Environmental correlates of severe clinical malnutrition and language development in survivors from kwashiorkor or marasmus. *Nutrition, the nervous system and behavior*. Washington, D. C.: Pan American Health Organization, 1972.

Cravioto, J., & DeLicardie, E. Longitudinal study of language development in severely malnourished children. In G. Serban (Ed.), *Nutrition and mental functions*. New York: Plenum Press, 1973. Pp. 143–191.

Cravioto, J., & Robles, B. Evolution of adaptive and motor behavior during rehabilitation from kwashiorkor. *American Journal of Orthopsychiatry*, 1965, 35, 449–464.

Davies, P. A., & Tizzard, J. P. M. Very low birthweight and subsequent neurological defect (with special reference to spastic diplegia). *Developmental Medicine and Child Neurology*, 1975, *17*, 3–17.

DeLicardie, E. R., & Cravioto, J. Behavioral responsiveness of survivors of clinically severe malnutrition to cognitive demands. In J. Cravioto, L. Hambraeus, & B. Vahlquist (Eds.), *Symposia of the Swedish Nutrition Foundation (Vol. XII): Early malnutrition and mental development*. Stockholm: Almqvist & Wiksell, 1974.

Evans, D., Moodie, A., Hansen, J. Kwashiorkor and intellectual development. *South African Medical Journal*, 1971, *45*, 1413–1426.

Fisher, M. M., Killcross, M. C., Simonsson, M., & Elgie, K. A. Malnutrition and reasoning ability in Zambian school children. *Transactions of the Royal Society of Tropical Medicine and Hygiene*, 1972, 66, 471–478.

Fitzhardinge, P. M., & Steven, E. M. The small-for-date infant. II. Neurological and intellectual sequelae. *Pediatrics*, 1972, *49*, 50–57.

Geber, M., & Dean, R. F. A. The psychological changes accompanying kwashiorkor. *Courrier*, 1956, 6, 3–14.

Gomez, F., Ramos, R., Frenk, S., Cravioto, J., Chavez, R., & Vasquez, J. Mortality in second and third degree malnutrition. *Journal of Tropical Pediatrics*. 1956, 2, 77–83.

Graham, G., & Adrianzen, B. Late "catch-up" growth after severe infantile malnutrition. *The Johns Hopkins Medical Journal*. 1972, *131*, 204–211.

Graham, G. C., & Morales, E. Studies in infantile malnutrition. I. Nature of the problem in Peru. *Journal of Nutrition*, 1963, 79, 479–487.

Graves, P. L. Nutrition, infant behavior and maternal characteristics: A pilot study in West Bengal, India. *American Journal of Clinical Nutrition*, 1976, 29, 305–319.

Hertzig, M. E., Birch, H. G., Richardson, S. A., & Tizard, J. Intellectual levels of school children severely malnourished during the first two years of life. *Pediatrics*, 1972, *49*, 814–823.

Jelliffe, D. B. Effect of malnutrition on behavioral and social development. In *Proceedings of western hemisphere nutrition congress*. Chicago: American Medical Association, 1965. Pp. 24–27.

Kanawati, A., Darwish, O., & McLaren, D. Failure to thrive in Lebanon. III. Family income, expenditure and possessions. *Acta Paediatrica Scandanavia*, 1974, 63, 108–112.

Klein, R., Lester, B., Yarbrough, C., & Habicht, J. On malnutrition and mental development: Some preliminary findings. In A. Chavez (Ed.), *International congress of nutrition 9th*. New York: S. Karger, 1975.

Lester, B. M. Cardiac habituation of the orienting response to an auditory signal in infants of varying nutritional status. *Developmental Psychology*, 1975, *11*, 432–442.

Lester, B., Klein, R., & Martinez, S. The use of habituation in the study of the effects of infantile malnutrition. *Developmental Psychobiology*, 1975, *8*, 541–546.

Levinson, F. J. *Morinda: An economic analysis of malnutrition among young children in rural India.* Cambridge, Massachusetts: Cornell/MIT International Nutrition Policy Series, 1974.

Marcondes, E., Lefevre, A., Machado, D., Garcia de Barros, N., Cavallo, A., Gazal, S., Quarentei, G., Setian, N., Valente, M., & Barbieri, D. Neuropsychomotor development and pneumoencephalographic changes in children with severe malnutrition. *Environmental Child Health*, 1973, *19*, 135–139.

McCance, R. A., & Widdowson, E. M. Protein deficiencies and caloric deficiencies. *The Lancet*, 1966, *2*, 158–159.

McLaren, D. S. A fresh look at protein-calorie malnutrition. *The Lancet*, 1966, *2*, 485–488.

McLaren, D. S., Yaktin, U. S., Kanawati, A., Sabbagh, S., & Kadi, Z. The subsequent mental and physical development of rehabilitated marasmic infants. *Journal of Mental Deficiency Research*, 1973, *17*, 273–281.

Monckeberg, F. Effect of early marasmic malnutrition on subsequent physical and psychological development. In N. Scrimshaw & J. Gordon (Eds.), *Malnutrition, learning and behavior.* Cambridge, Massachusetts: MIT Press, 1968.

Nelson, W. E., Vaughn, V. C., & McKay, R. J. *Textbook of pediatrics.* (9th ed.) Philadelphia: Saunders, 1969.

Pollitt, E. Behavioral correlates of severe malnutrition in man. In W. Moore, M. Silverberg, & M. Read (Eds.), *Nutrition, growth and development of North American Indian children.* Washington, D. C.: DHEW, 1973. Pp. 72–76 (Publication No. (NIH) 72-26).

Pollitt, E., & Granoff, B. Mental and motor development of Peruvian children treated for severe malnutrition. *Revista Interamericana de Psicologia*, 1967, *1*, 93–102.

Rao, N., Pralhad, Darsham Singh, & Swaminathan, M. C. Nutritional status of preschool children of rural communities near Hyderabad city. *Indian Journal of Medical Research*, 1969, *57*, 2132–2346.

Richardson, S. A. The background histories of school children severely malnourished in infancy. *Advances in Pediatrics*, 1974, *21*, 167–195.

Richardson, S. A., Birch, H. G., & Hertzig, M. E. School performance of children who were severely malnourished in infancy. *American Journal of Mental Deficiency*, 1973, *77*, 623–632.

Richardson, S., Birch, H., & Ragbeer, C. The behaviour of children at home who were severely malnourished in the first two years of life. *Journal of Biosocial Science*, 1975, *7*, 255–267.

Scrimshaw, N. S. & Behar, M. Protein malnutrition in young children. *Science*, 1961, *133*, 2039–2047.

Stickney, R. E., Beghin, I. D., Urrutia, J. J., Mata, L. J. Arenales, P., Habicht, J-P., Lechtig, A., & Yarbrough, C. Systems analysis in nutrition and health planning: Approximate model relating birth weight and age to risk of deficient growth *Archivos Latino Americanos de Nutricion.* (Submitted for publication.)

Waterlow, J.C., & Alleyne, G.A.O. Protein malnutrition in children: advances in knowledge in the last ten years. *Advances in Protein Chemistry*, 1971, *25*, 117–241.

Waterlow, J. C., & Rutishauser, H. E. Malnutrition in man. In J. Cravioto, L. Hambraeus, & B. Vahlquist (Eds.), *Symposia of the Swedish Nutrition Foundation (Vol. XII): Early malnutrition and mental development.* Stockholm: Almqvist & Wiksell, 1974.

Winick, M., Meyer, K., & Harris, R. Malnutrition and environmental enrichment by early adoption. *Science*, 1975, *190*, 1173–1175.

Winick, M., & Rosso, P. Head circumference and cellular growth of the brain in normal and marasmic children. *Journal of Pediatrics*, 1969, *74*, 774–778.

World Health Organization. Malnutrition and mental development. *WHO Chronicle*, 1974, *28*, 95–102.

Wray, J. D., & Aguirre, A. Protein-calorie malnutrition in Candelaria, Colombia. 1. Prevalence: Social and demographic causal factors. *Journal of Tropical Pediatrics*, 1969, *15*, 76–98.

Yaktin, U. S., & McLaren, D. S. The behavioral development in infants recovering from severe malnutrition. *Journal of Mental Deficiency Research*, 1970, *14*, 25–32.

3

The Role of the Thyroid in the Development of the Human Nervous System

JOHN B. STANBURY

Massachusetts Institute of Technology

The thyroid gland synthesizes, stores, and secretes the two thyroid hormones triiodothyronine and thyroxine. These contain three and four atoms of iodine, respectively. In order to maintain a normal flow of hormones and to avoid goiter, it is necessary that an adult obtain a daily intake of at least 40–50 μg of iodine in his food and drink. Requirements during infancy and childhood are not much less. The thyroid hormones make their appearance at the 12th week of fetal life and thereafter play an important role in differentiation, development, and growth.

The paragraphs that follow summarize the control of thyroid function and the role of iodine deficiency in limiting the availability of thyroid hormones. The relationship between the thyroid and endemic thyroid disease, especially cretinism, is explored. The concept is developed that the deleterious impact of iodine deficiency extends well beyond overt cretinism and may have important implications for social and economic development.

THYROID CONTROL

The thyroid gland functions in an intimate, negative feedback-coordinated control system with the anterior pituitary (Figure 3.1). The thyrotrophin-secreting cells of the pituitary are governed in part, at least, by a tripeptide-releasing factor from the hypothalamus. It probably performs as a regulator of the setpoint of the control system but is probably not involved in its finer tuning. When the concentration of thyroid hormone in the peripheral blood falls for any reason, this is sensed by the thyrotrophic cells, which increase their synthesis and secretion of thyrotrophic hormone. If the iodine that is available in the diet falls below 40–50 μg per day, the control system responds in such a way as to increase sharply the secretory rate of thyrotrophic hormone. This stimulates the thyroid to increase its clearance of iodide from the blood and to synthesize and secrete hormone. It also induces growth and increased vascularity in the gland. The quantity of iodide that is present in the thyroid is also a regulatory factor in thyroid function in that the sensitivity of the thyroid to thyrotrophin increases as the iodine of the gland falls.

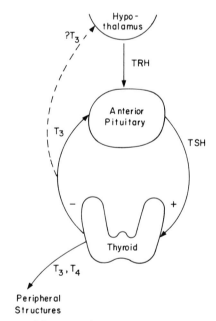

Figure 3.1.   Diagram of the control system of the thyroid gland. T_4: thyroxine. T_3: triiodothyronine. TRH: thyrotropin-releasing hormone. TSH: thyrotropin.

The thyroid system is able to compensate for large changes in iodine supply over long periods of time. There is enough stored hormone in the normal gland to meet physiological needs for many weeks even if no hormone is synthesized. On the other hand, a reduction in iodine supply below minimal needs evokes growth of the thyroid. If the changes are early and limited in magnitude, partial or complete involution and restoration of normal glandular architecture may be achieved by restoration of normal iodine supply. If the growth stimulus is strong, and if it extends over a long period of time, not only may the thyroid become quite large, but nodule formation and degenerative changes may appear. Also, if iodine deficiency is severe and protracted, it may be impossible to achieve a normal secretory rate of the thyroid hormones even with intense hyperplasia of the gland, and the patient may then become hypothyroid.

The thyroid gland may attempt to compensate in still another way for a reduction in iodide supply. It does this by shifting synthesis away from thyroxine and toward triiodothyronine. The latter requires less iodine in its chemical structure and is a more potent hormone. Thus, examination of the iodinated amino acids in the iodide-deficient thyroid discloses that the ratio of the hormone precursor monoiodotyrosine to diiodotyrosine is increased as is the ratio of triiodothyronine to thyroxine. Similarly, there may be maintenance of a normal concentration of triiodothyronine in the peripheral blood even when the concentration of thyroxine has fallen as a result of severe iodide deficiency.

IODINE SUPPLY

Iodine, which is an essential element in the diet of all vertebrates, is sparsely and irregularly scattered over the surface of the earth (Goldschmidt, 1954, p. 602). Nowhere does it exist naturally in high concentration. Principal commercial sources are from the nitrate deposits of northern Chile, from distillation of seaweeds, and as a byproduct of the petroleum industry. It can also be obtained from sea water, but the process is expensive. It tends to be somewhat more abundant in soils that are old and those that acquire iodine as a result of fallout from sea mists. It seems to be particularly wanting in recent soils, such as those that have been laid down following late Pleistocene glaciations. Most of the iodine in the human diet comes from food, while only a small fraction of the daily intake is in water.

Iodine readily crosses the placenta. The nursing infant acquires its iodine in breast milk, and since the breast is less efficient than the thyroid in clearing iodide from the blood, the infant is at a disadvantage when there is a limited supply. Hypothyroid mothers may give birth to normal infants if iodide supply is normal. On the other hand, the fetus without a thyroid is dependent on transplacental transfer of thyroid hormones, which is limited in man. Such infants are often born with retarded bone age, but early recognition and treatment usually permits catch-up growth and normal development, although the universality of this rule is by no means established.

ENDEMIC GOITER

Endemic goiter, the response of man to iodine deficiency, is an extremely widespread disorder. It has been estimated that there may be as many as 200 million people in the world with significant enlargements of their thyroids. The disease was highly prevalent in the Great Lakes district and in the Pacific Northwest of this country two generations ago, before the introduction of preventive measures. At the present time, it is an important and frequent disorder throughout the entire Andean world; in the central regions of South America; in the Alps, where iodide prophylaxis has not yet been instituted; in the Middle East, including Iran, Iraq, and Afghanistan; throughout the arc of the Himalayas; in New Guinea and New Zealand; and in a great band that extends across the heart of Africa (Langer, 1960, p. 9). There are doubtless foci of endemic goiter in central Russia and in China, but only limited information is available from these regions. Endemic goiter is not confined to mountainous regions; for example, it has been until recently a problem in the Low Countries, where iodide intake is still considerably below that in the United States. It has also been reported along the coastal regions of Panama.

Wherever appropriate measurements have been made, almost without exception, endemic goiter has been associated with a mean daily estimated iodine intake of less than 40–50 μg. An exception appears to be the region near Cali, Colombia, where Gaitán and his co-workers (Gaitán et al., 1968) have observed persisting goiter in a region where iodine deficiency prevailed until the early or middle 1950s but has now been corrected by prophylactic administration of iodized salt. Nevertheless, Gaitán and his colleagues have observed goiter in children with ample iodide intake and have also obtained evidence for the presence in water of a goitrogenic agent (Gaitán, 1973). Even in that region, however, there was a sharp and dramatic reduction in the incidence and severity of goiter when prophylactic administration of iodized salt began. In Idjwi Island in eastern Zaire, Ermans, Delange, and their colleagues (Delange, 1974; Delange & Ermans, 1971; Ermans, Delange, van der Velden, & Kinthaert, 1972) have found that iodide deficiency exists throughout the island but that goiter is much more severe in the northern half. These investigators have suggested that there is a second factor in addition to iodide deficiency that is responsible for the expression of the disease in that region.

The clinical pattern of endemic goiter varies from one region to another, depending, at least in large part, on the severity of iodine deficiency and its duration. When the disease is most severe, the majority of the population group may have visible goiters, and many of these will be nodular, especially in adults (Figure 2). Particularly in severely affected regions, even preadolescent children will have nodular thyroids. On the other hand, in a region of mild endemicity, one may be able to demonstrate modest enlargement of the thyroid in only 20–30% of periadolescent children. In general, when the disorder is mild, more girls than boys are affected. With advancing age, the goiter tends to persist in the female and to become smaller or disappear in the male.

Cultural and economic events are important in the epidemiology of endemic goiter. Maisterrena observed a virtual disappearance of endemic goiter over the course of a few years in a Mexican village when a new road opened possibilities for increased social mobility and the importation of dietary items from other parts of the country (Maisterrena, Tovar, & Chávez, 1969, p. 397). Pharoah, on the other hand, found evidence for a sharp increase in the manifestations of iodide deficiency in New Guinea when the traditional sources for salt, which

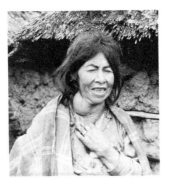

Figure 3.2.   Large nodular goiter in an adult woman from the region of Tocachi, Ecuador.

proved to be high in iodine content, were abandoned as a highly refined iodide-free salt became available commercially (Pharoah & Hornabrook, 1974).

While it may be that factors other than iodide deficiency, such as goitrogens in foods, may contribute to endemic goiter, without exception the introduction of iodide prophylaxis has been followed by a dramatic reduction or elimination of endemic goiter. This has been strikingly true in the United States where recent surveys have failed to disclose the presence of a focus of endemic goiter (Matovinovic, Child, Nichaman, & Trowbridge, 1974, p. 67). It has also been observed in Switzerland, Guatemala, Colombia, New Zealand, and elsewhere. The most efficient technique of prophylaxis has been the distribution of iodide through iodization of salt. Where salt is not distributed through commercial channels, or where iodization is not practical, prophylaxis has been effectively implemented through administration of iodized poppyseed oil. The iodide is slowly released from the oil and gives protection for 2 to 4 years. Programs with iodized oil have been highly successful in Central Africa (Thilly, Delange, Goldstein-Golaire, & Ermans, 1973), New Guinea (Hetzel & Pharoah, 1971), Peru (Pretell et al., 1969), and Ecuador (Fierro-Benítez, Ramírez, Estrella, Jaramillo, Díaz, & Urresta, 1969).

In the past few decades, there has been a tendency for the intake of iodide to rise in the developed countries. In the United States, since the early 1950s, the average intake of iodine has risen from approximately 150 μg per day to approximately 500 μg per day. The reason for this is the wide use of iodide in a variety of industries. For example, iodine is widely used in the baking industry as a dough conditioner. It is also used as iodophores in a variety of sterilization processes, such as in the milk industry. It finds its way into a number of widely used food colorings and vitamin preparations.

Endemic goiter is a disease of the undeveloped populations of the world. Thus, it is found most often in association not only with iodide deficiency but with borderline or overt malnutrition, monotonous diets, and other evidence of impoverishment. Accordingly, it becomes difficult to disentangle the role that various factors may play in growth and development when not only is there iodide and perhaps thyroid deficiency but also protein and calorie deficiency, poor clothing, exposure to cold and other environmental stresses, frequent infections, heavy parasitism, and so on. Formal and informal education may be severely limited and may compound the difficulty in assessing possible limitations on intellectual growth caused by iodide deficiency and goiter.

SPORADIC CONGENITAL HYPOTHYROIDISM

Among populations with ample iodine intake, approximately 1 newborn in every 8,000 has congenital hypothyroidism. The majority of these have an absence of the thyroid gland. Some either have a small remnant of thyroid tissue at the root of the tongue or along the track of the embryonic descent of the thyroid (Bauman, Bode, Hayek, & Crawford, 1976). A few are congenitally hypothyroid because of a genetic absence of an enzyme or a structural or transport protein intimately involved in the synthesis or control of thyroid function (Stanbury, 1972, p. 223). It has not yet been established whether complete absence of the thyroid causes permanent and irreversible damage if there is not thyroid replacement medication beginning at birth, but the evidence favors the view that more often than not there is permanent damage but that a considerable degree of catch-up can be achieved (Smith, Blizzard, & Wilkins, 1957). Those patients who have remnants of functioning thyroid tissue have a better outlook.

If untreated, the congenitally athyreotic child inevitably develops severe retardation in statural, neurological, and intellectual development. The changes are classically described. They include short stature, permanent changes in the structure of the hip, causing a waddling gait, severe intellectual retardation, and, in the postnatal period, persistent jaundice, poor feeding, hypothermia, and often an umbilical hernia.

Animal models of the congenital athyreotic state in man have been produced in the rat, lamb (Hollingsworth, Belin, Packer, Moser, & McKean, 1975), and monkey. Thus, destruction of the fetal thyroid with radioactive iodine or by administration of an antithyroid drug such as methimazole causes delayed growth and impaired myelination in the central nervous system. These changes have been carefully studied in several laboratories (Balázs, Cocks, Eayrs, & Kovács, 1971; Kerr, Allen, Scheffler, & Couture, 1974, p. 221; Legrand & Bout, 1970, p. 1199; Pickering, 1968, p. 182; Rosman, Malone, Helfenstein, & Kraft, 1972). Balázs et al. (1971), have shown that in the orderly development of the rat nervous system, there are migrations of groups of cells to their appropriate positions and a shift when thyroid hormone becomes available from proliferation to differentiation in certain cell groups. These processes are severely disrupted if thyroid hormone is not available at the appropriate time. In thyroid deficiency, the arborization of nerve cells and development of synapses are retarded, the interconnections between cells are reduced, and myelination is impaired. Glial cell number is reduced as well.

Changes induced by thyroid deficiency have been studied particularly in the cerebellum of the developing rat. Rosman has shown that the myelination delay was not dependent on poor nutrition in his hypothyroid rats. The changes in the rat brain must be corrected before postnatal day 14, or they are irreversible. This probably corresponds to the early postnatal period in man. The result of these changes may be permanent impairment in muscular coordination and ability to learn, which may not be apparent unless considerable demand is placed on the subject of the experiment (Eayrs, 1971).

It is interesting to note that in experimental animals fetal hypothyroidism induced by fetal thyroidectomy or by antithyroid drugs causes permanent changes in hearing (Deol, 1973, p. 235), whereas fetal hypothyroidism in man is not accompanied by deafness. On the other hand, hypothyroidism engendered by severe iodide deficiency during fetal and postnatal life in man is often accompanied by deafness. There appears to be no satisfactory explanation for these phenomena.

ENDEMIC CRETINISM

Severe endemic goiter is almost always accompanied by the appearance of a number of individuals in the community who have certain distinctive features in common and are clearly distinguishable from the rest of the population. They are characterized by short stature, severe intellectual deprivation, some dysarthria or no speech at all, oftentimes by deafness, deformities of the hip, a shuffling gait, or, in extreme cases, an inability to walk, with severe contractures, and a rather characteristic facies. Dentition may be delayed and disordered. They often, but not always, have large nodular goiters. They have classically been called "cretins" and have been likened to the congenitally hypothyroid subject of nonendemic regions.

In the course of studies on endemic goiter and endemic cretinism in northern India in the first decade of this century, McCarrison described two somewhat overlapping types of endemic cretinism; one type he designated as the neurological form and the other the myxedematous form (McCarrison, 1908, p. 1275). Patients with the neurological form had predominantly deafmutism, awkward gait and movement, squint, and spastic neurological signs (Figure 3.3). The myxedematous form, on the other hand, tended to be shorter in stature, not to be deaf, and to have primarily the signs of hypothyroidism (Figure 3.4). McCarrison was careful to point out that these were not

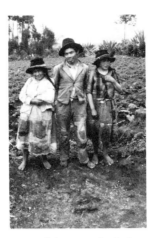

Figure 3.3.   Three cretins of the neurological type from rural Ecuador.

mutually exclusive diagnoses and that there were intermediate forms. The large majority of his patients belonged to the neurological form of the disease, and that is the form that has been most commonly encountered in the Andes, North India, Switzerland, Australia, and New Guinea (Fierro-Benítez, Peñafiel, DeGroot, & Ramírez, 1969, p. 296). On the other hand, the predominant type of cretinism in Zaire is the myxedematous form (Bastenie, Ermans, Thys, Beckers, van den Schrieck, & Visscher, 1962, p. 187). There, the typical retarded subject in the endemic goiter region has very short stature, markedly delayed

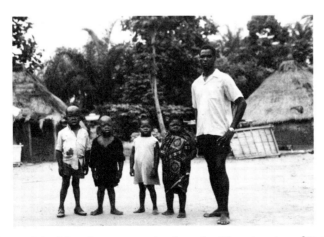

Figure 3.4.   Myxedematous cretins from the Ubangi region of Zaire.

bone age, and displays sexual infantilism and the full clinical and laboratory panoply of severe hypothyroidism.

Studies in New Guinea, Indonesia, Central Africa, and Ecuador have all demonstrated severe iodide deficiency in association with endemic cretinism. There has, however, often been evidence of partial or complete compensation for the hypothyroid state in the neurological cretin; thus, often, the plasma concentrations of thyroid hormones, including thyroid stimulating hormone (TSH), may be normal or nearly normal. Presumably, in those individuals, the structural and functional damage occurred during an earlier phase in development, whereas by the time of study sufficient iodide had become available for partial or complete compensation. Nevertheless, by that time, permanent structural damage had already occurred.

The causes behind the differences between the neurological and the myxedematous forms of the disorder are not known, nor is it known why one form should predominate in one part of the world and another elsewhere. Clearly, in the myxedematous cretin of central Africa, there has been damage to the thyroid gland at some stage in development. These subjects have thyroid glands that are no larger than normal, or scarcely larger, but they are in normal position. They have extremely high plasma levels of thyrotrophic hormone, but their thyroids do not respond to this stimulation as usual with hyperplasia. Specimens of these thyroids have not yet become available for histological studies. The neurological cretin of Indonesia or the Andes achieves better growth and bony development because his thyroid is able to use more efficiently the available iodine, at least in certain stages of development, and accordingly he escapes some of the features that characterize the myxedematous cretin of central Africa (Bastenie et al., 1962, p. 187; Djokomoeljanto, 1974). There may be other dietary factors in the pathogenesis of myxedematous cretinism, such as ingestion of cassava, which contains large amounts of cyanogenic glycoside. This possibility has been explored by Ermans and his colleagues (Delange & Ermans, 1971, p. 1354).

Perhaps the strongest evidence favoring iodide deficiency as the principal etiologic factor in endemic cretinism is its virtual disappearance when iodide prophylaxis is introduced. The disorder has long since disappeared from Switzerland. Controlled studies in Ecuador (Ramírez et al., 1972, p. 223) and Africa (Delange, personal communication) have indicated a sharp reduction or disappearance with iodized oil prophylaxis, and this has also been documented in New Guinea (Pharoah, Butterfield, & Hetzel, 1972, p. 201).

The incidence of endemic cretinism in any particular endemia is uncertain for several reasons, among them most particularly because of the problem of precise definition and ascertainment. There is no satisfactory definition of cretinism, and there are no precise criteria for diagnosis in the individual subject. Furthermore, the diagnosis is generally not made until at least 1 year of age, and by this time the death rate among affected infants has probably been higher than that of their peers. Later, the death rate is presumably higher among cretins than in the general population, but information on this point is lacking. One can only report that at any one time there is a certain prevalence of patients who conform to such diagnostic criteria as he would like to employ. Thus, prior to the iodized oil prophylaxis program in two villages in rural Ecuador, the prevalence of cretinism was approximately 8% (Fierro-Benítez et al., 1969, p. 306). On Idjwi Island in eastern Zaire, Dumont, Delange, and Ermans (1969, p. 91) found a rate of approximately 1%. On the other hand, villages have been observed in the Ubangi region of northwestern Zaire in which 4.2% of the population conformed to the customary pattern of myxedematous cretinism (Thilly, Delange, Camus, Berquist, & Ermans, 1974, p. 121), and similar figures have been reported by Ibbertson in Nepal (Ibbertson, Gluckman, Croxson, & Strang, 1974, p. 129) and by Querido and his colleagues in remote villages in Indonesia (Querido, Djokomoeljanto, & van Hardeveld, 1974, p. 8).

Considerable light has been thrown on the pathogenesis of myxedematous cretinism by the studies of Delange, Ermans, and their colleagues in the Ubangi region of northwestern Zaire (Thilly et al., 1974, p. 121). They found evidence of hypothyroidism in mothers whose newborn proved to be cretinous. High plasma levels of thyrotrophic hormone and low levels for triiodothyronine and thyroxine characterized these mothers. Maternal hypothyroidism and iodide deficiency place the fetus and neonate at considerable risk. During pregnancy, the fetus would be denied iodide because the maternal thyroid has a high avidity for iodide, thereby denying iodide to the fetus. Furthermore, with a low plasma level of thyroid hormone there would be relatively limited possibility for transplacental transfer, which, at best, is very limited. During the nursing period, the maternal thyroid again would compete effectively for the available iodide, and with low plasma levels of thyroid hormones, there would be a relatively limited transfer of these into the milk. Thus, the nursing infant would be denied iodide for synthesizing hormone and also hormone that it obtains under normal circumstances through the milk.

Any goitrogenic substance in the diet might further impair thyroid function by impeding transfer of iodide across the placenta during pregnancy and into the milk during lactation and might also reach the thyroid and impair its function directly.

ENDEMIC THYROID-RELATED RETARDATION

In any severe endemic, one can readily identify the cretins in the community because of their striking appearance. It may sometimes be necessary to search them out because they are often kept inside their homes and not exposed to public view. An important consideration is whether there also exists in such a community a substantial number of persons who have lesser degrees of retardation but who are not so readily identified for lack of physical features or developmental impairment and who blend into the community. This important question has been explored by several investigators. Fierro-Benítez and his colleagues administered a battery of tests of intellectual function to a cross-section of children in two villages in rural Ecuador, in which endemic goiter has been severe (Fierro-Benítez, Ramírez, Estrella, & Stanbury, 1974, p. 135). The mothers of some of these children had been given prophylactic doses of iodized oil prior to or during pregnancy. Performance in these children was compared with that of age- and sex-matched children from the same villages. Those whose mothers had been treated with iodized oil performed substantially better than those of mothers who·had not. Greene (1973, p. 119), working in the same villages, found that 17% of the "normal" population showed clear signs of neurological deficit in visual–motor perception. Querido and Swabb (1975) have supporting data from villages in central Java where it was found that children residing in areas of endemic goiter but without overt endemic cretinism were substantially behind those of control villages, although both groups were racially, ethnically, and culturally identical. They demonstrated that many children in these iodine-depressed regions may have evidence of hypothyroidism on close examination. Using the Raven test, they found that 19% of noncretinous children in the iodine-deficient village scored below the 10th percentile, whereas 6.6% were below this level in the control village.

Both these studies clearly indicate that the endemic cretin is at one end of a spectrum of retardation that extends all the way from the typical severe classic cretin to the individual who, through circumstance, has had enough thyroid hormone to escape impaired development. Thus, the societal impact of endemic goiter takes on a new dimension. The disorder is more than a trivial cosmetic problem; it is more than a disorder that occasionally is responsible for the appearance in the community of a severely retarded individual. The societal cost of the latter in a subsistence agrarian economy is probably not large, particularly in view of the high death rate among them. What may be devastating to the social and economic evolution of a society is the presence of a large subgroup of persons who are mildly to moderately retarded in their intellectual abilities, physical skills, and learning capacities. The cost of an effective prophylactic program is trivial indeed when compared with the economic burden imposed by endemic goiter.

Little enough is known about the critical timing of thyroid deficiency that produces the varied manifestations of the spectrum of endemic retardation induced by iodine deficiency. It is not yet known what salvage is possible if one could begin therapy at or shortly after birth. Restoration of function and growth is probably achievable in most instances of sporadic congenital hypothyroidism, but in these subjects, by and large, the mother has been normal, and the pregnancy has been normal. As Ermans and his colleagues have shown, this is not the case with the endemic cretin, and it is entirely possible that irreversible damage has already been done during fetal life (Thilly *et al.*, 1974, p. 121).

Fierro-Benítez and his colleagues have extensively studied the effects of restoring normal iodide intake on growth and development of preschool and school-age children in an endemic goiter region (Fierro-Benítez *et al.*, 1974, p. 135). The children chosen had no overt evidence of hypothyroidism. Over a period of several years, these investigators were unable to demonstrate any noteworthy effect on linear growth, skeletal maturation, dentition, or other criteria of somatic development. As already noted, however, these observers found that children of mothers who were given iodized oil prior to the fourth fetal month performed substantially better on a battery of tests of intellectual function than did matched controls from the same village.

SUMMARY

The thyroid hormones are critically important in statural growth and in the orderly development of the central nervous system. Hormone deficiency in the early phases of development extending into the postnatal period causes impaired development and, if untreated, leads to retardation. If treatment is delayed, the changes are irreversible. Endemic goiter, an exceedingly common disaster in many parts of the world, is the response to iodine deficiency and perhaps also in some instances to dietary goitrogens. When severe, it is accompanied by cretinism. Recent studies indicate that in addition to overt cretinism, many persons in a region of endemic goiter may have milder and less apparent degrees of retardation as a result of the prevailing thyroid deficiency.

REFERENCES

Balázs, R., Cocks, W. A., Eayrs, J. R., & Kovács, S. Biochemical effects of thyroid on the developing brain. In M. Hamburgh & E. J. W. Barrington (Eds.), *Hormones in development.* New York: Appleton-Century-Crofts, 1971.

Bastenie, P. A., Ermans, A. M., Thys, O., Beckers, C., van den Schrieck, H. G., & Visscher, M. de. Endemic goiter in the Uele region. III. Endemic cretinism. *Journal of Clinical Endocrinology and Metabolism*, 1962, 22, 187–194.

Bauman, E. A., Bode, H. H., Hayek, A., & Crawford, J. D. [99m]Technetium pertechnetate scans in congenital hypothyroidism. *Journal of Pediatrics*, 1976, 89, 268.

Delange, F. *Endemic goiter and thyroid function in Central Africa.* Basel: Karger, 1974.

Delange, F., & Ermans, A. M. Role of a dietary goitrogen in the etiology of endemic goiter on Idjwi Island. *American Journal of Clinical Nutrition*, 1971, 24, 1354.

Deol, J. An experimental approach to the understanding and treatment of hereditary syndromes with congenital deafness and hypothyroidism. *Journal of Medical Genetics*, 1973, 10, 235–242.

Djokomoeljanto, R. The effect of severe iodine deficiency. (A study on a population in Central Java, Indonesia). Dissertation. Semarang: Universitas Diponegoro, 1974.

Dumont, J. E., Delange, F., & Ermans, A. M. Endemic cretinism. In J. B. Stanbury (Ed.), *Endemic goiter.* Pan American Health Organization Scientific Publication No. 193, Washington, D.C., 1969.

Eayrs, J. T. Thyroid and developing brain: Anatomical and behavioral effects. In M. Hamburgh & E. J. W. Barrington (Eds.), *Hormones in development.* New York: Appleton-Century-Crofts, 1971.

Ermans, A. M., Delange, F., van der Velden, M., & Kinthaert, J. Possible role of cyanide and thiocyanate in the etiology of endemic cretinism. In J. B. Stanbury & R. L. Kroc (Eds.), *Human development and the thyroid gland: Relation to endemic cretinism.* New York: Plenum, 1972.

Fierro-Benítez, R., Peñafiel, W., DeGroot, L. J., & Ramírez, I. Endemic goiter and endemic cretinism in the Andean region. *New England Journal of Medicine*, 1969, 280, 296–303.

Fierro-Benítez, R., Ramírez, I., Estrella, E., Jaramillo, C., Díaz, C., & Urresta, J. Iodized oil in the prevention of endemic goiter and associated defects in the Andean region of Ecuador. I. Program design, effects on goiter prevalence, thyroid function, and iodine excretion. In J. B. Stanbury (Ed.), *Endemic goiter.* Pan American Health Organization Scientific Publication No. 193, Washington, D.C., 1969.

Fierro-Benítez, R., Ramírez, I., Estrella, E., & Stanbury, J. B. The role of iodine in intellectual development in an area of endemic goiter. In J. T. Dunn & G. A. Medeiros-Neto (Eds.), *Endemic goiter and cretinism: Continuing threats to world health.* Pan American Health Organization Scientific Publication No. 292, Washington, D.C., 1974.

Gaitán, E. Water-borne goitrogens and their role in the etiology of endemic goiter. *World Review of Nutrition and Dietetics,* 1973, *17,* 53–90.

Gaitán, E., Wahner, J. W., Correa, P., Bernal, R., Jubiz, W., Gaitán, J. E., & Blancos, C. Endemic goiter in the Cauca Valley: I. Results and limitations of twelve years of iodine prophylaxis. *Journal of Clinical Endocrinology and Metabolism,* 1968, *28,* 1730–1746.

Goldschmidt, V. M. The geochemistry of iodine. In A. Muir (Ed.), *Geochemistry.* New York: Oxford Univ. Press (Clarendon), 1954.

Greene, L. S. Physical growth and development, neurological maturation and behavioral functioning in two Ecuadorian Andean communities in which goiter is endemic. I. Outline of the problem of endemic goiter and cretinism. Physical growth and neurological maturation in the adult population of La Esperanza. *American Journal of Physical Anthropology,* 1973, *38,* 119–134.

Hetzel, B. S., & Pharoah, P. O. D. (Eds.). *Endemic cretinism.* Chipping Norton, New South Wales, Australia: Surrey Beatty, 1971.

Hollingsworth, D. R., Belin, R. P., Packer, J. C., Jr., Moser, R. J., & McKean, H. Experimental cretinism in lambs: An intrauterine model with thyroid evaluation in surviving lambs. *Johns Hopkins Medical Journal,* 1975, *137,* 116–122.

Ibbertson, H. K., Gluckman, P. D., Croxson, M. S., & Strang, L. J. W. Goiter and cretinism in the Himalayas: A reassessment. In J. T. Dunn & G. A. Medeiros-Neto (Eds.), *Endemic goiter and cretinism: Continuing threats to world health.* Pan American Health Organization Scientific Publication No. 292, Washington, D.C., 1974.

Kerr, G. R., Allen, J. R., Scheffler, G., & Couture, J. Fetal and postnatal growth of rhesus monkeys (*M. mulatta*). *Journal of Medical Primatology,* 1974, *3,* 221–235.

Langer, P. History of goitre. In *Endemic goitre. World Health Organization Monograph Series, No. 44,* Geneva, 1960.

Legrand, J., & Bout, M. C. Influence de l'hypothyroidisme et de la thyroxine sur le development des epines dendritiques des cellules de Purkinje dans le cervelt de jeune Rat. *Compt. Rend. Acad. Sci. Paris,* 1970, *271,* 1199.

Maisterrena, J. A., Tovar, E., & Chávez, A. Endemic goiter in Mexico and its changing pattern in a rural community. In J. B. Stanbury (Ed.), *Endemic goiter.* Pan American Health Organization Scientific Publication No. 193, Washington, D.C., 1969.

Matovinovic, J., Child, M. A., Nichaman, M. Z., & Trowbridge, F. L. Iodine and endemic goiter. In J. T. Dunn & G. A. Medeiros-Neto (Eds.), *Endemic goiter and cretinism: Continuing threats to world health.* Pan American Health Organization Scientific Publication No. 292, Washington, D.C., 1974.

McCarrison, R. Observations on endemic cretinism in Chitral and Gilgit Valleys. *Lancet,* 1908, *ii,* 1275.

Pharoah, P. O. D., Butterfield, J. H., & Hetzel, B. S. The effect of iodine prophylaxis on the incidence of endemic cretinism. In J. B. Stanbury & R. L. Kroc (Eds.), *Human development and the thyroid gland: Relation to endemic cretinism.* New York: Plenum, 1972.

Pharoah, P. O. D., & Hornabrook, T. W. Endemic cretinism of recent onset in New Guinea. *Lancet,* 1974, *ii,* 1038–1039.

Pickering, D. E. Thyroid physiology in the developing monkey fetus (Macaca mulatta). General Comparative Endocrinology, 1968, 10, 182–190.

Pretell, E. A., Moncloa, F., Salinas, R., Kawanu, A., Guerra-Garcia, R., Gutierrez, L., Bereta, L., Pretell, J., & Wan, M. Prophylaxis and treatment of endemic goiter in Peru with iodized oil. Journal of Clinical Endocrinology and Metabolism, 1969, 29, 1586.

Querido, A. Djokomoeljanto, R., & van Hardeveld, C. The consequences of iodine deficiency for health. In J. T. Dunn & G. A. Medeiros-Neto (Eds.), Endemic goiter and cretinism: Continuing threats to world health. Pan American Health Organization Scientific Publication No. 292, Washington, D.C., 1974, p. 8.

Querido, A., & Swabb, D. F. (Eds.). Brain development and thyroid deficiency. Amsterdam: North-Holland, 1975.

Ramírez, J., Fierro-Benítez, R., Estrella, E., Gomez, A., Jaramillo, C., Hermida, C., & Moncayo, F. The results of prophylaxis of endemic cretinism with iodized oil in rural Andean Ecuador. In J. B. Stanbury & R. L. Kroc (Eds.), Human development and the thyroid gland: Relation to endemic cretinism, 1972.

Rosman, N. P., Malone, M. J., Helfenstein, M., & Kraft, E. The effect of thyroid deficiency on myelinisation of brain: A morphological and biochemical study. Neurology, 1972, 22, 99–106.

Smith, D. W., Blizzard, R. M., & Wilkins, L. Mental attainments of hypothyroid children: Review of 128 cases. Pediatrics, 1957, 19, 1011–1022.

Stanbury, J. B. Familial goiter. In J. B. Stanbury, J. B. Wyngaarden, & D. S. Fredrickson (Eds.), The metabolic basis of inherited disease. New York: McGraw-Hill, 1972.

Thilly, C. H., Delange, F., Camus, M., Berquist, H., & Ermans, A. M. Fetal hypothyroidism in endemic goiter: The probable pathogenic mechanism of endemic cretinism. In J. T. Dunn & G. A. Medeiros-Neto (Eds.), Endemic goiter and cretinism: Continuing threats to world health. Pan American Health Organization Scientific Publication No. 292, Washington, D. C., 1974.

Thilly, C. H., Delange, F., Goldstein-Golaire, J., & Ermans, A. M. Endemic goiter prevention by iodized oil: A reassessment. Journal of Clinical Endocrinology and Metabolism, 1973, 36, 1196–1204.

4

Hyperendemic Goiter, Cretinism, and Social Organization in Highland Ecuador

LAWRENCE S. GREENE

University of Massachusetts/Boston

INTRODUCTION—MALNUTRITION AND BEHAVIOR

Anthropologists have traditionally been concerned with the description of the biological and sociocultural variation that exists between different human populations, and in recent years there has been an increased interest in the biological basis of behavioral variation (Bolton, 1973; Foulks, 1972; Katz & Foulks, 1970; Wallace, 1961). This work has attempted to demonstrate how environmental stresses and endogenous factors influence behavior in human populations and how the behavioral variation so produced can have an effect on the sociocultural characteristics of human communities.

This chapter is a continuation and expansion of these research interests in its concern with the effects of iodine and protein–calorie malnutrition (PCM) on nervous system development and behavior in two human populations. The fundamental purpose of this study is to demonstrate that extreme nutritional stress early in life can limit the full expression of the genetically coded potential for nervous system development among members of human populations. It is assumed

that there are genetically based differences in neurological potential
between individuals; however, this paper will suggest that in areas in
which iodine and PCM (as well as other serious nutritional stresses)
are widespread and severe, a *significant portion* of the individual
variation in behavioral capacity can be accounted for by the differential effect of nutritional stresses on nervous system development.

In a more general sense, this study is concerned with the interrelatedness of environmental, biological, and sociocultural systems. It
demonstrates how two particular environmental stresses affect an aspect of endocrine function, neurological development, and consequently, behavior in a biological system (a human population) and
then shows how these changes in the biological system profoundly
affect certain basic aspects of the sociocultural system. These interrelationships are outlined diagramatically in Figure 4.1.

Figure 4.1 is a heuristic model similar to those of Katz and Foulks
(1970, 1972), Foulks (1972), and Katz (1973). Its exact form is somewhat variable, and the model presented here has been simplified for
the sake of clarity. Its basic purpose is to suggest that environmental,
biological, and sociocultural systems are interrelated and to help indicate how factors affecting one of the component systems have an

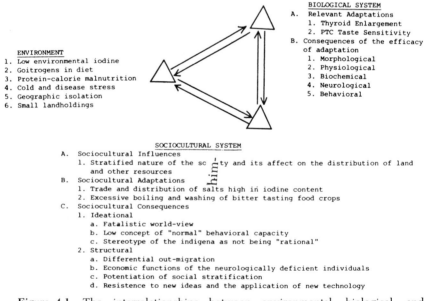

Figure 4.1. The interrelationships between environmental, biological, and
sociocultural systems (after Greene, 1976).

influence on the other systems. The variables within each system that are most relevant to the present problem are indicated. Given the environmental characteristics of the populations under study (Fierro-Benítez, Penafiel, De Groot, & Ramírez, 1969), this investigation has focused on the effects produced in the biological system by these nutritional and other environmental stresses.

In this model, behavioral capacity is viewed as the final common pathway of biological adaptation. The consequences of the effectiveness of morphological, physiological, and neurological adaptation are all reflected in the behavioral capacity of individuals. Since the locus of culture is the individual, it becomes important that anthropologists consider the possibility that some communities contain significant numbers of neurologically deficient and behaviorally limited individuals who may be carriers and transmitters of an extremely limited range of the full informational content and behavioral repertoire of the culture. This, plus the effect of significant numbers of behaviorally deficient individuals on economic and other aspects of social organization, should be describable if not measurable.

Although a major theoretical focus of this study concerns the interrelatedness of these three systems, it should in no way be construed as a thesis advocating a rigorous environmental, or biological, determinism of social organization. The impact of cultural factors on personality integration (Benedict, 1934; Kardiner, 1945; Mead, 1935) and possibly on some structural and functional aspects of nervous system maturation during child growth and development (Rosenzweig, Bennett, & Diamond, 1972; Walsh & Cummins, 1976) is certainly accepted. What this study attempts to show is that specific nutritional stresses can affect nervous system development, thus placing *limits* on the biological system *within which* cultural factors may then work.

The study that is to be described is presented within the context of the conceptual model outlined in Figure 4.1. Occasional reference to this model will help the reader become oriented to the various issues under discussion. The same model will be considered in greater detail in the concluding section.

THE CHOICE OF STUDY POPULATIONS—PROTEIN-CALORIE VERSUS IODINE MALNUTRITION

The basic goal of this study was to evaluate the effect of some widespread nutritional stress on neurological maturation and behavior in a human population. At first, it appeared that a population living in an area in which PCM was prevalent would be the best object of investigation. This type of malnutrition is quite common in many parts of the world and has been the subject of an extensive medical literature. However, the problem posed by iodine malnutrition, goiter, and cretinism, although somewhat less common, offers certain methodological advantages. This nutritional stress is easily quantifiable and affects almost all individuals in areas in which goiter is hyperendemic. The dietary deficiency of iodine is due to geochemical characteristics of the environment that show little or no variation over long periods of time; thus, iodine deficiency and behavioral deficits in *adults* can reasonably be imputed to iodine deficiency early in life in studies done retrospectively.

Perhaps the greatest advantage to working with a population in which goiter and cretinism are endemic is that there is an easily definable group of neurologically deficient individuals (deaf-mute "cretins") and an unquestionable relationship between thyroid function and nervous system development (Balázs, Kovács, Treichgraber, Cocks, & Eayrs, 1968; Bass & Netsky, 1969; Bass & Young, 1973; Eayrs, 1960, 1961; Eayrs & Taylor, 1951). Therefore, possibly the best human model system for evaluating the effect of a widespread nutritional stress on nervous system development, behavior, and social organization is an area in which iodine intake is extremely low, in which dietary factors may be interfering with the utilization of even the small amounts of iodine coming into the system, and in which there is a high prevalence of cretinism. The *parroquias* of La Esperanza and Tocachi in the Andean region of Ecuador embody these characteristics.

ENDEMIC GOITER AND CRETINISM IN HIGHLAND ECUADOR

Stanbury (this volume) has discussed the worldwide distribution of endemic goiter and cretinism and its relationship to low levels of environmental iodine. In Ecuador, epidemiological surveys (Fierro-Benítez & Recalde, 1958) found that endemic goiter was a significant health problem in some parts of the Andean region. Prevalence of goiter varied sharply between adjacent villages and was not reported at locations above approximately 3200 m. Deaf-mute mentally retarded individuals were present in significant numbers and showed classic signs of cretinism except that they were usually not hypothyroid. Studies of iodine metabolism indicated that dietary iodine deficiency was the principal factor causing the endemia. The prevalence of goiter was greatest in the highlands and lowest along the coastal plain. In the highlands, prevalence was higher in the northern and central provinces (above 30%) and lower in the southern provinces (10–20%) near Peru.

The central and northern Andean area, in which prevalence is highest, is distinguished from the southern Ecuadorian Andes and the

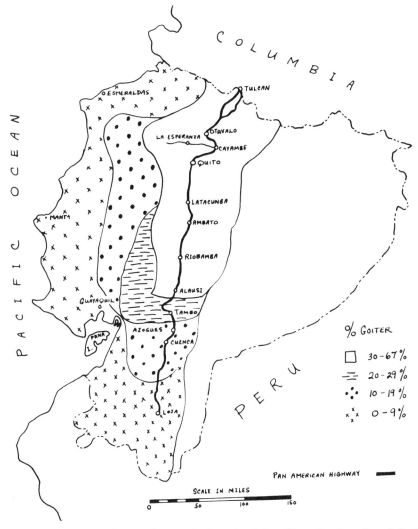

Figure 4.2. Prevalence of goiter in Ecuador (after Fierro-Benítez, Penafiel, De Groot, & Ramírez, 1969). Reprinted, by permission, from the *New England Journal of Medicine,* 1969, *280,* 298.

Peruvian Andean region in being located at a far greater distance from the Pacific Ocean. The Ecuadorian Andean provinces with the highest prevalence of goiter all lie due east of a coastal plain that is from 150 to 200 km wide, while the southern Ecuadorian and Peruvian Andes are only separated from the sea by some 30 km. Goldschmidt (1958) has demonstrated that the iodine content of soils decreases in proportion to distance from the sea; therefore, this geographical factor may contribute to the particularly high prevalence of goiter encountered in the north and central highland area.

A second study reported by Fierro-Benítez et al. (1969a) made a rather complete evaluation of virtually the total populations in 8 rural Andean villages in the central and northern region in which the prevalence of goiter was high. In 6 of the communities, crude sea salt containing 0.24 μg/gm iodine was consumed and goiter was endemic, ranging in prevalence from 12.4 to 54.4% of the total population. The iodine content of the local drinking water ranged from 0.50 to 1.50 μg/liter. In these populations, the average urinary iodide excretion was between 7.7 and 22.5 μg/day. In the 2 other communities, both called Salinas, a locally produced salt high in iodine content was consumed. Here, the prevalence of goiter was below 5%, and urinary excretion of iodide was high. The socioeconomic levels of the eight communities were generally comparable.

One finding of this study was that the prevalence of nodular goiter differs between communities with similar levels of total goiter. There was also a change in the sex ratio of goiter with increasing prevalence. Whereas the frequency of goiter was much greater among females than males at lower prevalence (about 8:1), at high prevalence, such as occurred in Tocachi, the frequencies were about equal (1:1). The frequency of cretinism rose as the prevalence of goiter, especially nodular goiter, increased; however, there was no difference in the prevalence of total, nodular, or diffuse goiter in families with or without cretins. The prevalence of cretinism was as high as 8.2% in Tocachi and 6.0% in La Esperanza. Hypothyroidism was uncommon even in the cretin subjects.

Fierro-Benítez and his colleagues focused their studies on Tocachi and La Esperanza (Dodge, Palkes, Fierro-Benítez, & Ramírez, 1969; Estrella Aquirre, 1974; Fierro-Benítez, Ramírez, Carlucci, Estrella, & Suárez, 1974; Fierro-Benítez, Ramírez, Estrella, Jaramillo, Díaz, & Urresta, 1969; Fierro-Benítez, Ramírez, Garcés, Jaramillo, Moncayo, & Stanbury, 1974; Fierro-Benítez, Ramírez, & Suárez, 1972; Fierro-Benítez, Stanbury, Querido, De Groot, Alban, & Cordova, 1970; Ramírez, Fierro-Benítez, Estrella, Jaramillo, Díaz, & Urresta, 1969;

Stanbury, 1972b). This chapter is primarily concerned with the community of La Esperanza, although some data from Tocachi will also be presented. This work is an extension of the studies of Dr. Rodrigo Fierro-Benítez and his group with whom I worked from December 1970 until January 1972.

GENERAL SCOPE AND OBJECTIVE OF THE STUDY

Severe Nutritional Stress and the Continuum of Neurological and Behavioral Deficit

The primary goal of this study was to empirically demonstrate that the large number of deaf-mute "cretins" in La Esperanza (6.0% of the population according to Fierro-Benítez et al., 1969a, b) were not the only individuals with neurological deficits and behavioral limitations in this population. Instead, I hypothesized that these individuals merely represent one end of a continuum of effect ranging from deaf-mute cretins with severe neuromotor abnormalities and extreme behavioral limitations, to individuals with moderate neurological deficits and behavioral limitations, to people with slight neurological deficits and no behavioral limitations, to normal individuals. I was suggesting that on careful study human populations in which goiter and cretinism are hyperendemic will be found to contain a surprisingly large number of individuals with some degree of neurological deficit and consequent behavioral limitation.

Figure 4.3, which is adapted from a previous publication (Greene, 1973), indicates how our medical experience with sporadic cretinism in industrialized societies has, until recently, clouded our conception of the breadth of neurological deficit in populations living in areas in which goiter and cretinism are endemic. Sporadic cretinism occurs at extremely low frequencies in all societies and is primarily caused by a congenital absence of the thyroid gland or genetically based abnormalities in thyroid enzyme systems (Stanbury, 1972a). If these people do not receive replacement therapy with thyroid hormones early in life, they will develop into the typical cretin individual. The top figure shows the relationship between thyroid function and neurological development in most industrialized societies, with sporadic cretins being the only group showing neurological deficits as a result of abnormalities in thyroid function.

The bottom diagram in Figure 4.3 shows the relationship between thyroid function and neurological development in a population in

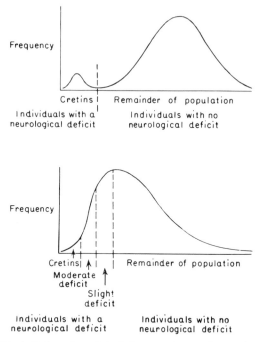

Figure 4.3. *(Top)*. Rejected model of the prevalence of neurological damage in a population in which goiter and cretinism are endemic. *(Bottom)*. Proposed model of the prevalence of neurological damage in a population in which goiter and cretinism are endemic.

which dietary iodine intake is very low and goiter and cretinism are endemic. This model suggests that under these environmental conditions the deaf-mute cretin group is merely the most obvious part of a continuum of neurological deficit due to thyroid stress. If the environmental stress is great enough to lead to the production of a high prevalence of deaf-mute cretins, then we would certainly expect many other individuals in these populations to show more moderate or slight neurological deficits.

The Effect of the High Prevalence of Neurologically Deficient and Behaviorally Limited Individuals on Social Organization

The second goal of this study is to show the impact of the large numbers of behaviorally limited individuals on the sociocultural characteristics of the community of La Esperanza. To this end, I collected data on the behavioral capacities, social roles, and economic functions of almost all of the deaf-mute individuals and a smaller, but significant, number of moderately retarded individuals. These data form an empirical basis for an understanding of how a community containing such individuals is organized and how it functions.

BACKGROUND: A HIGHLY STRATIFIED SOCIAL SYSTEM

The present study is concerned with the effect of nutritional stress on nervous system development, behavior, and social organization in a human population. However, the life circumstances of any population, or segment of a population, is to a great extent a product of its position in an existing social system. The rules and values of the sociocultural system determine how the environment is to be divided up, so to speak, thus affecting the resource base of subpopulations in a very real sense. An appreciation of the sociocultural milieu of a population is thus important if we are to truly understand how the essential aspects of the environment are filtered through the sociocultural system and differentially distributed to component subpopulations. Since a social system at one point in time, the present, is a product of its past, it behooves us to consider the historical setting of the present study in some detail. Seen with the context of the past, the present will certainly be more explicable.

Historical Dimensions

The history of Ecuador has been enormously influenced by two major military–political impositions: the Inca and the Spanish. Both of these events had a lasting influence on the indigenous culture and an even more profound effect on the structural aspects of the emerging Ecuadorian national society. A brief review of the history of the colonial and republican periods is thus quite important for an understanding of the contemporary Ecuadorian reality.

The Inca Conquest

The Inca imposition lasted for only about 60 years in south and central Ecuador and for no more than about 10–20 years in the northern portion of the country prior to the Spanish conquest in 1534 (Rowe, 1946). Nevertheless, due to their superb organizational skill, the Inca had a profound effect on the indigenous Ecuadorian society. When the Inca empire fell to the conquistadores, it left a structure of political unification over which the Spaniards readily grafted their own institutions, and the imposition of Quechua over the 10 isolated intermontone basins provided a linguistic unification that was utilized by the Spanish Crown and the Catholic Church as the language of administration and evangelization at the local level.

The Inca empire was extremely authoritarian, a factor that had important consequences in predisposing the indigenous population to the Spanish imposition. The Inca divided the conquered lands of local communities into three parts (Rowe, 1946, p. 265). The first portion went to the state religion; the second portion went to the Inca himself; and the third part was made available to the local inhabitants as communal land that was owned by the state but to which they had usufruct rights.

The Inca did not impose any property tax on the population, but the people were subject to two major taxes, which were paid in labor. One of these consisted of obligations to cultivate the lands owned by the state. The second labor tax, called the *mita,* involved annual obligations of service to the state in the military, in public works projects, in the mines, in the postal system, as well as service to the nobility. The Inca empire, although authoritarian, was not extractive and used its highly centralized governmental structure to integrate an empire that provided for the basic needs of its citizens—whether they were irrigation, communication, protection, or relief from local crop failure.

The Spanish Conquest

Following the Spanish conquest, the indigenous territories were organized on the basis of *encomiendas,* which were somewhat similar to the Inca system of labor obligation to the state, a fact that probably facilitated its implementation. The *repartamiento* and *encomienda* were grants of Indians, their land, and their labor to individual conquistadores or to institutions such as the various orders of the Catholic Church. The labor of the *indigenas* supported the *encomenderos,* who were their overseers, and provided the agricultural tribute that went to the crown. Indian labor obligations *(mita)* in the mines also provided tribute to Spain's treasury.

The number and extent of these landholdings was enormous. In her study of Hacienda Pesillo, approximately 50 km northeast of La Esperanza, Crespi (1968, p. 45) notes that "by the end of the 18th century, estates of different religious orders virtually monopolized all of what is today Cantón Cayambe. Little if any vacant land intervened between neighboring haciendas."

The Spanish colonization and its institutions, such as the *en-*

comienda, were essentially extractive measures designed to enrich the Spanish crown and the conquistadores, with little interest in the local populations except for the ways in which they could be used to meet these ends.

The Emerging Stratified Social System

The Spanish conquest created a social hierarchy, with the conquistadores on top and the indigenous population at the bottom. In the colonial period, a new social hierarchy emerged that was primarily based on the increasingly complex "racial" characteristics of the population. At the apex of this social pyramid were Whites who had been born in Spain or in the colony. Those born in Ecuador were called *criollos* and had second-class White status until after independence from Spain. Interracial matings led to a multiplicity of mixtures of Indian, Negro, and White parentage. These individuals were ranked both genetically and socially in a series of *castas,* or racial categories, which reflected alleged descent. In addition to the *blanco,* these categories included the *mestizo,* the result of Indian and white matings; the *cholo,* the offspring of *mestizo* and Indian unions; the *mulatto,* an offspring of Negro and White unions; the *zambo,* the result of Negro and *mulatto* matings; and the *indígena.* In the social, economic, and political spheres of life, *casta* membership was quite important, with those *castas* with the greater degree of White ancestry having the higher status. No *casta* occupied a lower position than the *indígena,* and in the colonial period these categories were literally racial.

The Republican Period

With independence from Spain in 1822 the Ecuadorian-born White—*criollos*—assumed the mantle of government and power. The revolution had little or no effect in restructuring the pyramidal social hierarchy except that *criollo* status was elevated with respect to foreign-born Whites. At the level of the community, landowners representing the Spanish Crown were replaced by Whites born in Ecuador who continued the same extractive practices except that the proceeds went to their own enrichment rather than to the Spanish treasury. Tributary payment to the central government was eventually abolished, but payment to the Church continued.

Under the Republic, the affiliation of the *indígena* to land was essentially the same as it had been throughout the colonial period. As noted above, land was concentrated in the hands of the state, the church, and *blanco* large landowners. The *indígenas* obtained usufruct rights to small plots of *hacienda* lands (called *huasipungos*) by providing labor to the *hacienda* and were called *huasipungueros*.

In 1906, legislation empowered the government to confiscate much of the vast landholdings of the Catholic Church and established an agency, now known as the *Asistencia Social*, with responsibility for managing these expropriated *haciendas*. However, change in ownership led to little or no betterment for the *huasipungero* residents of these *haciendas* but merely signified a change in power and wealth from Church to State. The basic structure of the *hacienda* stayed intact. Only the owners changed, and little or none of the proceeds reaped by the *Asistencia* filtered down to the rural indigenous population.

This essentially feudal relationship between the land-rich *blanco* and *mestizo* sociocultural segment and the land-poor indigenous half of the society continued unchanged until the Agrarian Reform Law of 1963 bestowed the *huasipungos* on public and private *haciendas* to the *huasipungueros* for past services rendered.

The Contemporary National and Local Sociocultural Setting

The contemporary national and local sociocultural setting is very much a product of the historical antecedents just described. Ecuador is still a highly stratified society; however, the stratification is now primarily based on ethnic affiliation and behavior rather than on purely physical characteristics. About 45% of the population are *indígenas* who live in rural areas or are recent urban migrants (Republica del Ecuador, 1964). Most of these rural inhabitants are landless or extremely land-poor despite the agrarian reform. There is no ideology of equality, and the *indígenas* occupy the very lowest social position. Both the *blanco* and *mestizos* view the *indígena* primarily as a source of cheap and easily manipulatable labor, which forms the economic basis of their relative comfort.

Government at the local level is highly centralized and nondemocratic. The local civil administrative official in the *parroquia* is not elected but is appointed by the authorities in Quito. Thus, predominantly indigenous communities like La Esperanza (78% *indígena*) are dominated by the *blanco* minority and their representatives in Quito. Although not quite as bad off as they were in the not too distant past (10–15 years ago), the rural land-poor, predominantly indigenous population lies at the very bottom of the social pyramid.

THE STUDY COMMUNITY: LA ESPERANZA

The *parroquia* of La Esperanza is an extremely isolated community located in the northeastern portion of the province of Pichincha (Fig. 4.2). Studies by Fierro-Benítez *et al.* (1969*a,b*) have shown that 52.8% of the total population had goiters and that 6.0% of the inhabitants were deaf-mute "cretin" individuals. The community is situated on the southern flank of Mt. Mojanda (4300 m) approximately 2 km north of the equator. Its central nucleated *barrios* lie at an altitude of 2850 m, while the lower more rural *anejos* extend across a broad plain to reach the banks of the Pisque river at about 2550 m. Three large *haciendas,* 2 state-owned and the other owned by a large beer company, are located above the central nucleated zone and extend to the crest of Mojanda. These landholdings are each well over 1500 acres in size and account for about half of the arable land in the *parroquia*. The *haciendas* contain 3 *anejos,* which are a part of the community and are located between 2900 and 3050 m. The productive *hacienda* agricultural lands lie between 2900 and 3300 m, above which are cold *páramo* grasslands, which are used for grazing sheep and some cattle.

The *parroquia* of La Esperanza, which is the smallest legal civil administrative unit, is actually composed of nine separate *barrios* and *anejos,* the inhabitants of which are more closely related to one another by bonds of kinship than they are to inhabitants of the other *barrios* and *anejos*. These social units, which are somewhat similar to the autochthonous *ayllu,* all have some degree of informal organization. The location of the various *barrios* and *anejos* are shown in Figure 4.4.

Based on an unofficial census taken in 1971, there were 1872 people living in 368 households. However, many individuals listed in the census were actually working and residing in Quito; thus, the actual population of the *parroquia* was closer to 1600 permanent residents. This population is distributed over more than 30 km² exclusive of the additional 35 km² of *páramo* grasslands above 3300 m.

The ethnic composition of the *parroquia* is 78% *indígena* and 22% *blanco* and *mestizo,* based on data in the Registro Civil and an ethnic classification of surnames. In reality, the *mestizo* category is not used in the local classificatory system; one is either *blanco* or *indígena*. The indigenous segment of the population is concentrated in the rural *anejos* (Guaraquí, Mojanda, Tomalon, Cuvinche, Chimburlo), while the *blancos* primarily live in the nucleated central *bar-*

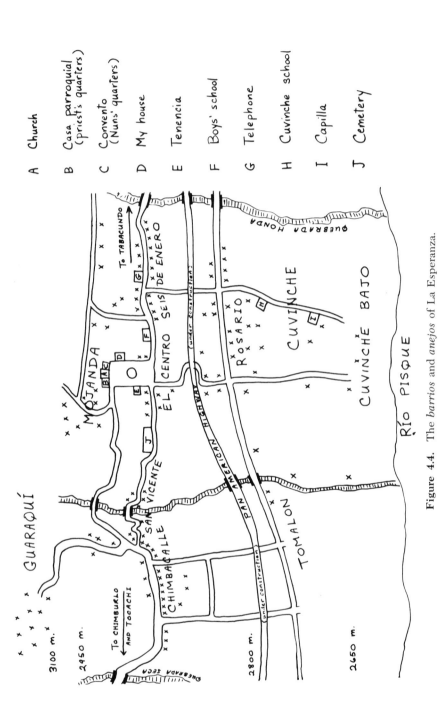

A   Church

B   Casa parroquial
    (priest's quarters)

C   Convento
    (Nuns' quarters)

D   My house

E   Tenencia

F   Boys' school

G   Telephone

H   Cuvinche school

I   Capilla

J   Cemetery

Figure 4.4. The *barrios* and *anejos* of La Esperanza.

68

rios (Seis de Enero, El Centro, Chimbacalle, Rosario). The main focus of the indigenous sociocultural segment is their *anejo*, in which they have strong ties of kinship and their lands *(los terrenos)*. *Anejo* endogamy has been and still is the preferred form of marriage. The less numerous *blancos* are more oriented toward the *parroquia* and its institutions (the civil government, the church, the school, the credit and weaving cooperatives), which they dominate.

In addition to the three large *haciendas*, there is a single smaller privately owned *hacienda* of about 150 acres. Five *blanco* families each own between 20 and 40 acres of land each, most of which is scattered in several different parcels. Beyond this, the great majority of these primarily indigenous rural peasants are extremely land-poor. A survey of 119 of the 368 households in the community indicated that the average amount of land owned was 2.5 acres. Forty-two percent of the households surveyed owned no land at all; 37.8% of the population, mostly those who are landless, were involved in sharecropping arrangements averaging 4.7 acres.

Most households are semisubsistence agriculturalists—pastoralists who grow corn, potatoes, peas, beans, and squash for domestic consumption. Wheat and barley are grown both for domestic consumption and, among households with larger landholdings, as a cash crop. Herding sheep and cattle is carried out at a significant level by about 16% of the population. Households involved in herding are mainly those *indígenas* affiliated with the *haciendas* who has rights of pasture in the *páramo* grasslands.

Opportunities for wage labor are extremely limited in La Esperanza. There are 6 paying positions in the local governmental apparatus, all of which are occupied by *blancos*. Monthly salaries in 1971 averaged 450–650 *sucres* ($18–26). Five positions in the local school system were filled by individuals with a secondary school education, half of whom were from outside the *parroquia*. The only form of wage labor available to *indígenas* was on the *haciendas* where approximately 70 adult males had full-time work earning from 15 to 17 *sucres* daily (60–68 cents) 5 days a week. Occasional wage labor was also available from the *blanco* and *mestizo* small landowners. This will be discussed more fully below.

The data to be presented in the following sections evaluate the effect of iodine and PCM on nervous system development and behavior among the population of La Esperanza. Hopefully, the extensive historical background has illuminated some aspects of the national sociocultural setting in which this population has existed. In the final sections, the characteristics of the sociocultural system of La

Esperanza will be discussed more fully within the content of the biological data that will now be presented.

NEUROLOGICAL MATURATION AMONG THE ADULT
POPULATION OF LA ESPERANZA

The basic objective of this study was outlined above but merits restatement at this point. Briefly, this work attempts to demonstrate that there are *large numbers* of individuals with moderate neurological deficits and describable behavioral limitations living in areas in which various type of malnutrition are widespread. It is suggested that these individuals exist in addition to a smaller number of individuals with severe neurological deficits and behavioral limitations whose existence in these populations is more apparent and generally recognized. The data that are now presented evaluate this hypothesis in the Ecuadorian Andean community of La Esperanza, in which goiter and cretinism are endemic.

The Bender Gestalt Test

Neurological maturation in visual–motor perception was evaluated using the Bender Gestalt Test (Bender, 1938). The test consists of nine figures that the subject is shown and asked to reproduce. Each card is presented separately and is kept in front of the subject at all times. There is no time limit for reproducing the figures.

The Bender productions were scored using the Developmental Bender Scoring System (Koppitz, 1964), which measures the number of errors made in the reproduction of the Gestalt figures. The normal child's ability to reproduce these figures correctly is a function of the process of maturation in the visual-motor perceptive function of the central nervous system. Younger children make more errors and older children fewer errors until an asymptote (plateau) of 1.5 ± 2.0 errors is reached at about 9.5 years of age in North American children. The test can thus distinguish those *adult* individuals who, due to a neurological injury, are functioning below the level of a 9.5-year-old North American child in terms of their visual–motor perceptive ability.

I have used the mean Bender score of the 9.5-year-old North American Standardization sample (1.5 ± 2.0 errors) as a rough standard for complete visual–motor maturation in an adequately nourished and medically healthy population. Those *adult* individuals in La Esperanza with scores more than 2 standard deviations below this mean have been considered suspect of showing some degree of neurological deficit. These are individuals 15–54 years of age who have Bender Gestalt error scores of 5.5 or greater. Such scores place these individuals below the third percentile among 9.5-year-old North American children.

The Bender test is extremely simple and relatively "culture free." The test only evaluates a limited aspect of neurological development involving visual–motor perception; however, in populations living under chronic, extreme nutritional stress, damage to the nervous system tends to be diffuse, and individuals showing deficits in one area of cerebral functioning are often deficient in other areas as well. The behavioral data to be presented in the later sections are essentially a validation of the more concrete neurological data. A more extensive discussion of the rationale for the use of the Bender Gestalt Test in this population has been presented elsewhere (Greene, 1973, 1974, 1976).

The Study Sample

The first part of the study sample consists of 44 of the 51 deaf-mute "cretin" individuals in La Esperanza. These individuals were recognized by the community as people who did not speak or hear and were individuals who showed varying degrees of neuromotor and behavioral limitations, which will be described more fully below. The Bender Gestalt Test was administered to these subjects in their family compound by the author and his assistant, who was a well-known and liked person from the community. All except the most severely retarded subjects were able to understand the nonverbal instructions and demonstrations and attempted to reproduce the figures. Those productions that were so poor that they were unscorable were arbitrarily assigned a score of 20.

The second portion of the study sample consists of 275 of the approximately 677 adults between 15 and 54 years of age. These individuals were volunteers from all *barrios* and *anejos*, ethnic and socioeconomic strata in the community. The Bender Gestalt Test was administered to these subjects by the author and his assistant over a period of about 3 weeks. The subjects were seated in comfortable chairs and worked on an ample table with a smooth surface. The tests were administered in the school in Guaraquí in the upper altitudinal zone, in a side building of the church in the middle altitudinal zone, and in the school in the *capilla* in the lower altitudinal zone.

The Deaf-Mute Group

Table 4.1 shows the mean Bender Gestalt scores and the frequency distribution of errors for the adult deaf-mute "cretins" in La Esperanza. The mean Bender scores of this group were more than 4 SDs standard deviations below the North American referent, thus indicating that these individuals are generally as retarded in visual–motor maturation as they are in language and auditory development. The mean scores of the female deaf-mutes are much poorer than those of the males.

The distribution of the Bender scores indicates that there is a considerable degree of variation in the extent of the neurological deficits in this group. Seventy-six percent of the males and all of the female deaf-mutes showed moderate to severe deficits in visual–motor perception. Extreme deficits (> 15 errors) were much more common among the female (55%) than the male (20%) "cretins." Surprisingly, 2 deaf-mute males (8%) made fewer than 3 errors, thus indicating normal visual–motor perceptive functioning, and 4 deaf-mute males (15%) made between 4 and 6 errors, suggesting no more than slight to moderate deficits in visual-motor perception. These 6 individuals did

TABLE 4.1

Mean Number of Errors and the Frequency Distribution of Error Scores on the Bender Gestalt Test. Deaf-Mute "Cretin" Group

Deaf-Mute "cretins"	Males	Females
$\overline{X}$	9.8	15.9
SD	5.7	4.6
N	25	20

Number of errors	Male		Female	
	N	%	N	%
0	1	4.0	0	0
1–3	1	4.0	0	0
4–6	4	16.0	0	0
7–9	12	48.0	3	15.0
10–12	0	0	4	20.0
13–15	2	8.0	2	10.0
>15	5	20.0	11	55.0
	25	100	20	100

not present neuromotor abnormalities and were included in the Group I deaf-mute category, which will be described below.

These data indicate that the deaf-mute "cretin" group is far from homogeneous; rather, they represent a fairly wide spectrum of neurological deficit. All of these subjects have apparently experienced an intrauterine hypothyroid stress that has a deleterious effect on the development of the middle and perhaps inner ear (Bargman & Gardner, 1972; Costa, 1972; Koenig & Neiger, 1972). Whether this stress must take place in the first trimester or shortly thereafter is, at present, uncertain. The variability in neuromotor development, visual–motor perception, and more complex cognitive abilities within this group is undoubtedly a function of differences in the time, duration, severity, and chronicity of these stresses in the different individuals. Differential experience with PCM may also contribute to the observed variation in neurological development.

We can speculate that the two highest scoring male deaf-mutes may only have experienced a limited intrauterine stress, after which thyroid function, both pre- and postnatally, may have been within normal limits. These two individuals, plus the four males in the 4–6 error category, really seem to be a much less severely affected group than the remainder (> 7 errors) of the male and female deaf-mute group combined.

Based on a total population of 1600 resident individuals, of which 900 are over 15 years of age, the 51 deaf-mute individuals represent 5.7% of the total adult population. Two and one-tenth percent of the adult population of this community are individuals 15–54 years of age who made more than 15 errors on their Bender Gestalt Test. Visual–motor perceptive functioning in this group is below that level that is characteristic of 5-year-old North American children.

The "Normal" Population

Sex Differences

The mean Bender Gestalt scores and the frequency distribution of errors in the sample from the "normal" adult population 15–54 years of age in La Esperanza is shown in Table 4.2. There are striking and statistically significant sex differences ($F = 40.3$, $df = 1/268$, $p < .001$) in these data, with the females showing a mean error score (3.8) more than twice that of the males (1.8). A much lower percentage of the females made no errors compared to the males. There were almost

TABLE 4.2

Mean Number of Errors and the Frequency Distribution of Error Scores on the Bender
Gestalt Test in a Sample of 275 "Normal" Adult Individuals between 15 and 54 Years of
Age

	Sample of the "normal" population	
	Males	Females
$\overline{X}$	1.8	3.8
SD	2.1	2.9
N	110	165

Number of errors	Males		Females	
	N	%	N	%
0	42	38.2	21	12.8
1–3	49	44.6	65	39.4
4–6	14	12.7	53	32.1
7–9	5	4.5	17	10.3
10–12	0	0	8	4.8
13–15	0	0	1	.6
>15	0	0	0	0
Total	110	100	165	100

three times as many females as males who made 4–6 errors, and more
than five times as many females made greater than 7 errors.

These data indicate that under these environmental conditions (extremely low iodine intake) there is a much higher prevalence of
neurological damage among females than males. This is a function of
sex-specific, hormonal-dependent differences in adaptation to low
iodine intake and is not a product of sex differences in role expectations on such a task (Greene, 1973). The sex differences in Bender
scores were present among children 6–15 years of age in La Esperanza but were totally absent in the adjacent population of Tocachi,
in which the children had received supplementary injections of
iodine in oil (Greene, 1976).

Total Bender Error Scores

In the section on the Bender Gestalt Test, I have outlined the
rationale for using 5.5 errors (1.5 ± 2.0) as the cutoff point beyond
which normal human variation should be considered to end and at
which the definition of neurological deficit in visual–motor perception should begin. This is a rather low criteria for normalcy. To qualify

as having a neurological deficit in visual–motor perception, these adult individuals 15–54 years of age must obtain Bender Gestalt scores that fall below the third percentile of 9.5 North American children.

Table 4.3 shows the number of La Esperanza adults who have Bender scores that were categorized as indicative of deficits in visual-motor perception. This amounted to 17.4% of the total adult sample. Another important finding was that the indigenous members of the population scored significantly more poorly than did the members of the *blanco* sociocultural segment ($F = 5.63$; $df = 1/213$, $p < .05$).

"Brain Damage" Scores

Of the 31 scoring criteria used in the Koppitz Developmental Bender Scoring System, 10 are considered to be "highly significant" indicators of brain damage. Using these criteria, the deaf-mute group had a mean brain damage score of 1.9; the group considered likely to be brain damaged on the basis of their total score had a "brain damage" score of 1.5; and the remainder of the "normal" population had a mean "brain damage" score of .25. Therefore, the group defined as being suspect of cerebral injury on the basis of their total Bender scores also made a large number of errors that are significant indicators of "brain damage." The mean number of "highly significant" errors among these individuals closely approximates that of the

TABLE 4.3

"Normal" Adult Individuals 15–54 Years of Age with Bender Gestalt Error Scores More than Two Standard Deviations (5.5 Errors) and Four Standard Deviations (9.5 Errors) below the Mean of 9.5-Year-Old North American Children

	Male		Female	
	N	%	N	%
Number of errors 6–9 (>2 SD)	8	7.3	31	18.8
More than 10 (>4 SD)	0	0	9	5.5
Total	8	7.3	40	24.2

deaf-mute group and is considerably greater than that of the remainder of the "normal" population.

The Continuum of Neurological Effect

All of the "normal" males with neurological deficits (7.3% of the sample) were between 2 and 4 SDs of the referent mean, as were 31 (18.8%) of the "normal" females with deficits. These individuals can be considered to have *moderate* neurological deficits in visual–motor perception. Sixteen (35.6%) of the deaf-mute "cretins" show a similar degree of deficit. Nine "normal" females (5.5% of the sample) were more than 4 SD below the referent mean. These individuals show severe deficits in visual–motor perception that place them among the lower half of the deaf-mute "cretin" group.

Figure 4.5 graphically shows the overlap of the scores of the deaf-mute "cretin" group and the "normal" population. The columns indicate the ratio of deaf-mute "cretins" to members of the "normal" *sample* achieving scores within each score range. Although the "cre-

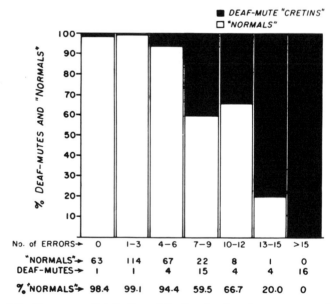

Figure 4.5. Frequency distribution of the Bender Gestalt error scores of the deaf-mute and "normal" samples. Percentage deaf-mute and "normal" individuals in each error score category. Sexes combined.

tins" represent 100% of the individuals with greater than 15 errors, there is a considerable degree of overlap in the 7–15 error range. Over 60% of the individuals in the 7–12 error range are *not* deaf-mutes, and 20% of the scores falling in the 13–15 error range belong to "normal" individuals.

These data demonstrate quite conclusively that the deaf-mute "cretin" group is part of a continuum of neurological deficit that affects a large portion of the total population. The major distinguishing feature of the deaf-mute group is that they manifest nervous-system damage that has affected the development of hearing and speech; some show neuromotor abnormalities; and some show extreme deficits in visual-motor perception. A strikingly large portion of the "normal" population show deficits in visual–motor perception that are quite comparable to those shown by the majority of the deaf-mutes.

It is thus a valid conclusion that the empirically gathered data support the proposed model for the prevalence of brain damage in this population.

Causal Factors

Inbreeding in La Esperanza, as measured by isonymy, is considerably lower than in the Hutterite population and no higher than those figures reported from several isolated communities in Switzerland, Italy, and Peru that do not show such high rates of retardation (Greene, 1976). Thus, there is no reason to believe that the deleterious effects of inbreeding account for the high prevalence of behavioral limitation in La Esperanza. Iodine malnutrition (low environmental iodine plus the ingestion of naturally occurring antithyroid compounds of plant origin) and PCM are the major environmental factors producing the high prevalence of neurological and behavioral deficits (Fierro-Benítez *et al.*, 1969 a,b; Greene, 1976; Stanbury, this volume).

Greater taste sensitivity to phenylthiocarbamide (PTC) appears to function as an avoidance mechanism for the rejection of naturally occurring goitrogens (antithyroid compounds) of plant origin (Greene, 1974). Under the environmental conditions that exist in La Esperanza, PTC taste sensitivity is a significant predictor of neurological maturation in children and appears to be an important determinant of who is, or is not, likely to be retarded (Greene, 1974, 1976). Socioeconomic status (reflecting differential nutritional and experiential components) is a second significant predictor of neurological development among children in this community (Greene, 1976).

BEHAVIORAL CAPACITIES OF THE DEAF-MUTE
"CRETIN" AND MODERATELY AFFECTED
"NORMAL" GROUP

This section evaluates the behavioral capacities of the deaf-mute
"cretins" and the non-deaf-mute individuals who have moderate
neurological deficits in visual–motor perception as demonstrated in
the previous section. I was particularly interested in the economic
functions of these individuals and how their presence in such large
numbers might affect the economic organization of the community.
The data for this section consist of a study of 33 individuals from the
deaf-mute group (15 females and 18 males) and 14 persons (10 females
and 4 males) from among those individuals with moderate neurological deficits. Observations of these individuals and interviews with the
members of their households provided the basic source of information. I encountered some of these individuals quite routinely during
the year that I lived in La Esperanza and was thus able to observe
them in different contexts and in a number of formal and informal
situations. The data and conclusions were discussed with my assistant, Merdado Albuja, who knew all those subjects quite well.

The Deaf-Mute "Cretins"

The deaf-mutes were placed in one of four categories based on their
physical development and behavioral capacities. Group I consists of
those deaf-mute individuals whose physical growth was within the
normal range for this population but who all showed slight to moderate deficits in visual–motor perception and some degree of cognitive
limitation (Figure 4.6). Their physical abilities were often equal to those
of normal adults of their own sex, but their mental abilities were more
like those of local children 8–10 years of age. Fifty-two percent of the
deaf-mutes were placed in this group. The behavioral capacities of
this and the other deaf-mute groups are summarized in Table 4.4.
    Group II consists of deaf-mute individuals who had slight
neuromotor abnormalities producing some limitations in their physical abilities. They all had moderate deficits in visual-motor perception
(7–12 errors) and greater cognitive limitations than those individuals
placed in Group I. As a group, these individuals were approximately
equivalent in behavioral capacities to like-sex children 6–7 years of
age. Eighteen percent of the deafmutes were placed in this group.
    Group III are deaf-mute individuals who showed moderate physical
and neuromotor abnormalities that greatly limited their ability to do

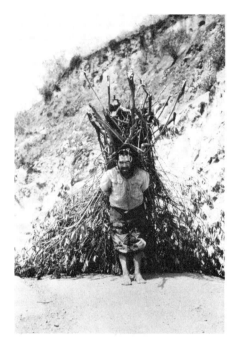

Figure 4.6.   Group I deaf-mute "cretin."

any type of useful work. These individuals showed severe deficits in visual-motor perception (13–20 errors). As a group, they demonstrated behavioral capacities that were generally equal to those of local children between 4 and 5 years of age. This group accounted for 12% of the total deaf-mute population. (Figure 4.7).

Group IV contains the most severely retarded deaf-mutes (Figures 4.8 and 4.9). These subjects were all under 120 cm in stature and had severe abnormalities in visual–motor perception and neuromotor functioning. These individuals demonstrated behavioral capacities equivalent to local children who were under 3 years of age. Half of these subjects were incapable of normal bipedal locomotion, and one moved by crawling on all fours. Eighteen percent of the deaf-mute subjects were placed in this category.

The following material is taken directly from my field notes and represents a portion of my first visit with the households of two deaf-mute individuals. This description, perhaps more than the tabulated data, should provide the reader with some sense of the life situation of these people. Proper names have been changed.

TABLE 4.4

Behavioral Capacities of Individuals with Moderate Neurological Deficits and the Deaf-Mute "Cretin" Group[a]

Individuals with moderate neurological deficits		Behavioral capacities
Estimated total number in La Esperanza	183	Capable of speech and hearing but ability to communicate with language is greatly limited. Capable of most agricultural and pastoral tasks except plowing (uncertain). Capable of most or all domestic tasks. Many engage in periodic wage labor but receive a lower remuneration than normal subjects. Some have formed independent households and borne or fathered children.

Deaf-mute "cretins"	N	Percentage of "cretin" group	Behavioral capacities
Group I	17	52	Speech and hearing greatly limited or absent. Capable of most agricultural and pastoral tasks except plowing, planting seeds, and herding cattle. Can often cook and sew a little. Capable of some wage labor. No independent households. Travel throughout the *parroquia*.
Group II	6	18	Speech and hearing greatly limited or absent. Slight neuromotor abnormalities producing limitations in physical labor. Can weed, *desgranar maíz*, collect small loads of wood and water. Care for small number of sheep or posted cattle. Not much cooking or sewing. Not capable of wage labor. No independent households. Travel throughout *barrio* or *anejo*.
Group III	4	12	Speech and hearing greatly limited or absent. Moderate neuromotor abnormalities. Weed, feed *cuyes*, watch posted cattle and corralled sheep. Restricted to family compounds or nearby.
Group IV	6	18	Speech and hearing entirely absent. Severe neuromotor abnormalities. Many incapable of bipedal locomotion. Gather weeds for *cuyes*. Restricted to family compound.

[a] After Greene (1976).

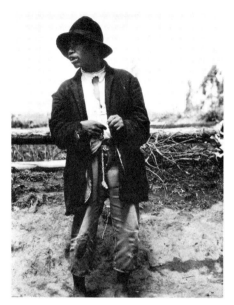

Figure 4.7. Group III deaf-mute "cretin."

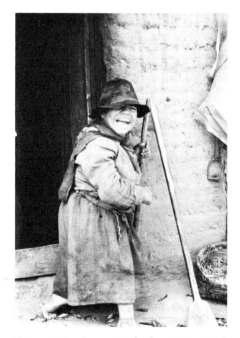

Figure 4.8. Group IV deaf-mute "cretin."

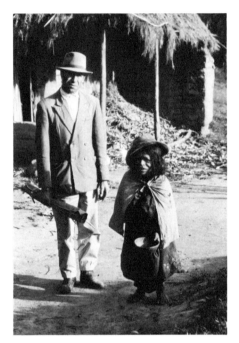

Figure 4.9. Group IV deaf-mute "cretin" and normal adult.

Isabel—Group III (almost Group IV)

Juan José Chanta lives in Tomalon at approximately 2,800 m. Isabel Imba is a deaf-mute about 20 years old who lives with him. She does not speak and hears only a very little. She is hardly capable of walking. Isabel is Señora Chanta's cousin and has lived with them since her father died when she was 6 years old.

Isabel does not understand much. She doesn't know how to plant seeds even though Juan José has tried to teach her. She is able to slowly harvest grains, but not very much at all. She can remove the kernels of corn from the cob, but again only at a very limited rate of speed. Isabel can watch the gentle posted cattle and corralled sheep, but she cannot move or pasture them. She walks with difficulty and cannot carry loads. Isabel rarely leaves the immediate vicinity of the family compound.

She does not know how to weed. Isabel cannot cook, peel potatoes, or wash her clothes. The main things that Isabel does are cut alfalfa for the cattle; gather weeds for the guinea pigs; and put wood in the hearth. Isabel was breast-fed until 2 years of age.

Miguel—Group I

Miguel is a deaf-mute of about 50 years of age who lives in the household of Alberto Segundo Ralla. Miguel was born and grew up in Chimbacalle, but when his father died about 7 years ago, he was left without a house or land. Since about that time, he has lived in Guaraquí, first in the house of Martin Luga and now here.

Miguel does not speak, but hears a little bit. He is capable of doing almost all agricultural tasks. While living with Señor Ralla, he pastures the animals almost all of the time. These include two cows, two bulls, and two calves. The Ralla's do not have sheep. Miguel can plant, harvest grains, weed, and remove the kernels from the corn cob. He can also carry heavy loads of wood and buckets of water. Miguel does not appear to be able to plow with a team of oxen.

Miguel can go to the store in Chimbacalle and buy salt and some other simple items. He knows that he is being cheated if he only gets one or two pieces of bread instead of the normal five for 1 *sucre* but does not object if he is given three or four pieces.

Miguel can sew and cook a bit and can clean his own clothes. He can also peel potatoes and shell peas, although he does not do many of these domestic tasks in the Ralla household.

When I was taking a photo of the entire household, I was having difficulty getting the 4-year-old child to stand in front of the group with his face to the camera. Miguel put his hand on the child's shoulder and turned him toward me while at the same time indicating with his other hand for the child to look toward me.

One outstanding feature of these data was the degree to which Group I individuals were reported to be able to perform the large majority of domestic and agricultural tasks. "*¡Hace todo!*" ("He does everything!") was a frequent reply from members of the household when asked what those individuals could or could not do. Most routine tasks, except plowing and occasionally planting, were easily mastered by the Group I individuals if given an adequate amount of time. The fact that they did not spontaneously initiate activities and had trouble sequencing different routines was not considered to be a negative attribute. As most agricultural, pastoral, and household work is quite routine, these individuals were highly valued for being good workers who followed instructions without question or resistance.

Routine tasks were easily mastered by Group I individuals, many of those in Group II, and some in Group III. These individuals demonstrated a range of capabilities that permitted them to do much of the routine work in this agricultural–pastoral economy. Although truly quantitative data are lacking, it is quite apparent that the cost to a household for maintaining the deaf-mute individuals was much below that of the economic benefits derived from their daily labor. This is especially true of the individuals in Group I. The expected daily cost of wage labor in 1971 was 10–15 *sucres* (40–60 cents) for normal *indígenas* and 5–8 *sucres* (20–40 cents) for those with moderate neurological deficits. The deaf-mute "cretin" individuals, especially those in Group I, were capable of most work that was performed by normal individuals and were available on a 24-hour basis and at a much lower cost. The deaf-mutes were also extremely docile and accepted unpleasant work, like sleeping in the fields with the animals or pasturing sheep all day in the cold *páramo*.

More than half of the Group I deaf-mutes that I studied were primarily involved in pasturing sheep. Four of these individuals were *apegados* in households in Guaraquí. The *indígenas* of this *anejo* have rights of pasture in the *páramo* grasslands of the *hacienda* and thus own fairly large flocks. These individuals were not members of the families with whom they lived but were given a place to sleep and food for their services, which was mostly pasturing sheep and sometimes cattle. In this community, more than half of the people who habitually pastured sheep were either deaf-mute "cretins" or individuals, often adolescent girls, with moderate neurological deficits.

Children between 6 and 10 years of age usually pastured sheep; however, the local governmental authorities were pressuring the *indígenas* to send their children to school when they reached 6 years of age. The *indígenas* themselves had begun to place a greater value on education, and a school had recently been built in Guaraquí. A certificate of graduation from the sixth grade was now a requirement for many jobs in Quito. These factors worked toward creating a situation in which fewer children were available for pastoral activities, and there was a veritable demand for deaf-mute "cretins" to fill this need as inexpensively as possible.

Individuals with Moderate Neurological Deficits

Many of the "normal" individuals who showed moderate neurological deficits on their Bender Gestalt Tests manifested behavioral characteristics similar to those of a number of local inhabitants with whom I had fairly routine contact, but on whom I did not have neurological data. These individuals were not deaf-mutes, were of normal stature, and had no apparent neuromotor abnormalities but had impressed me as being exceptionally "simple" and difficult to understand. When five of these impressionistically "simple" individuals between 30 and 45 years of age were given the Bender Gestalt Test, four achieved scores greater than 5.5, and one received an error score of 5. It thus appeared as though a significant number of these impressionistically "simple" individuals showed indications of moderate neurological deficits in visual–motor perception. Neurological deficits in one area of cerebral functioning are likely to covary with the presence of deficits in higher cerebral functions under these environmental circumstances. Therefore, these data strongly supported my suspicion that there was a neurological basis to the behavioral "simplicity" characteristic of this group of individuals with whom I had face-to-face relationship on an almost daily basis.

While some of the deaf-mute "cretins" had *blanco* surnames, the great majority of the individuals with moderate neurological deficits were *indígenas*. Behavioral observations were made on 14 of these individuals (4 males and 10 females) who had shown moderate neurological deficits in visual-motor perception (7–12 errors) on the Bender Gestalt Test. Three of the males and six of the females had formed their own households, while the others remained in their parental households or with siblings. The male members of this group who were living in conjugal unions had fathered slightly fewer children than normal males of their age, while the women members of this group had borne significantly fewer children than "normal" women. This was true of the 6 living in conjugal unions as well as the 4 who did not have stable unions.

These individuals were capable of most agricultural and pastoral tasks; however, they invariably worked under the guidance of someone who told them what to do and sequenced their activities for them. Most were able to plant, an activity that many Group I deaf-mutes were not capable of. All were capable of working for wage labor, and many of them did this routinely. These individuals usually received wages in produce *(por raciones)*, earning the equivalent of 4–6 *sucres* (16–24 cents) in produce for a day's labor, and some of these individuals made up to 8 *sucres*. Normal female *indígenas* earned the equivalent of 6–8 *sucres* for the same work, while the male *indígenas* made 15–17 *sucres* for a day's work on the *haciendas*.

Many individuals who impressionistically fit into this moderately affected group were those who supplied much of the labor to the *blanco* and *mestizo* landowners and occasionally also to other *indígenas*. Payment for agricultural labor is usually in produce and is somewhat at the discretion of the landowner. Both my assistant and I agreed that many of the individuals with moderate neurological deficits were systematically underpaid by the *blanco* and *mestizo* landowners.

BEHAVIOR AND SOCIAL ORGANIZATION

Consequences of the Presence of the Behaviorally Limited Individuals

Ideational

Adaptations. The presence of large numbers of behaviorally limited individuals in La Esperanza (5.7% deaf-mute "cretins" and 17.4% moderately retarded individuals) has a profound effect on the sociocultural characteristics of the community. The primary adaptation to the high prevalence of retardation is ideational. The definition of normality is considerably lowered, and the deaf-mute "cretin" group is the basic referent for what is normal or abnormal. Any individual who has more than minimal language and hearing capacity is excluded from this group and is considered to be "normal." Most agricultural and pastoral activities are rather routine, and even 82% of the deaf-mute group are capable of some economically useful tasks. Therefore, these people do not make the distinction that some of the "normal" individuals (the moderately deficient group) are somewhat limited in their capacity to perform some agricultural work and in their ability to initiate tasks and properly sequence work routines without help.

Besides their economic usefulness, there are two other cultural factors that help integrate these behaviorally limited individuals into the community. The first is the overwhelming fatalism of the Catholic religion. The existence of a deaf-mute "cretin" within both the family and the community is regarded as reflecting "God's will," which must be accepted as such. Fatalism is certainly one form of adaptation to extreme poverty and low social position, and this attitude is much stronger among the poor *indígenas* and *mestizos* than among the *blancos.*

A second cultural factor that helped integrate the deaf-mute "cretins" into the community was the familial nature of Hispanic culture and the Catholic religion. In a sense, the community of La Esperanza is conceived of as a large family, the relationships between the members of the community being familial. The deaf-mute individuals fit into this familial context and are treated as unfortunates but still members of the communal family. Their status, both within their households and in the community, is that of children of varying ages, depending on their capacities. Their social roles are thus somewhat equivalent to those of children who are not attending school. Only the

Group IV deaf-mutes lie outside of this network of affect. These individuals are so grossly retarded that they are almost regarded as stigmata. Individuals in this group are rarely allowed outside of their family compounds and are thus an unseen dimension of the community.

Rationalizations. The presence of such a large number of obviously retarded individuals in these predominantly indigenous rural communities has provided the empirical basis for a stereotyped view of the *indígena* as not being *racional* (rational). The *blancos* and *mestizos* view the *indígena* as a member of an inferior *raza* (race) that is only capable of providing brute labor. The members of the *blanco* and *mestizo* sociocultural segments see the frequent behavioral limitations and low social position of the *indígena* in terms of this group's purported genetic inferiority, thus effectively rationalizing the highly stratified nature of the social system. They do not view these phenomena as possibly being neurologically based behavioral deficits produced by nutritional factors that themselves have been caused, to a considerable extent, by the stratified nature of the social system and the uneven distribution of essential resources.

Structural

Outmigration. During the past 20 years, the population of La Esperanza has undergone a precipitious expansion, primarily as a result of a marked decrease in the infant-mortality rate. The increase in population has produced enormous pressure on the small amount of land and has led to an increased outmigration, primarily to Quito. The first to leave were mainly *blancos* and *mestizos* in the 1950s, but by the early 1960s many *indigenas* were seeking wage labor in Quito, which, if they were successful, was often a first step in the direction of emigration. Those individuals who emigrate are invariably people who have the behavioral capacity to procure wage-labor positions in the highly competitive labor market (oversupply of labor in relation to demand) in Quito. Many of these individuals have finished their primary schooling (Grade 6), a legal prerequisite for many types of governmental and nongovernmental employment.

Individuals who remained in La Esperanza were those people who had adequate amounts of land and/or were able to gain wage labor on the *haciendas* and the large number of behaviorally limited individuals who would not have been capable of procuring wage labor in Quito or elsewhere. The extreme conservatism of these individuals and their tie to familiar surroundings and stereotyped routines made outmigration unlikely even if employment were available. The result of this situation was that La Esperanza and similar communities, such as Tocachi, were losing a large number of their more capable inhabitants and becoming communities disproportionately populated by individuals with significant behavioral limitations. Thus, differential outmigration has been an important factor in the decline and involution of La Esperanza.

Community culture. The presence of so many retarded individuals, most of whom were *indígena*, resulted in a community containing a large number of docile inhabitants whose behavior was very conservative and tended to be extremely stereotyped. Cultural factors certainly contributed to this mental set, as the *indígena* held himself in very low self-esteem compared to the *blancos*. However, these cultural factors overlay real neurologically based behavioral limitations on the part of many indigenous members of the community.

Many of these individuals walked and talked normally and looked normal but were carriers and transmitters of an extremely limited aspect of the community culture. They dressed like members of their community; thus, they were conveyers of that material aspect of their cultural tradition. They spoke—to varying degrees; thus, they were participants in the language community, yet their linguistic participation was at a most concrete level. Conceptualization and generalization seemed to be beyond the capacity of many of these individuals. In essence, the community had a real dearth of adults capable of more complex social behavior and a huge surfeit of members with cognitive capacities not exceeding those of children 5–10 years of age.

At all levels of the community, the social fields were dominated by a rather limited number of individuals, while the great majority of people were exceptionally passive. It was striking how few individuals took more than passive roles in the ritual life of the community; how a small number of *blancos*, almost by default, made virtually all decisions concerning the *parroquia;* how in each *barrio* and *anejo* no more than two or three informal leaders were responsible for almost all organization; and how many inhabitants (certainly the deaf-mutes and most moderately retarded individuals) fell outside the field of *compadrazgo* relationships (ritual kinship) and were thus excluded from an important network of affect and an even more important community-wide and interethnic system of social and economic obligation.

That the local *blanco* minority (22% of the population) could politically dominate the indigenous majority and the ability of the *blanco*-dominated national government to maintain absolute authority in primarily or totally indigenous communities are both strong manifestations of the docility of the indigenous populations. I am suggesting that there is a biological basis to at least some portion of this passivity.

Effects on economic organization. The greatest impact of the large number of behaviorally limited, primarily indigenous individuals was the creation of a large pool of cheap labor that mainly benefited the *blanco* and *mestizo* landowners. The more capable deaf-mutes and the large number of moderately deficient individuals supplied most of this labor. The payment for labor, except on the *haciendas,* was almost always in produce, and these docile individuals, most of whom were *indígenas,* were easily manipulated and exploited within the context of the *patrón–peon* relationship.

The deaf-mutes and the moderately affected individuals were frequently from land-poor households that were obligated in some way to the *blanco* landowners, often because they or their households were *apegados* to the *blanco* (had a hut but no fields on his property) or because he was their *padrino de matrimonio* (godfather of marriage). Payment for these obligations was in labor, for which these *indígenas* received a very minimal payment in produce.

Other land-poor *indígenas* in the moderately deficient group who did not have such obligatory labor debts to the *blanco* and *mestizo* landowners also sought wage labor from this group. Such employment, although not between landowner and tenant, displayed another dimension of the *patrón–peon* relation. It is a relationship between the provider of work, the *patrón,* and a particular individual, the *peon,* to whom he gives employment. The relationship is relatively stable, with the *patrón* providing work to *particular peones,* as opposed to other individual *peones.* Because work of any kind is extremely scarce, and the supply of alternative laborers is great, the *peones* accepted a rather poor wage, which is paid *por raciones* (in produce). That the wage is paid in produce, as opposed to money, makes it easy for the *patrón* to further manipulate and "shortchange" these docile and behaviorally limited individuals.

These exploitative economic relationships are paralleled by extreme displays of affection by the *patrón* for his *peones.* In essence, the docile individuals are cajoled, flattered, and manipulated into accepting *"más cariño y menos raciones"* (more affection and less produce). To a behaviorally limited *indígena,* who is usually looked down upon and mistreated by *blancos* in everyday life and is excluded from the network of affect in the *compadrazgo* relationship, this source of affect from the high-status *patrón* is a potent reinforcement for the continuation of this exploitative relationship.

The more capable *indígenas* have greater options for labor and are able to procure a *somewhat* more symmetrical source of affect through the *compadrazgo* relationship (ritual kinship), from which the deaf-mutes and moderately affected individuals are excluded. They were thus less likely to enter into the highly exploitative *patrón–peon* economic relations.

SUMMARY

The Republic of Ecuador has a highly stratified social system that is the product of its unique history and the fact that the country's population remains divided into virtually two halves, the indigenous and the nonindigenous. The nonindigenous (*blanco* and *mestizo*), primarily urban, sociocultural segment controls the reins of government and most of the natural wealth, including land. The *indígenas* are concentrated in the rural areas. They are extremely land-poor (as are the poor *mestizos* in the rural areas), and until recently (the mid-1960s), many of these indigenous populations were virtual serfs *(huasipungeros)* on large state and private landholdings. Because the "rules" of the national sociocultural system are that of a society highly stratified along ethnic lines, the primarily rural indigenous population has a very constricted resource base on the most marginal and inhospitable lands. This situation has placed these populations under considerable nutritional and disease stress, with both of these factors having an effect on nervous system development.

The present study has evaluated an aspect of nervous system development and behavioral capacity in an Ecuadorian Andean community in which iodine malnutrition is severe and goiter and cretinism are endemic. PCM is also common, but is less severe and widespread. It has shown that in addition to the 5.7% of the adult population who are deaf-mute "cretin" individuals, there is another 17.4% of the population that show more moderate neurological deficits and behavioral limitations. These data support the hypothesis that the deaf-mutes are not the only retarded individuals but merely the most severe end of a continuum of neurological deficit and behavioral limitation.

The presence of such a disproportionate number of behaviorally limited primarily indigenous individuals (23% of the adult population) has a marked effect on the sociocultural characteristics of the community of La Esperanza. The numerically less numerous *blancos* dominate all of the community's institutions, to which the *indígenas* relate only passively. Most importantly, the large number of land-poor, behaviorally limited *indígenas* provide a pool of inexpensive and easily manipulatable labor that is utilized by the *blanco* landowners. This labor pool forms the economic basis of this highly stratified society, and the behavioral limitations of this group of individuals assures the landowners that their labor will be docile and unlikely to be able to find economic alternatives.

CONCLUSIONS

The nutritional stress and the highly stratified nature of the social system were both extreme in this study, thus making the relationship between the environmental, biological, and sociocultural systems stand out more clearly. I am suggesting that the model developed in this work is somewhat applicable to many other "less developed" countries and to the lower socioeconomic strata in some industrialized countries. Although the nutritional stresses may not be as extreme under other circumstances, I believe that a careful evaluation will show that in many parts of the world significant segments of human populations show discernible neurological deficits and behavioral limitations.

In general, a reasonable portion of the observed inter- and intrapopulation variation in behavior in these populations can probably be explained in terms of the effect of nutritional and disease stress on nervous system development. The recognition of the importance of these relationships should prompt us to ask questions that have not yet been asked about sociocultural organization and change historically, prehistorically, and for that matter, throughout human evolution.

REFERENCES

Balázs, R., Kovács, P., Treighgräber, W. A., Cocks, W. A., & Eayrs, J. T. Biochemical effects of thyroid deficiency on the developing brain. *Journal of Neurochemistry,* 1968, *15,* 1335–1349.
Bargman, G. J., & Gardner, L. I. Experimental production of otic lesions with antithyroid drugs. In J. B. Stanbury & R. L. Kroc (Eds.), *Human development and the thyroid gland. Relation to endemic cretinism.* New York: Plenum, 1972. Pp. 305–323.
Bass, N. H., & Netsky, M. G. Microchemical pathology of adult rat cerebrum following neonatal nutritional deprivation and hypothyroidism. *Transactions of the American Neurological Association,* 1969, *94,* 216–219.
Bass, N. H., & Young, E. Effects of hypothyroidism on the differentiation of neurons and

glia in developing rat cerebrum. *Journal of the Neurological Sciences*, 1973, *18*, 155–173.

Bender, L. *A visual motor gestalt test and its clinical use.* American Orthopsychiatric Association, *Research Monographs No. 3*, 1938.

Benedict, R. *Patterns of culture.* Boston: Houghton Mifflin, 1934.

Bolton, R. Aggression and hypoglycemia among the Qolla: A study in psychobiological anthropology. *Ethnology*, 1973, *12*, 227–257.

Costa, A. Embryogenesis of the ear and its central projection. In J. B. Stanbury & R. L. Kroc (Eds.), *Human development and the thyroid gland. Relation to endemic cretinism.* New York: Plenum, 1972. Pp. 291–303.

Crespi, M. K. *The patrons and peons of Pesillo: A traditional hacienda system in highland Ecuador* (Doctoral dissertation, University of Illinois, 1968). (University Microfilms, No. 69–1324).

Dodge, P. R., Palkes, H., Fierro-Benítez, R., & Ramírez, I. Effect on intelligence of iodine in oil administered to young Andean children—a preliminary report. In J. B. Stanbury (Ed.), *Endemic goiter.* Pan American Health Organization Scientific Publication No. 193. Washington, D.C.: World Health Organization, 1969. Pp. 378–380.

Eayrs, J. T. Influence of the thyroid on the central nervous system. *British Medical Bulletin*, 1960, *16*, 122–126.

Eayrs, J. T. Age as a factor determining the severity and reversibility of the effects of thyroid deprivation in the rat. *Journal of Endocrinology*, 1961, *22*, 409–419.

Eayrs, J. T., & Taylor, S. H. The effect of thyroid deficiency induced by methyl thiouracil on the maturation of the central nervous system. *Journal of Anatomy*, 1951, *85*, 350–358.

Estrella Aguirre, E. La acción de los mecanismos sociales sobre el estado de nutrición de una comunidad indígena de los Andes Ecuatorianos. Un proyecto de estudio. *América Indígena*, 1974, *34*, 807–827.

Fierro-Benítez, R., Penafiel, W., De Groot, L. J., & Ramirez, I. Endemic goiter and endemic cretinism in the Andean region. *New England Journal of Medicine*, 1969, *280*, 296–302. (a)

Fierro-Benítez, R., Ramírez, I., Carluci, M. A., Estrella, E., & Suárez, J. Biopatología andina y nutrición. *América Indígena*, 1974, *34*, 777–795.

Fierro-Benítez, R., Ramírez, I., Estrella, E., Jaramillo, C., Díaz, C., & Urresta, J. Iodized oil in the prevention of endemic goiter in the Andean region of Ecuador. I. Program design, effects on goiter prevalence, thyroid function, and iodine secretion. In J. B. Stanbury (Ed.), *Endemic goiter,* Pan American Health Organization Scientific Publication No. 193. Washington, D.C.: World Health Organization, 1969. Pp. 306–340. (b)

Fierro-Benítez, R., Ramírez, I., Garcés, J., Jaramillo, C., Moncayo, F., & Stanbury, J. B. The clinical pattern of cretinism as seen in highland Ecuador. *American Journal of Clinical Nutrition*, 1974, *27*, 531–543.

Fierro-Benítez, R., Ramírez, I., & Suárez, J. Effect of iodine correction early in fetal life on intelligence quotient. A preliminary report. In J. B. Stanbury & R. L. Kroc (Eds.), *Human development and the thyroid gland. Relation to endemic cretinism.* New York: Plenum, 1972. Pp. 239–247.

Fierro-Benítez, R., & Recalde, F. Estudios previos y planificación de los trabajos de investigación sobre bocio endémico en la Región Andina. *Revista de Facultad de Ciencias Médicas (Quito)*, 1958, *9–10*, 55–67.

Fierro-Benítez, R., Stanbury, J. B., Querido, A., De Groot, L., Alban, R., & Cordova, J. Endemic cretinism in the Andean region of Ecuador. *Journal of Clinical Endocrinology and Metabolism*, 1970, *30*, 228–236.

Foulks, E. F. *The arctic hysterias of the North Alaskan Eskimo*. Anthropological Studies. No. 10. Washington, D.C.: American Anthropological Association, 1972.

Goldschmidt, V. M. *Geochemistry*. New York: Oxford University Press (Clarendon), 1958.

Greene, L. S. Physical growth and development, neurological maturation and behavioral functioning in two Ecuadorian Andean communities in which goiter is endemic. I. Outline of the problem of endemic goiter and cretinism. Physical growth and neurological maturation in the adult population of La Esperanza. *American Journal of Physical Anthropology*, 1973, *38*, 119–134.

Greene, L. S. Physical growth and development, neurological maturation, and behavioral functioning in two Ecuadorian Andean communities in which goiter is endemic. II. PTC taste sensitivity and neurological maturation. *American Journal of Physical Anthropology*, 1974, *41*, 139–152.

Greene, L. S. *Nutrition and behavior in highland Ecuador* (Doctoral dissertation, University of Pennsylvania, 1976). (University Microfilms, 1976, No. 76-695.

Kardiner, A. *The psychological frontiers of society*. New York: Columbia Univ. Press, 1945.

Katz, S. H. Evolutionary perspectives on purpose and man. *Zygon*, *1973*, *8*, 325–340.

Katz, S. H., & Foulks, E. F. Mineral metabolism and behavior: abnormalities of calcium homeostasis. *American Journal of Physical Anthropology*, 1970, *32*, 299–304.

Katz, S. H., & Foulks, E. An ecosystems approach to health in the arctic. *Acta sociomedica Scandinavica (supplementum)*, 1972, *6*, 185–194.

Koenig, M. P., & Neiger, M. The pathology of the ear in endemic cretinism. In J. B. Stanbury & R. L. Kroc (Eds.), *Human development and the thyroid gland. Relation to endemic cretinism*. New York: Plenum, 1972. Pp. 325–333.

Koppitz, E. M. *The Bender Gestalt test for young children*. New York: Grune & Stratton, 1964.

Mead, M. *Sex and temperament in three primitive societies*. New York: Morrow, 1935.

Ramírez, I., Fierro-Benítez, R., Estrella, E., Jaramillo, C., Díaz, C., & Urresta, J. Iodized oil in the prevention of endemic goiter and associated defects in the Andean region of Ecuador. In J. B. Stanbury (Ed.), *Endemic goiter*. Pan American Health Organization Scientific Publication No. 193. Washington, D.C.: World Health Organization, 1969. Pp. 341–359.

Republica del Ecuador. Junta Nacional de Planificación y coordinación Económica. *Segundo censo del población y primer de vivienda: 1962*. Quito: División de Estatística y Censos, 1964.

Rosenzweig, M. R., Bennett, E. L., & Diamond, M. C. Brain changes in response to experience. *Scientific American*, 1972, *226*, 22–30.

Rowe, J. H. Inca culture at the time of the Spanish conquest. In J. H. Steward (Ed.), *Handbook of South American Indians*. Vol. 2. *The Andean civilizations*. Washington: U.S Government Printing Office, 1946. Pp. 196–330.

Stanbury, J. B. Familial goiter. In J. B. Stanbury, J. B. Wyngaarden, & D. S. Frederickson (Eds.), *The metabolic basis of inherited disease*. (3rd ed.). New York: McGraw-Hill, 1972. Pp. 223–265. (a)

Stanbury, J. B. The clinical pattern of cretinism as seen in highland Ecuador. In J. B.

Stanbury & R. L. Kroc (Eds.), *Human development and the thyroid gland. Relation to endemic cretinism*. New York: Plenum, 1972. Pp. 3–17. (b)

Wallace, A. F. C. Mental illness, biology and culture. In F. Hsu (Ed.), *Psychological anthropology*. Homewood, Illinois: Dorsey Press, 1961.

Walsh, R. N., & Cummins, R. A. Neural responses to therapeutic environments. In R. N. Walsh & W. T. Greenough (Eds.), *Environments as therapy for brain dysfunction*. New York: Plenum, 1976. Pp. 171–200.

5

Malnutrition and Human Performance

MERRILL S. READ[1]

National Institute of Child Health and Human Development

The papers that have been presented in this volume represent a unique blend of the behavioral, biomedical, and sociopolitical facets of malnutrition. All focus primarily on the consequences of severe malnutrition. Thus, Suskind (this volume) has provided us with a comprehensive view of the origin and characteristics of protein–calorie malnutrition (PCM) with clear implications for long-term consequences in terms of child health and development. Thomson and Pollitt (this volume) have taken this topic further in their thoughtful review concerning the behavioral–intellectual implications for those children unfortunate enough to experience severe PCM early in life. Their conclusion that the behavioral impact of severe malnutrition, particularly kwashiorkor, that occurs after the first year of life may not necessarily be irreversible is important and encouraging. The companion papers by Stanbury (this volume) and Greene (this volume) again deal with severe malnutrition, in this case iodine deficiency, which afflicts a sizable number of the world's people.

It is important to note that there are other specific deficiency problems of comparable magnitude in the world that might be equally well

[1] Division of Family Health/Nutrition, Pan American Health Organization.

discussed here, particularly deficiencies of vitamin A and iron. Although the conclusions for health and development might differ in detail, certainly neither the urgency nor the philosophy would change should these other nutritional problems be examined in detail.

In addition to the question of severity of malnutrition, these papers are concerned with the timing of the insult. In both PCM and iodine deficiency, the earlier the insult, the more likely for the consequences to be permanent and nonremedial. Pregnancy emerges as a particularly vulnerable period. However, duration of malnutrition also is of major concern. This has been forcefully reinforced by the elegant retrospective study by Stein, Susser, Saenger, and Marolla (1975) of the consequences of famine during pregnancy as occurred during the Dutch famine of World War II. The relative lack of impact of the famine on intellectual development of the survivors undoubtedly was due in large measure to the brevity of the severe restriction, the generally good health of the mothers at the outset of deprivation, and the comparatively rapid return to satisfactory health and nutrition following the lifting of the siege. None of these conditions apply to the millions of the world's people who live with chronic undernutrition. This is the problem that I wish to address, with special reference to the consequences for functional competence of the individual within his society and in terms of costs to that society.

⁎ Thomson and Pollitt and Suskind have referred to the incidence of PCM in Asia, Africa, and Central America. Whereas severe clinical PCM may afflict up to 20% of the children, chronic moderate malnutrition may be experienced by up to three or four times as many. Without prompt nutritional rehabilitation, severe PCM most often leads to death. Moderate malnutrition generally results in marked growth retardation and in increased susceptibility to diseases. ⁎

MALNUTRITION AND CHILD DEVELOPMENT

Let us now turn our attention to the impact of this widespread chronic malnutrition on behavioral and intellectual development. Unfortunately, there are fewer published studies of such children, and the results are more confusing than the data for severe PCM. It would be anticipated that the effects, if any, would be less serious and therefore harder to measure. Furthermore, moderate or chronic undernutrition must be viewed in the context of the malnourished child's social and familial environment, many parts of which also shape behavioral development. Finally, nearly all the studies on chronic undernutrition have been retrospective in nature, with no detailed information concerning the type, severity, or duration of prior malnutrition other than that inferred from anthropometric measurements and dietary assessments at the time of clinical examination. For a detailed review of these studies, see the papers by Read (1973a, b, 1975a, b); only recently published material not previously cited in these reviews will be referenced in the current report.

Despite the problems inherent in retrospective research, a number of studies in Mexico, India, Africa, and the Caribbean have shown that chronically undernourished children tend to lag behind their well-nourished counterparts in terms of behavioral development. The primary deficits appear to involve motor-integrative performance, reading ability, concentration, and motivation rather than the more cognitive (problem solving) processes. Even within the same family, those children who were more poorly nourished did less well on behavioral tests and in school than did their better nourished brothers and sisters. Whether these differences disappear as a result of extended school experience remains an unanswered question.

The best way to determine the impact of nutritional status on development is to measure what an individual eats over time, while at the same time assessing developmental characteristics. Recent studies have taken this longitudinal approach. Generally, one group of participants is nutritionally supplemented while another group from the same environment is not. All participants in these projects receive previously unavailable medical care.

The largest and most thorough of these studies is presently being conducted in rural Guatemala. The study design involves four small villages roughly comparable in socioeconomic status. All villages are provided a unique and effective clinic-centered medical-care system that is very low in cost ($1–2 per clinic visit including staff training, salaries, facilities, and medicines) when compared to others reported in the literature (Habicht, 1973). The identification of illness is further complemented by regular biweekly home visits. In this way it is possible to determine the nature and duration of the frequent but relatively minor illnesses that may interfere with food intake and with growth. The biweekly home visits also permit early identification of missed menses so that the onset of pregnancy can be estimated within 15 days for most women. A midwife attends all births, most of which occur in the home. Birth weight is recorded within 24 hr of birth by trained staff members. A total sample of 1083 children is under study,

671 of whom were born during the 4-year enrollment period and 412 children who were under 3 years of age when the study started in 1969.
⋆ Two supplements are being provided. One is a protein–calorie vitamin–mineral mixture called "atole" containing 50% milk solids plus 50% Incaparina (cottonseed meal, corn flour, lysine, yeast, vitamins, and minerals). The other is called "fresco" and has about one-third the calorie level plus the same vitamins and minerals. Each supplement is provided ad libitum in a central facility with the consumption measured accurately. Special attention is given in the supplementation program to reaching the pregnant and lactating women as well as children up through 7 years of age. Home dietary surveys are done quarterly. An extensive psychological test battery has been developed for this population that is used for testing all children at regular intervals. Measures of socioeconomic status and of home-teaching concepts are also performed. ⋆
⋆ Nutritional supplementation has increased birth weight, which tends to be low in these populations. On the average, 30 gm of additional birthweight were associated with each additional 10,000 calories consumed during pregnancy (Lechtig, Habicht, Delgado, Klein, Yarbrough, & Martorell, 1975). Babies of women who regularly participated fully in the supplementation program were about 125 gm heavier than those of women who participated poorly or not at all. A similar difference in birth weight was found in successive births to mothers who were well supplemented during one pregnancy and poorly supplemented during a following pregnancy. Interestingly enough, the beneficial effect on low birth weight appeared to be due primarily to calorie ingestion and was not enhanced by the additional protein available in the atole supplement. ⋆

Nutritional supplementation also has been related to better growth of children at age 3 years (Klein, Delgado, Engle, Lechtig, Martorell, & Yarbrough, 1976). The data suggest that about half the difference in growth rate between these Guatemalan children and United States growth standards may be due to nutrition; the remainder appears to be associated with morbidity during childhood and, to an unknown extent, to genetic influences. Calorie supplementation presently appears to be the major nutritional contributor to improved growth, but the importance of added protein is being carefully explored.

By 15 months of age significant relationships between supplement ingestion and performance on the psychological tests were observed that have remained consistent up to 4 years of age (Klein *et al.*, 1976). Item analyses of the individual scales suggest that the impact is more closely associated with the more motoric and manipulative items in contrast to the linguistic or cognitive items, at least at the earlier ages. The studies are continuing to determine whether these patterns remain as the children approach the age for school entry.

The Guatemalan investigators are attempting to account for nonnutritional, nonmedical contributors to mental development in the village setting. The impact of these is sizable even under the low socioeconomic conditions encountered in the study villages (Engle, Klein, Yarbrough, Lasky, & Lechtig, 1974). Nevertheless, they believe that the behavioral differences they are reporting are to a considerable extent related to the improved nutritional status resulting from the supplements. In other settings with a wider range of social and environmental differences, the latter may contribute importantly to behavioral retardation sometimes attributed to malnutrition. Certainly socioeconomic factors have repeatedly been shown to contribute to performance as seen when physically comparable children from different social strata were compared; those from lower socioeconomic families generally did less well on psychological tests.

Christiansen, Vouri, Mora, and Wagner (1974) have reported on studies of malnourished children and their families in the poor areas of Bogota. They note that the mothers of malnourished children "had lower educational and occupational aspirations for their children, tended to play less, give less verbal reinforcement and to do less direct teaching in regard to their children; in addition, they tended more often to give primary child-rearing responsibility to other children in the family." These investigators are now studying the impact of specific mother-training programs, with and without nutrition intervention, on behavioral development of these children.

Chavez and his colleagues (Chavez, Martinez, & Yashine, 1975) have been particularly innovative in exploring the relationship between malnutrition and parent-infant interaction. They have studied 17 children born to mothers living under "normal" low socioeconomic conditions in a rural Mexican community. A similar number of other mothers from the same community received supplements from Day 45 of pregnancy through lactation, and their infants were supplemented from weaning. The supplemented children did better on all aspects of the Gesell test through 2 years of age. By 1 year of age, the physical activity was significantly greater in the supplemented children; a sixfold difference was observed by 2 years. The unsupplemented children spent more time in their cribs or beds and less time exploring, were kept or chose to stay in their houses for the majority of the time, and were held more often during the first year of life. The supplemented children clearly were more exploratory, active, and expressive. As the supplemented children grew more rapidly, they received more attention and care from the other family members. The mothers themselves were more active and more involved with their children. Even more surprising, the fathers paid much more attention to their child and clearly demonstrated pride in the child's progress; this is a rare phenomenon with children of this age in this culture.

Other recent studies further emphasize the importance of the environment in terms of outcome. These derive from cases of severe malnutrition but are worthy of note in the context here. One intriguing study (Lloyd-Still, Hurwitz, Wolff, & Schwachman, 1974) involved babies, many of whom had cystic fibrosis, a disease that leads to failure of intestinal absorption. All of these babies were well fed by their middle-class families, but they failed to grow due to malabsorption problems. After treatment they grew normally. Siblings were used for controls on the behavioral testing. Follow-up tests indicated some behavioral retardation through the first 5 years of life. After that the retardation gradually disappeared, presumably because the children were raised in a favorable social environment. Ellis and Hill (1975) similarly report no adverse effects on IQ or wide-range achievement tests at 7–10 years of age in cystic fibrosis cases known to have had 20–40% weight deficits at some point during infancy; cystic fibrosis patients who had not been exposed to such malnutrition were used for controls in this study.

In another study (Winick, Meyer, & Harris, 1975), Korean children known to have had severe malnutrition early in life were adopted by families in the United States. By 7 years of age the children were normal in performance as shown by standardized IQ and achievement scores provided by their schools. Other Korean children who had never been malnourished and who were also adopted by American families were similarly investigated; they were above normal in IQ and performance. These observations suggest that the stimulation of the adopted environment facilitated normal behavioral development but that the malnourished children may not have achieved their full intellectual potential.

MALNUTRITION AND WORK CAPACITY

It is clear from the material reviewed that chronic moderate malnutrition affects the activity level of the growing child. Implicit in some of the reports is the suggestion that malnutrition decreases the energy and activity level of the mother as well. Extending this thought further, what do we know about the impact of chronic undernutrition on activity level and work performance of men? Any appreciable decrease in the work capacity of the male head of the household could, in turn, reduce family income, decrease ability to purchase an adequate diet, and in the long run adversely affect the nutritional status and health of all the family members. Such a situation would be most expected to be encountered in preindustrialized agricultural areas in which the production of food and of other goods depends directly on heavy physical activity, often near the level of maximal effort.

There are surprisingly little quantitative data on malnutrition as it may relate to adult human work capacity. A few studies were conducted during and after World War II on the consequences of severe caloric restriction in healthy United States males. Among these are the classic studies of starvation in previously well-nourished human volunteers reported by Keys, Brozek, Henschel, Michelsen, and Taylor (1950). The subjects' spontaneous activity and capacity to perform hard physical activity decreased as the period of caloric restriction was prolonged; performance capability was restored upon rehabilitation. Subsequent studies (Taylor, Buskirk, Brozek, Anderson, & Grande, 1957) showed that young men subsisting on low-calorie diets for relatively short periods of time reduced their work output during hard physical activity.

Only in the past decade or so has serious attention been given to the work capacity of chronically undernourished workers. Current studies are focusing on two types of widespread nutritional problems: (1) restricted energy intake, which might be expected to decrease energy output, work capacity, and the ability for sustained hard labor; and (2) iron deficiency anemia, which might limit blood oxygen transporting capacity with adverse effects on work capacity.

Protein–Calorie Malnutrition

Viteri (1971) and Viteri and Torun (1975), working with healthy rural Guatemalan workers, have shown that the energy requirements for performing agricultural tasks remained relatively constant regardless of variations in caloric intake. On the other hand, a limited calorie intake below the level required for sustained work apparently puts a ceiling on total energy expenditure and therefore on total productivity. They cite data from two different populations: one consuming 2700 calories per person per day and the other 3500 calories. The daily

800 calorie difference in intake was reflected in an equivalent decrease in calorie expenditure in various activities. In detailed studies
of the energy costs of agricultural activities, this group (Viteri, Torun,
Galacia, & Herrera, 1971) has shown that rural workers spend all of
the calories they ingest in daily activities, at least within the "normal"
calorie consumption range in Guatemala.

Spurr, Barac-Nieto, and Maksud (1974, 1975) have used maximal
ability to consume oxygen (V_{O_2} max) as one measure of physical work
capacity in Columbian adult male agricultural workers. They consider
V_{O_2} max to be one of the most direct measures available for assessing
physical fitness. They also included direct productivity measures
wherever suitable. The Columbian subjects were chronically undernourished as determined by low blood albumin, total protein, and
cholesterol levels; a battery of other clinical and anthropometric measures were also taken. Spurr et al. did not find that the biochemical or
clinical indications of malnutrition could be related to high or low
work output (e.g., tons of sugarcane cut per day). The low-productivity
workers did have lower V_{O_2} max and were somewhat shorter and
lighter, with less lean body mass than the high producers. The
maximum oxygen consumption differences were found consistently
regardless of whether the data were expressed in terms of height or
weight. This suggests that the low producers may have had a history of
prolonged chronic malnutrition. In support of the idea that malnutrition affects performance and fitness, these investigators also have
shown that patients with clinically severe malnutrition exhibited low
aerobic power (maximum), which was markedly improved by protein
repletion. However, after full rehabilitation, the V_{O_2} max values were
still below those obtained from comparable adequately nourished
subjects.

Anemia

What about anemia? Does it affect adult work performance? Certainly the available evidence from animal models and from studies
with children suggest that anemia might decrease work capacity or
sustained physical activity (Read, 1975b; Pollitt & Leibel, 1976).

In studies of otherwise well-nourished adult subjects, Anderson and
Barkve (1970) found that iron-deficiency anemia impaired working
capacity and lengthened the time required for cardiorespiratory function to return to normal following standardized exercise. Similarly,
Sproule, Mitchell, and Miller (1960) reported differences in respira-

tory function and a variety of cardiovascular tests between iron-deficient anemic and normal subjects in response to exercise.

Viteri (1973; Viteri & Torun, 1974), working on a Guatemalan coffee plantation in which anemia is prevalent, has reported that 62 adult male workers with hemoglobins between 4 and 8 gm% and with packed cell volumes (PCV) below 30% exhibited markedly reduced work capacity. Furthermore, scores on the Harvard Step Test decreased roughly proportional to the reduction in hematologic values. Therapy with elemental iron with or without folic acid resulted in rapid recovery (1–2 months) of hematologic values, work capacity, and Step Test scores; subjective improvement in a sense of well-being also was reported by these workers. It may be of value to note that 72% of the workers who had or achieved PCV values greater than 40% had fair to excellent performance scores.

A recent report (Gardner, Edgerton, Barnard, & Bernauer, 1975) summarizes data from 13 male and 16 female adult workers in rural Venezuela. Heart rate, blood lactate, and oxygen consumption data were obtained in conjunction with muscular strength tests and Step Test exercise. Intramuscular iron coupled with treatment for hookworm infestation were used to correct anemia. Within 80 days after treatment, hemoglobin levels increased from 7.7 to 12.4 gm% for the women and from 7.1 to 14.0 gm% for the men. Iron treatment did not affect hand grip or shoulder adductor strength. Peak exercise heart rates and ventilation were significantly higher in the anemic subjects. No differences were found in oxygen consumption in response to the Step Test, although the investigators calculated that a mean of 15% more oxygen was delivered per pulse in the iron-treated subjects than in the placebo group. Blood lactate levels were significantly lower following performance testing of the nonanemic subjects. Unfortunately, no assessment of work performance under normal hard physical labor was obtained. Nevertheless, the authors emphasize that their data "clearly support the concept that performance requiring high oxygen delivery is significantly affected by hemoglobin levels."

Basta and Churchill (1974) also have been investigating the impact of iron deficiency anemia on the work performance of male Indonesian construction and plantation workers. A hemoglobin level less than 12.9 gm% was taken as an indication of anemia; this is described as roughly equivalent to a PCV value of 37–38%. The two populations had a prevalence of 42–45% anemia by these definitions. Hookworm infestation was widespread and closely associated with anemia. In the nearly 600 construction workers and the 300 plantation workers, a significant correlation was found between the degree of anemia and performance on the Harvard Step Test. A daily intervention of 100 mg of elemental iron was provided to half of the plantation workers. Iron treatment over a 60-day period significantly increased serum iron, transferrin saturation, and TIBC levels; hemoglobin levels increased to more than 15 gm%. The iron-treated group performed significantly better than the anemic subjects on the Step Test. In addition, work output on such tasks as latex collecting was increased by 19–20% as a consequence of iron treatment for the anemic men. A similar difference in weeding (cultivating) performance was recorded when anemic and nonanemic workers were compared. These authors have extended their observations to show that there was an almost linear correlation between hemoglobin levels and monthly payments to latex tappers for output beyond the daily quota. Based on the cost of treatment and the sales value of the latex at the time of this study, they estimated that the benefit:cost ratio for correcting iron deficiency could run as high as 260:1! Even at much lower benefit ratios, the impact on both family and community is almost staggering in its implications.

It is amply apparent that nutritional status is closely associated with work performance, at least in those populations subsisting on marginal intakes in which maximal work is required daily.

DISCUSSION

There can be little doubt from the data summarized briefly here that nutrition, health, and human performance are intimately intertwined. This is further reinforced by the growing awareness of the interrelationship between malnutrition and infection, as discussed by Suskind. Not only is the ability to withstand infectious diseases or infestations decreased by chronic or acute malnutrition, but food consumption and nutrient utilization are adversely effected during episodes of infection or diarrhea. The combination leads to decreased environmental interaction for the child and to poorer performance for adults.

When the head of the household is undernourished, he will tend to be absent from work more often, to work fewer hours, or to perform less efficiently. When pay is on a piecework basis, this will seriously decrease income for the family as a unit. The likelihood of malnutrition in other family members will correspondingly increase.

If the mother is malnourished, she will tend to have smaller babies with higher risk of developmental retardation. She herself will be less energetic and less able to adequately care for her children. The undernourished child will be less active and demanding. The interaction of poorly nourished mother and undernourished child will in turn contribute to a less fully developed child who may grow up to be more lethargic, less well motivated, and unable to contribute to his community or to care for a family of his own. This sets up a cycle wherein poor environment leads to malnutrition, which in turn shapes behavior to perpetuate poverty, intellectual disability, and malnutrition.

It is highly unlikely that this vicious pattern can be reversed quickly or by a simple single intervention. Major attention must be given to a combination of public-health programs to decrease disease, family-planning programs to decrease the number of mouths to feed, and nutritional interventions aimed at the most vulnerable target groups. Ultimately, the goal is more adequate income for families so that they can feed and provide for themselves.

An exciting array of innovative programs for families and small communities has recently been described (UNICEF 1975a,b). Further careful thought should be given to the role of nutrition in work capacity and performance to see whether limited interventions at the breadwinner level would have a significant rippling effect of benefit not only to the worker but to his family and children as well.

REFERENCES

Anderson, H. T., & Barkve, H., Iron deficiency and muscular work performance. *Scandinavian Journal of Clinical Laboratory Investigation*, 1970, 25, Suppl. No. 114.

Basta, S. S., & Churchill, A. Iron deficiency anemia and the productivity of adult males in Indonesia. *Staff Working Paper No. 175*, International Bank for Reconstruction and Development, Washington, D.C., 1974.

Chavez, A., Martinez, C., & Yashine, T. Nutrition, behavioral development, and mother-child interaction in young rural children. *Federation Proceedings*, 1975, 34, 1574–1582.

Christiansen, N., Vouri, L., Mora, J. O., & Wagner, M. Social environment as it relates to malnutrition and mental development. In J. Cravioto, L. Hambraeus, & B. Vahlquist (Eds.), *Early malnutrition and mental development*. Uppsala, Sweden: Almqvist & Wiksell, 1974. Pp. 186–199.

Ellis, C. E., & Hill, D. E. Growth, intelligence, and school performance in children with cystic fibrosis who have had an episode of malnutrition during infancy. *Journal of Pediatrics*, 1975, 87, 565–568.

Engle, P., Klein, R. E., Yarbrough, C., Lasky, R. E., & Lechtig, A. Efecto de la desnutricion sobre el desarrollo mental. In *Organizacion de Servicios para el Retrasado Mental*. Scientific Publication No. 293, Pan American Health Organization, Washington, D.C., 1974. Pp. 73–80.

Gardner, G. W., Edgerton, V. R., Barnard, R. J., & Bernauer, E. M. Cardiorespiratory, hematological, and physical performance responses of anemic subjects to iron treatment. *American Journal of Clinical Nutrition*, 1975, *28*, 982–988.

Habicht, J. P. Delivery of primary care by medical auxiliaries: Techniques of use and analysis of benefits achieved in some rural villages in Guatemala. In *Medical care auxiliaries*. Scientific Publication No. 278, Pan American Health Organization, Washington, D.C., 1973. Pp. 24–37.

Keys, A., Brozĕk, J., Henschel, A., Michelsen, O. & Taylor, H. L. *The biology of human starvation* (Vol. 2). Minneapolis: Univ. of Minnesota Press, 1950.

Klein, R. E. Malnutrition and human behavior: A backward glance at an ongoing longitudinal study. In D. A. Levitsky (Ed.), *Malnutrition and mental retardation: An assessment of current research*. Ithaca, New York: Cornell University Press, 1977 (forthcoming).

Lechtig, A., Habicht, J. P., Delgado, H., Klein, R. E., Yarbrough, C., & Martorell, R. Effect of food supplementation during pregnancy on birthweight. *Pediatrics*, 1975, *56*, 508–520.

Lloyd-Stills, J. D., Hurwitz, I., Wolff, P. H., & Shwachmann, H. Intellectual development after severe malnutrition in infancy. *Pediatrics*, 1974, *54*, 306–311.

Pollitt, E., & Leibel, R. L. Iron deficiency and behavior. *Journal of Pediatrics*, 1976, *88*, 372–381.

Read, M. S. Malnutrition, hunger, and behavior. I. Malnutrition and learning. *American Journal of Dietetics*, 1973, *63*, 379–385. (a)

Read, M. S. Malnutrition, hunger, and behavior. II. Hunger, school feeding programs, and behavior. *American Journal of Dietetics*, 1973, *63*, 386–391. (b)

Read, M. S. Behavioral correlates of malnutrition. In M. A. B. Brazier (Ed.), *Growth and development of the brain*. New York: Raven Press, 1975. Pp. 335–353. (a)

Read, M. S. Anemia and behavior. *Modern Problems in Paediatrics*, 1975, *14*, 189–202. (b)

Sproule, B. J., Mitchell, J. H., & Miller, W. F. Cardiopulmonary physiological responses to heavy exercise in patients with anemia. *Journal of Clinical Investigation*, 1960, *39*, 378–388.

Spurr, G. B., Barac-Nieto, M., & Maksud, M. G. Clinical and subclinical malnutrition: Their influence on the capacity to do work. *Annual Progress Report*, Contract No. AID/CSD 2943, May 1974. U.S. Agency for International Development.

Spurr, G. B., Barac-Nieto, M., & Maksud, M. D. Energy expenditure cutting sugarcane. *Journal of Applied Physiology*, 1975, *39*, 990–996.

Stein, Z., Susser, M., Saenger, G., & Marolla, F. *Famine and human development: The Dutch hunger winter of 1944/45*. New York: Oxford University Press, 1975.

Taylor, H. L., Buskirk, E. R., Brozĕk, J., Anderson, J. T., & Grande, F. Performance capacity and effects of caloric restriction with hard physical work on young men. *Journal of Applied Physiology*, 1957, *10*, 421–429.

Winick, M., Meyer, K., & Harris, R. C. Malnutrition and environmental enrichment by early adoption. *Science*, 1975, *190*, 1173–1175.

Unicef. Fighting childhood malnutrition: Part I. *Unicef News*, 1975, *85*, 3–30. (a)

Unicef. Fighting childhood malnutrition: Part II. *Unicef News*, 1975, *86*, 3–31. (b)

Viteri, F. E. Considerations on the effect of nutrition on the body composition and physical working capacity of young Guatemalan adults. In N. S. Scrimshaw & A. M. Altschul (Eds.), *Amino acid fortification of protein foods*. Cambridge, Massachusetts: MIT Press, 1971. Pp. 350–375.

Viteri, F. E., Physical fitness and anemia. In N. Shimazono & T. Arakawa (Eds.),

Malnutrition and functions of blood cells: Proceedings of an international symposium. Tokyo: National Institute of Nutrition, 1973. Pp. 559–583.

Viteri, F. E., & Torún, B. Anaemia and physical work capacity. *Clinics in Haematology,* 1974, *3,* 609–626.

Viteri, F. E., & Torún, B. Ingestión calórica y trabajo físico de obreros agrícolas en Guatemala. Efecto de la supplementación alimentaria y su lugar en los programas de salud. *Boletin de la Oficina Sanitaria Panamericana,* 1975, *78,* 58–74.

Viteri, F. E., Torún, B., Galicia, J. C., & Herrera, E. Determining energy costs of agricultural activities by respirometer and energy balance techniques. *American Journal of Clinical Nutrition,* 1971, *24,* 1418–1430.

6

Nutritional Stress and Postcontact Population Decline among the Maring of New Guinea[1]

GEORGEDA BUCHBINDER

Queens College, City University of New York

INTRODUCTION

During the 1960s, the Maring, a previously isolated New Guinea Highlands population experienced a population decline that was due primarily to a high mortality rate from introduced infectious disease. It appeared that influenza and other respiratory diseases followed by pneumonia were the most common causes of death during this period. The effects of these repeated epidemics were not uniform throughout the entire Maring population, but varied in their severity from one local group to the next. In the Simbai valley, the northwesternmost local Maring groups suffered the highest mortality, and their population size continued to decrease until 1974, the time of the last census. In contrast, the southeasternmost groups experienced lower mortality,

[1]The research on which this chapter is based was carried out between 1966 and 1974 and was supported by grants from the National Institute of Mental Health, Columbia University, The Faculty Research Awards Program of City University of New York, and the Wenner Gren Foundation.

and between December 1968 and August 1974, their numbers began to increase.

I will show that the differences in response to the stress of introduced infectious disease encountered among the various Maring populations in the Simbai Valley was related to differences in their nutritional status with regard to energy and protein, both prior to and during the course of my study. I will explore the possibility that previously existing as well as ongoing nutritional stress adversely affected the ability of a newly contacted New Guinea Highlands fringe population to cope with the stresses that followed culture contact. In particular, I will show that where the previous levels of nutritional stress were highest, the introduced stresses proved to be most lethal. I will also show that a relationship exists between a population's biological and behavioral response to stress and that this relationship takes the form of a positive feedback or amplification loop. That is to say, malnutrition adversely affects a population's ability to cope with disease stress, and the additional disease stress adversely affects the population's ability to feed itself, thus in turn worsening both the malnutrition and the disease.

I will begin by presenting a brief ethnographic sketch of the Maring and then describe the population decline that occurred among them in the 1960s. I will then discuss the health and nutritional status of the various Simbai Maring local populations, based on evidence derived from clinical and anthropometric studies. From there I will move to a discussion of the Maring diet and show that differences in nutritional status and in response to introduced disease are directly related to differences in the intake in both calories and protein. Finally, I will discuss some of the correlates in both individual and group behavior to different levels of nutritional and disease stress.

THE MARING

The Maring are swidden horticulturalists who occupy a territory of about 100 square miles in the central Simbai and Jimi Valleys in the Bismarck Mountains on the northern fringe of the central New Guinea highlands. Their total population numbers about 7000, with about 5000 living in the higher and more open Jimi and about 2000 in the lower, steeper, and more heavily forested Simbai (Figure 6.1).

Studies of the ecological and biological adaptations of the Maring began in 1962 and still continue. These studies have involved anthropologists, geographers, and various kinds of health workers. My

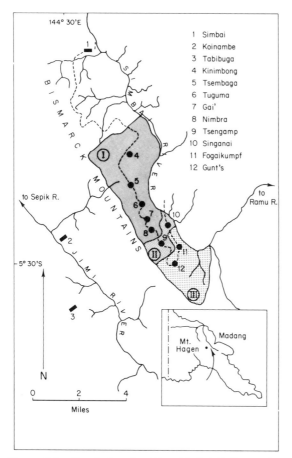

Figure 6.1. Population densities, Simbai Valley region.

Key: ● Government rest house; ▬ airstrip, --- walking track. I = more than 60 persons per square mile; II = 30–60 persons per square mile; III = less than 30 persons per square mile. The arrow in the insert indicates the location of the Simbai Valley.

own research among the Maring began in 1966. Between then and 1974, I have spent a total of about 30 months in the field, specifically investigating the interaction of nutrition and population dynamics among the 2000 Maring who inhabit the south wall of the Simbai valley.

The Maring are divided into 20 or more autonomous local groups, which range in size from slightly less than 100 to about 900 members. The composition of these groups is somewhat variable. Generally, each group consists of two or more putatively patrilineal exogamous

clans, but in a few instances, the entire local population claims descent from a common patrilineal ancestor. Although clan exogamy is
the rule, local-group endogamy is strongly favored, and as many as
50% of spouses may come from within the local group. The remainder
come from adjacent nonenemy groups on the same side of the range or
from friendly groups across the range. Prior to contact, these latter
marriages were important in facilitating trade of Simbai-produced salt
for Jimi-produced stone axes, for affines were frequently trading
partners. They still function in the movement of valuables, pork and
baby pigs, all of which may figure in affinal payments. Some marriages
were also contracted with non-Maring speakers to the north across the
Simbai and to the south across the Jimi, thus extending the trade
network.

Linguistic and cultural evidence suggests that the Maring are most
closely related to peoples to the south in the Central Highlands, and it
is likely that they entered their territory from the south or southeast,
occupying the upper-middle Jimi valley first and later spilling over
into the Simbai. It is not known how long they have been in their
present territory, but the high degree of genetic and linguistic variation that exists among local populations suggests an occupation of at
least several centuries; or alternatively, that they settled their present
territory in several waves. To the north and west of Maring territory
are distantly related Gainj and Karam speakers. To the east and northeast, Maring territory borders on a vast tract of uninhabited virgin
forest.

The Maring region differs from the New Guinea highlands proper
in being somewhat lower, steeper, and more heavily forested. Perhaps
because of this, the Maring engage in a classic form of bush-fallowing
horticulture rather than in a variant of the more intensive gardening
regimes followed by the more centrally located highlands groups.
Thus, new gardens are cut each year in the secondary forest that
covers the slopes between the altitudes of 2000 and 5500 ft. above sea
level. These gardens yield crops for from 14 to 26 months and are then
abandoned to fallow, which may last from about 8 to over 40 years.
Tuberous staples include taro, sweet potato, yams, and manioc. Taro is
the most important crop in the Simbai Valley, but sweet potatoes may
be more dominant in some of the higher Jimi Valley locations. Other
significant crops include sugar cane, bananas, *marita* pandanus (a tree
crop which provides the major source of fat in the Maring diet) and a
large variety of greens. Pigs, chickens, and some hunting dogs are
raised, and a few cassowaries and occasional hornbills and cockatoos
are kept. Hunting and gathering are also practiced, both in secondary

forest and in the primary forest above and below the range of cultivation. The numerous swift-flowing streams in Maring territory yield eels in the dry season, and, on occasion, catfish are taken from the much larger Simbai or Jimi rivers. Nonetheless, the Maring diet (at least during the late 1960s) comprises well over 95% vegetable matter. Game is scarce, and pigs and chickens, at least until very recently, were killed and eaten only on ceremonial occasions. Because of their largely vegetarian diet, the Maring are vulnerable to deficiencies in iodine and other trace elements as well as to protein malnutrition. It is a well-known ecological fact that such substances tend to be concentrated by living tissues and that the higher up in the food chain that an organism is, the greater the concentration of these substances in that organism. Thus, carnivores are much more likely to obtain an adequate supply of these nutrients from their normal food sources than are herbivores. Indeed, the Maring suffered an epidemic of endemic goitrous cretinism during the 1960s when their indigenous salt supply, which was highly iodized, was replaced by commercial trade salt that was not iodized (Buchbiner, 1974, 1976). The local groups, which were hardest hit by the iodine deficiency, were also the ones who suffered most from protein deficiency, and this fact may have compounded some of the adverse effects of protein malnutrition, but I will not go into detail about iodine deficiency in this paper, as it has been covered elsewhere (Buchbinder, 1976). Iodine deficiency was corrected by public-health measures in 1968, and no cretins have been born into the population since that time. The Maring diet will be discussed in greater detail in the next section of this chapter.

The Maring were first contacted by Australian administration patrols between 1956 and 1960. The government considered them pacified by 1962 when it opened their territory to outsiders such as missionaries and anthropologists. Prior to contact, warfare had been endemic among the Maring, with each local group participating as a major combatant on the average of every 8–12 years. Individuals probably fought more frequently than that, as there were elaborate systems of individual alliances. Maring warfare and its consequences have been exhaustively treated by others elsewhere (Rappaport, 1968; Vayda, 1971) and will not be discussed here except to point out that when the Maring were not fighting their neighbors, they were strictly avoiding contact with them, their territory, and any food grown on their territory. This avoidance probably acted as an effective method of quarantine and helped to slow down or prevent the spread of infectious disease from one local group to another. This avoidance behavior was disrupted by pacification, and missionaries encouraged the aggregation of large groups of people for religious services, probably facilitating the rapid transmission of disease.

Indirect contact, primarily in the form of trade, and possibly introduced disease occurred earlier. Thus, the first steel tools entered the area in the late 1930s, and by the time of direct contact, steel tools had replaced the indigenous stone tools. There is also evidence that the Maring were affected by the 1940s dysentery epidemic that swept through the New Guinea highlands, and they may also have been affected by a measles epidemic at the same time.

Although various Maringologists differ in their definition of what constitutes a local group, I will define local groups as being isomorphic with administration census units. These were de facto local groups during the time of my study.

In the Simbai Valley, there are nine such local Maring populations strung out along the valley wall going roughly from east to west. The environment of these groups varies, as does the population density and intensity and land use, and the availability of protein-rich foods (Figure 6.1). In general, the groups in the northwest are more crowded and have less access to protein-rich foods than do the groups in the east, which border on and exploit a vast tract of unoccupied forest. The northwestern groups, particularly Tuguma, Tsembaga, Gai, and Singanai are characterized by short stature, low weight, low hemoglobin values, and a high incidence of hypohaptoglobinemia (Table 6.1). The few cases of frank kwashiorkor and marasmus that occurred during my field work were also found among these northwestern groups. In addition, the percentage of children showing any signs of protein–calorie malnutrition (PCM) was higher here (Table 6.2). These groups also tended to exhibit lower fertility and higher mortality. The southeastern groups, particularly Nimbra, Tsangamp, and Gunt's, are characterized by increased stature and weight, higher hemoglobin levels, and a lower incidence of hypohaptoglobinemia (Table 6.1). In all instances, the differences between the most extreme local groups was highly significant $.05 > p > .01$. There were no instances of frank kwashiorkor or marasmus among the southeastern groups and the percentage of children with signs of PCM was lower than in the northwest (Table 6.2). Fertility is higher in the southeast and mortality lower. During the 1960s, the Maring experienced a population decline of slightly less than 1% per annum. This decline was due primarily to an excess of mortality rather than to outmigration. The excess mortality was most probably due to the effects of introduced disease, mainly influenza, which spread rapidly through the population as the previously existing boundaries to social intercourse between adjacent hostile groups were broken down by pacification. While all of the Simbai Maring local populations were affected by this population decline, they were not all affected equally. In general, the groups in the northwest, in which protein was relatively scarce and nutritional stunting had occurred, were much harder hit than were the groups in the southeast, in which protein resources were most plentiful and stunting was not as evident. Furthermore, a census taken in 1974 revealed that the southeastern groups were recovering from the decline and were indeed beginning to increase in number, while the northwestern groups were still declining or at best only holding their own.

I will now describe in greater detail the Simbai Maring population decline and then attempt to relate it to variation in the health and nutritional status of the component local populations.

THE DECLINE IN THE MARING POPULATION DURING THE 1960s

The demographic data on which my analysis of Maring population dynamics was made comes from a number of sources, including government censuses, censuses made by myself and other anthropologists, and reproductive histories and genealogies.

The Australian government began taking quasi-annual censuses in the Simbai Valley in 1960, and by about 1963 their figures were reasonably accurate. The 1963 census figures formed the basis of my demographic inquiries. In July 1966, A. P. Vayda censused the Maring population, and I recensused the Simbai Valley Maring again at the end of 1968 and in July 1974. In addition, while resident among the Tuguma in the western part of Simbai Maring territory, I maintained a birth and death register and collected complete genealogies for the more than 200 members of this group. Also, because of the limited time depth provided by census material, and because it was impossible to obtain complete genealogies from all 2000 Simbai Valley Maring, I collected reproductive histories from 418 women above the age of 17. This comprised almost the total cohort of women who were in or past the reproductive stage. I have detailed Maring demography and reproductive behavior elsewhere (Buchbinder, 1973); here I will only briefly summarize my findings.

By 1966, it was apparent from an examination of age–sex distribution pyramids that the Maring population was not replacing itself (Figure 6.2). In particular, the 0–4 and 5–9 age cohorts were severely

TABLE 6.1

Height, Weight, Hemoglobin, and Percentage Hypohaptoglobinemia of Adult Maring Males and Females by Local Group

Local	Height			Weight			Hemoglobin (gm/100 ml)			Hypohaptoglobinemia		
	Number	Mean	SD	Number	Mean	SD	Number	Mean	SD	Number	Deficient	Deficient (%)
Kinimbong												
Males	26	153.31	5.98	26	46.08	5.11						
Females	38	145.16	5.89	38	38.84	4.24						
Tsembaga												
Males	52	151.10	4.76	52	46.10	4.68	49	13.59	1.28	48	14	29.6
Females	46	141.93	4.88	46	38.91	4.49	52	12.86	1.19	53	8	15.1
Tuguma												
Males	60	151.65	4.95	60	45.82	7.54	52	12.79	1.54	49	8	16.3
Females	53	141.96	5.00	53	37.85	3.89	46	12.01	1.26	51	11	21.6
Gai												
Males	94	153.77	4.92	94	47.10	5.28	46	13.22	2.54	50	10	20.0
Females	78	144.72	6.03	78	40.95	6.43	67	12.99	1.34	71	8	11.2

Singanai												
Males	52	153.88	5.44	52	45.25	5.43				63	4	6.3
Females	40	144.15	6.86	40	38.33	5.25				55	0	0.0
Nimbra												
Males	83	155.08	5.71	83	48.86	5.94	55	14.48	1.27			
Females	80	145.70	4.75	80	40.21	5.79	53	13.54	1.27			
Tsengamp												
Males	50	154.70	5.40	50	46.61	5.50	59	14.22	1.51	59	7	11.9
Females	42	145.69	5.23	42	37.97	4.61	40	13.50	1.11	45	4	8.9
Fogaikumpf												
Males	31	155.29	4.58	31	49.16	5.38						
Females	27	146.41	5.55	27	42.11	4.92						
Gunt's												
Males	63	157.25	5.00	63	50.66	5.53	28	15.60	1.49	28	3	10.7
Females	74	147.35	5.04	74	42.46	4.19	12	14.03	0.86	12	0	0.0
Total												
Males	511	154.06	5.49	511	47.41	5.97	289	13.88	1.59	297	46	15.5
Females	478	144.89	5.71	478	39.94	5.31	270	13.03	1.23	286	31	10.3

TABLE 6.2

Simbai Maring Children Age 0–5 Years with Signs of Protein–Calorie Malnutrition in 1968, by Local Group from West to East

Local groups	Number of children examined	Number with signs	Percentage
Kinimbong	27	6	22.2
Tsembaga	41	9	22.0
Tuguma	34	8	23.5
Gai	63	9	15.9
Singanai	36	5	13.9
Nimbia	64	10	15.7
Tsengamp	44	7	15.9
Fogaikumpf	19	1	5.3
Gunt's	72	8	11.1

depleted. It is not clear whether this was due to excess mortality of children or to a lowered fertility during the time period involved. I suspect that the former was the most important cause, although elsewhere I have shown that Maring fertility is low in comparison to that of other highland New Guinea populations. Vital indicies computed for the interval between 1963 and 1966 revealed that the Simbai Maring population had been experiencing a decline due to an excess of deaths over births, which averaged over the whole population to a rate of −0.4% per year. This rate of change was by no means uniform throughout the valley but ranged from −3.4% in the northwest to +2.6% in the southeast. In general, the populations at the northwestern end of the valley were declining, as were those located at low altitude (Singanai and Fogaikumpf), while those located at the southeastern end of the valley were increasing.

By December 1968 the age–sex distribution of the population was beginning to normalize (Figure 6.3). By this I mean that the youngest cohort was somewhat replenished but still not enough for population replacement. Vital statistics computed for the 1966–1969 interval indicated that during this period the rate of population decline had doubled to an overall average rate of −0.8% per year, with a range of from −4.3% to +1.5%. Again the same pattern emerged. The western groups were declining in number, while the eastern groups were maintaining their numbers or increasing.

The census conducted in 1974 indicated that the Simbai Maring population was recovering from the decline that it had experienced during the 1960s. The age–sex distribution showed an increase in the

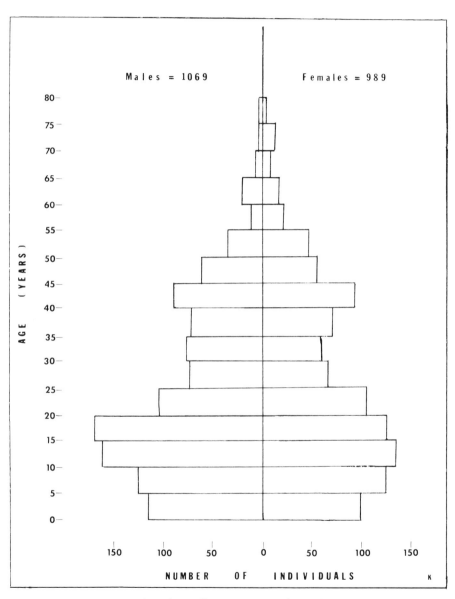

Figure 6.2. Total Simbai Valley Maring population (August 1966).

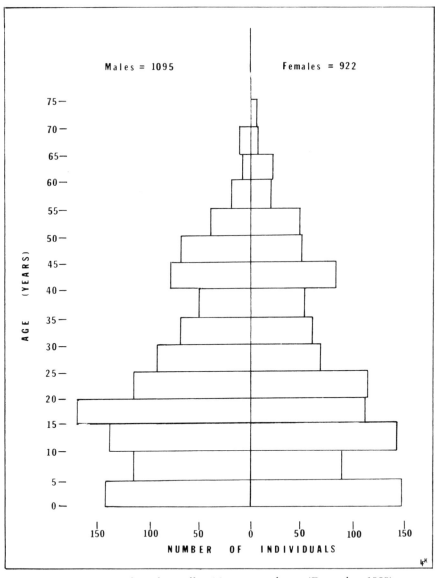

Figure 6.3. Total Simbai Valley Maring population (December 1968).

younger cohorts (Figure 6.4), and vital statistics revealed that in the interval between December 1968 and July 1974, the population was increasing at an overall average rate of .3% per year. However, once again the rate of change showed marked variation from one local group to the next. This time the variation ranged from −1.4% to +2.4% per year, and again it was the northwestern groups that were declining, while those in the southeast showed the greatest increase. It should be noted that throughout the course of this study, the groups that were declining most rapidly not only had higher than average mortality among the local populations but also lower than average fertility.

Wide variation in demographic indices among small populations during short periods of time is not unusual and may often be attributed to random events. The variation exhibited by the Simbai Maring local populations was patterned rather than random, and the pattern persisted for at least the 10-year time period during which this study was conducted. Moreover, an analysis of reproductive histories revealed a long-standing difference in the fertility of the women in the region. This difference amounted to an average of one pregnancy for women whose childbearing was completed. As might now be expected, the more fertile women were found in the southeast and the least fertile in the northwest. The survival rate of children was also relatively high among the southeastern groups. Women in the northwestern groups experienced an average of 3.5 pregnancies, and 75% of their children survived to adulthood. Women in the southeast experienced an average of 4.5 pregnancies, and 85% of their children survived to adulthood.

The encountered differences in fertility and mortality appear to be related to differences in the health and nutritional status of the various local Simbai Maring populations. In general, the groups characterized by short stature, high incidence of both protein and calorie malnutrition, and high levels of anemia (Tables 6.1 and 6.2) were also characterized by high mortality and low fertility.

In my opinion, the above figures do not reflect the magnitude of the population decline, at least as I observed it among the groups that were declining most rapidly. In August 1966, when I took up residence with the Taguma Maring in the western part of the Simbai Valley, they numbered 255 people. By the time I left in May 1969, 43 people or almost one-fifth of the population had died. To make matters worse, only 3 of the 12 infants born during that interval were still alive when I left, and 2 of them died subsequently. Most deaths resulted from an acute respiratory infection, most probably influenza followed

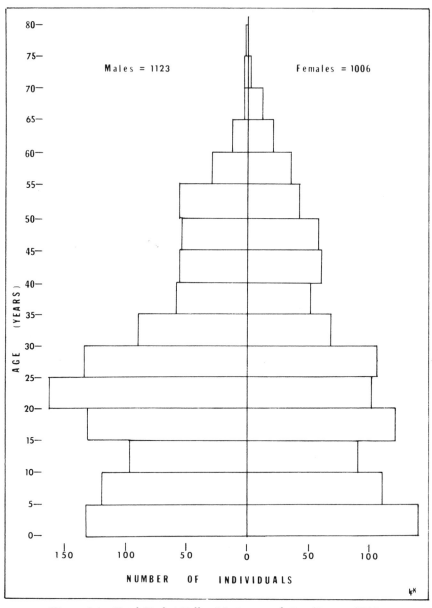

Figure 6.4. Total Simbai Valley Maring population (August 1974).

122

by pneumonia, and the course of the fatal illness was extremely rapid. Most of those who died of this infection did so within 24-48 hr after the onset of symptoms.

MARING HEALTH AND NUTRITIONAL STATUS

Three basic methods for evaluating the health and nutritional status of the Simbai Maring population were employed. The first was a clinical examination of virtually the entire population performed by an epidemiologist from the Department of Public Health. The second method consisted of an anthropometric survey of the entire population by the author. I measured heights, weights, skinfold thickness, and arm circumferences for each subject, and head and chest circumferences for children. I obtained these measurements on at least two occasions for most subjects between 1966 and 1968 and measured children again in 1974. Third, hemoglobin and haptoglobin values were determined for the 600 blood samples collected during the course of a genetic survey (Buchbinder & Clark, 1971). In addition, the records of the Anglican Mission's Maternal and Child Health Service were consulted.

Again, the results of these studies have been detailed elsewhere (Buchbinder, 1973, 1976; Buchbinder & Clark, 1971) and will only be summarized here.

Clinical examinations revealed a much higher incidence of PCM and of iodine deficiency among the western groups than among those in the east. While the incidence of malaria was higher in the east, the hemoglobin concentration of the western groups averaged 2 gm% lower than that in the eastern groups, and this difference was statistically significant at the .01 level. It is not known whether the anemia encountered in the west was due to protein or to iron deficiency. Hyperhaptoglobinemia, a condition associated both with malaria and with protein deficiency, was more prevalent in the west among the shortest and thinnest Maring. And its presence may be a further indication of the amount of nutritional stress to which these local populations are subject.

Anthropometric studies demonstrated significant variation in all measured parameters among the local populations. Once again, the people in the east were found to be taller, heavier, and fatter than the people in the west. The difference in stature amounted to 6.2 cm, and that in weight to 4.6 kg. In general, there was a gradual increase in both stature and weight from west to east (Table 6.2). I observed that the differences in the stature of adults were also present in children of all age groups and noted that the rate of growth, although slow for all Maring children, was much slower in the west.

All of these findings point to the fact that the western groups were under a greater amount of nutritional stress than were the eastern groups and that the nutritional stress took the form of protein–calorie deficiency. Also, because the differences in stature equally affected all age groups, it is likely that the differences in nutrient availability in the area had been long standing. I conducted detailed studies of the diets of the two most contrastive populations in order to determine the magnitude of the differences in nutrient intake. These data are presented below.

THE MARING DIET

To obtain information on the composition of the Maring diet, I conducted individual and household food-consumption studies at Tuguma in the western part of the Simbai Maring territory and at Gunt's in the far east of the territory. These two communities were chosen because they exhibited the greatest contrast in health, anthropometric, and demographic parameters. The food production and intake of the 45 members of 9 households, 2 at Gunt's and 7 at Tuguma, was measured for a period of time ranging from 1–2 weeks. Two of the Tuguma households were restudied at 6-month intervals. During the study period, all food brought into the household was weighed, and a determination of its intended allocation was made. In addition, each individual portion of food eaten by each member of the household was weighed on a portion scale.

Because of the tedious and time-consuming nature of direct dietary-intake studies, sample size was limited. In order to compensate for this limited sample size, I conducted surveys among the entire Simbai Maring population in order to determine the number of pigs killed in the year prior to the study and the amount of meat of any kind consumed in the week prior to the survey. In addition, because of the almost exclusive vegetable content of the Maring diet, staple crops were analyzed for their protein content. The results of these studies are presented below.

Composition of the Diet

The percentage composition of the diet of each household in the study has been computed and is presented in Table 6.3. Since dif-

TABLE 6.3

Composition of the Diet by Percentage Weight of Foods (1968)

	Mondo									Tababi		
	February	March			June		July	October	November	December		Overall average
Sweet potato	3.4	2.6	1.3	3.3	15.0	5.6	29.4	33.1	23.3	21.6	15.4	14.0
Taro (xanthosoma)	11.1	5.1	2.2		3.1	0.7	1.3	0.5		11.0	17.1	4.7
Taro (colacasia)	27.9	37.4	23.0	47.2	37.4	50.9	15.6	8.2	15.1	0.7	2.2	24.1
Manioc	1.3			1.9	9.6	0.7	4.1	0.5	4.4			2.0
Yams	12.8	19.8	12.1	24.7	9.9	7.4	11.9	3.0	7.0	0.6	0.5	10.0
Total roots	56.5	64.9	38.6	77.1	75.0	65.3	62.3	45.3	49.8	33.9	35.2	54.9
Banana	0.3			1.0	6.4	7.0	5.0	5.7	13.8	5.5	0.6	3.6
Other fruit	0.9		1.2	1.2	0.8	6.0	12.6	1.9		4.4		2.5
Miscellaneous vegetables	5.2	1.4	0.8	0.6	0.5	2.0	1.4	14.5	10.2	5.5	5.2	4.7
Marita pandanus	14.3	3.2		11.7		14.8		5.8	4.9	15.1	28.4	6.7
Leaves	7.6	13.0	6.32	11.7	9.9		10.7	14.1	2.3	12.8	15.0	10.7
Grasses	8.5	13.6	22.3	7.6	4.0	3.2	3.6	3.6	7.7	13.8	8.0	8.7
Sugarcane	6.6	3.8	30.8	2.2	3.4	1.7	3.8	9.3	11.2	9.9	8.0	8.2
Animal food	0.03						0.01			0.2		0.022

ferent households were studied at different times of the year, and since none of the households covered were considered to be atypical in terms of what they were eating, the variation in the percentage composition of the diet from household to household may be seen as representing seasonal differences in the availability of foods as well as purely individual preferences.

One of the most obvious and important facts to be noted from Table 6.3 is that the Maring are essentially vegetarians. Animal food, of any kind, appears in only 3 of the 11 studies, and in these it forms only a very minor constituent of the diet, from .03 to .02%.

As for all highland New Guineans, root crops form the major element of the diet, amounting to an overall average of 54.9%. This figure is much lower than that reported for Chimbu and other highland groups (Hipsley & Kirk, 1965, p. 80; Venkatachalam, 1962, p. 9) but is in line with figures reported by Rappaport (1968, p. 73) and Clarke (1971, p. 179) for other Maring groups. The actual percentage of tubers in individual family diets ranged from 33.9 to 77.1%. This variation reflects the seasonal availability of other high-calorie foods, notably of *marita* pandanus, and sugar cane.

The major root crops consumed by the Maring are: taro, sweet potato, yams, and manioc. Of these, taro is the most important, comprising 28% of the diet. Sweet potato is next in importance, comprising 14% of the diet. Yams constitute another 10.7%, while manioc appears to be a relatively minor food, forming only 2.0%.

The proportion of the various root crops appears to vary from season to season as well as from place to place. Everywhere, the Maring state a marked preference for taro and yams over sweet potatoes and manioc. The former are considered to be ceremonial food, the latter more fit for pigs. This is a very common New Guinea belief; it may be related to the fact that taro and yams are indigenous crops, while sweet potato and manioc are relatively recent introductions.

There is an inverse proportion in the percentage of taro and sweet potato consumed throughout the year. Thus, sweet potato is more important in the months of July to September when taro is relatively scarce.

Other important constituents of the Maring diet are leaves and grasses; together they comprise 19.4% by weight of the average total diet. Although the amount of these foods eaten by the individual families in the study varies, the variation is relatively small. Nonetheless, it appears that more of these vegetables are eaten when *marita* is available. This is not surprising since the two are often eaten together; greens mixed with *marita* sauce are a favorite Maring dish. Both

Rappaport (1968, p. 72) and Clarke (1971, p. 181) have commented on the importance of greens in the Maring diet. These foods are particularly good sources of vitamins and minerals, as well as protein, and this latter fact is important for people who are essentially vegetarians.

If we can take the 11 individual family studies to represent typical diets throughout the course of a year, then an interesting fact emerges; during the wetter months, the diet appears to be richer in protein, or at least in vegetable protein, than it is during the drier months. This is due not only to the increased consumption of greens and *marita* but also to the fact that during these months more taro is consumed than sweet potato and that the protein content of the former is considerably higher than that of the latter. In the dry season, there is a greater availability of animal protein in the form of game.

Protein Content of Root Crops

Because the Maring are essentially vegetarians and thus derive most of their protein from plant sources, it is important to know the protein content of the vegetables in their diet. Unfortunately, it was not possible to have all Maring foods analyzed for their protein content, and so the nutrient values of most of the foods consumed by the Maring in this study are derived from published values of the same or similar foods grown in other areas.

However, because of a generous offer from the Department of Public Health, I was able to have 86 samples of root crops (taro, yam, and sweet potato) grown at the same altitude on the territories of six Maring local groups (Tsembaga, Tuguma, Gai, Nimbra, Tsengamp, and Gunt's) analyzed for their protein content. The results of this analysis are presented in Table 6.4, and these values have been used in this paper to calculate the nutritive values of individual Maring diets.

While the sample size for each food from each location is probably too small to draw anything but tentative conclusions, some interesting facts emerge from these analyses that require comment. First, the average protein content of both taro and sweet potato falls well below the published values, while Maring-grown yams have a higher protein content. Thus, taro, the most important Maring staple, has an average protein content of only 0.95% by weight, as compared to the published range of values of from 1.4 to 1.9% protein by weight. This lower protein value of the most important food might be enough to make the difference between an adequate diet and one that is deficient in protein. A second fact needing comment is the amount and direction of variation in the protein content of taro grown in different Maring

TABLE 6.4

Protein Content of Root Crops Grown in Various Simbai Maring Locations

	Taro		Yams		Sweet potato	
Location	Number of samples	Protein (%)	Number of samples	Protein (%)	Number of samples	Protein (%)
Tsembaga	11	.975	5	2.04	5	.75
Mondo	5	.59	2	2.66	6	.705
Gai	4	1.24	2	2.62		
Nimbra	15	.90	5	2.18	1	.96
Tsengamp	6	1.03	2	2.75	2	.89
Gunt's	6	1.05	6	1.90	8	.875
Overall average	47	.95	22	2.32	22	.80
Range of published values		1.4–1.9		1.9–2.0		0.9–1.7

territories. The taro grown on Tuguma and Tsembaga territories in the northwest has half the protein content of that grown at Gunt's in the southeast, and this fact alone may be an important factor in accounting for the differences both in stature and in health of the two populations.

Results of Food Intake Studies

The energy and protein content of the diets of the two most contrastive Maring local populations are presented in Table 6.5 and they are compared with the 1973 FAO–WHO recommended intakes. Two levels of safe intake for protein are presented in this table, one for protein score of 70% the value of egg or milk protein and the other for 60%. The use of these values is somewhat arbitrary, as no amino acid analysis of Maring diets was performed, nor were biological assays done. Nonetheless, since practically all of the protein in the Maring diet is derived from plant sources, it is likely that the actual protein score of the diet does fall somewhere between 60 and 70% of the value of milk or egg protein.

On examination of Table 6.5, it becomes apparent that the Gunt's diet is more adequate in terms of both energy and protein than is the Tuguma, and although this finding is based on rather small samples, it is more than adequately confirmed by anthopometric, clinical, and demographic findings, which were presented earlier in this paper.

TABLE 6.5

Energy and Protein Value of Tuguma and Gunt's Diets Compared with 1973 FAO/WHO Standards[a]

| Consumers | | | Calories | | | Protein | | | |
Category	N	Average weight (kg)	Recommended intake	Actual intake	Kcal/kg	Recommended safe level 70%[b]	Recommended safe level 60%[b]	Actual intake	Gm/kg
Tuguma									
Adult men	13	45.4±3.8	2093	2311±493	50.9	37.0	43.2	34.6±13.0	0.8
Adult women	10	38.1±3.0	1524	2259±595	59.3	28.3	33.1	41.3±17.3	1.1
Boys 16–19	4	39.5±5.4	2135	1632±128	41.3	33.9	39.6	24.1± 4.8	0.6
Boys 13–15	2	28.7±3.9	2030	1789± 50	62.3	29.6	34.6	27.0±18.8	0.9
Boys 10–12	1	20.0±0.0	2600	1781± 0	89.1	23.7	27.1	14.7± 0.0	0.7
Girls 13–15	4	30.0±4.5	1722	1800±407	60.0	27.0	31.6	30.3± 8.0	1.0
Girls 10–12	1	16.5±0.0	2350	1011± 0	61.3	17.9	20.9	15.6± 0.0	0.9
Children 7–9	4	15.3±1.2	2190	1638±302	107.1	19.2	22.5	30.8± 8.4	2.0
Children 4–6	3	11.2±1.0	1830	1201±324	107.2	16.1	18.9	19.6± 4.4	1.8
Gunt's[a]									
Adult men	?	50.0	2300	2650	53.0	40.8	47.6	52.0	1.0
Adult women	1	42.0±0.0	1680	2860± 0	68.1	31.2	36.4	66.7± 0.0	1.6
Boys 16–19	2	52.2±9.6	2320	2382±195	45.8	44.6	52.1	61.6±25.9	1.2
Boys 10–12	2	23.3±0.4	2600	1719±339	73.9	27.0	31.5	32.2± 4.3	1.4
Girls 13–15	2	33.5±4.2	1898	2230±284	66.6	30.2	35.3	42.5± 1.9	1.3
Girls 10–12	1	22.4±0.0	2350	1114± 0	49.7	24.3	28.4	24.3± 0.0	1.1

[a] From Clarke (1971).

[b] These figures refer to the biological value of protein in relation to egg or milk protein, which is used as a standard and given the value of 100%.

In terms of energy requirements, the Tuguma diet is only adequate for adults. All other age and sex categories have either marginal or below recommended intakes. On the other hand, the Gunt's diet appears to provide enough energy for all but the youngest age categories in the sample. It should be noted that the FAO/WHO recommended energy intakes for children under 12 are not adjusted for body size, as the committee believes that small body size in adults in the population may be the result of nutritional stunting and that children should be provided with enough energy to allow for possible catch-up growth (FAO/WHO, 1973).

The Maring are a small people, particularly the Tuguma Maring, and while I believe that a large component of their diminutive stature is in fact due to nutritional stunting, some of it might also be genetic. If this were the case, then the recommended energy allowances for children might be exaggerated. But certainly energy deficits of the magnitude encountered could easily result in stunted growth and in poor utilization of the limited amount of protein in the diet.

If we compare the diets of the two local populations in terms of protein intake, the difference is even more striking. The Tuguma diet provides safe levels of protein only for adult women and for children between the ages of 7 and 9. It is deficient for all other groups. Actually, it may also be deficient for adult women, also, as the recommended safe protein-intake levels I have cited are for nonpregnant, nonlactating women, and one of the women in my sample was in her 9th month of pregnancy, and three others were lactating. The 1973 FAO/WHO report recommends that an additional 13–15 gm of protein be allocated to women in the latter part of pregnancy and an additional 24–28 gm be added for lactation. If this is done, it makes the protein intake of Tuguma women look marginal indeed.

The Gunt's diet provides adequate protein for all age and sex categories studied. Table 6.6 shows the amount of protein per 100 calories in the Tuguma and Gunt's diet by age and sex category, and again we can see the higher protein content of the Gunt's diet.

Intrapopulation Variation in Food Intake

An interesting finding of the food-intake studies, particularly at Tuguma, where my sample size was relatively large, and where I also had the opportunity to make nonquantitative observations over the course of several years, was the amount of variation in the food consumed by individuals within the same age and sex categories. Some people were literally eating twice as much as others. While we

TABLE 6.6

Composition of the Diet: Grams of Protein per 100 Calories Consumed by Various Age and Sex Groups at Tuguma and Gunt's

	Grams of protein per 100 calories	
Age–sex category	Tuguma	Gunt's
Adult men	1.50	2.37
Adult women	1.83	2.90
Boys 16–19	1.48	2.59
Boys 13–15	1.51	2.58
Boys 10–12	.83	2.65
Girls 13–15	1.68	1.91
Girls 10–12	1.54	2.18
Children 7–9	1.88	—
Children 4–6	1.63	—

are well aware of the variation in food consumption in our own society and in other large and differentiated societies, we are less aware or have given less attention to the fact that such variation can exist in small-scale homogeneous egalitarian populations. In theory, at least, and also likely in practice, any Maring can produce as much food as he needs, and no one need go hungry, as food is freely given for the asking. What, then, causes this variation in consumption levels?

Some of the variation in food intake was predictable on the basis of age and activity level. Older, less active people ate less than young adults, as did older unmarried adolescents who had few economic responsibilities. Anthropometric observations confirm this finding. For the Maring population, both total body weight and the amount of subcutaneous fat decreases with age after peaking in the early twenties (Buchbinder, 1973).

The two adult men in the sample who had the poorest diets actually died of influenza within several months of the time their diets were studied. One was a recent widower who was obviously distressed by the loss of his wife. The other was a shaman who was under a number of dietary restrictions, who was married to a woman much his junior, and who spent a lot of time helping her unmarried brothers in an adjacent local population with their gardening. She was also burdened with the care of a retarded cretin infant. Most of the other people with low intakes were single, and many were in mourning, quite possibly too depressed to make the effort to acquire food. In addition, it might be noted that one of the Maring mourning customs is the avoidance of the favorite food or cooking method of the deceased for periods of time up to 2 years. This practice might conceivably adversely affect the diet, particularly if several people are being mourned at once, and this was frequently the case among the Tuguma Maring in the 1960s when mortality in this population was high.

Others who had a low food intake complained of a number of vague physical symptoms, from mild fever to backache to colds. Maring tend to stop eating when they feel ill, and noticeable weight loss often accompanies even rather mild bouts of illness. Elderly persons were known, on occasion, to state that they had lived long enough and then retire to their homes, refuse food, and die. Anorexia often accompanies states of physical illness or emotional stress. Its consequences in previously well-nourished individuals may be minimal, but in poorly nourished people, the consequences are likely to be serious indeed.

Women in their last months of pregnancy are cautioned about eating too much. They are told that there is not enough room for both the food and the developing fetus and that if they eat too much the fetus would be squashed. The one pregnant woman in the Tuguma sample had a very low food intake and produced a low birth weight baby who died at the age of 6 or 7 months.

The household with the highest per capita consumption of both energy and protein was that of a very energetic and politically ambitious man of about 30 and his 2 wives. Not only did they eat more, but they produced significantly more food than did any other household in my sample. They had more pigs than any other household, and a number of retainers were frequently fed by them. Their greater production allowed them to contribute substantially to a number of feasts, and their prestige and influence rose accordingly.

The high degree of variance in food intake in this egalitarian society raises a number of points. In the first place, given an average per capita energy and protein intake that is, at best, only marginally adequate and is, in fact, below recommended values for most children and adolescents, the high degree of variance suggests that a fairly large proportion of the population may be under severe nutritional stress. Also, the patterns of variance in food consumption suggest that nutrient intake may very well be lowest in individuals who are already debilitated either because of illness or because of psychological stress, and these people are then more susceptible to infection, which would only worsen their nutritional status and lead to the familiar downward spiral of the synergism of infection and malnutrition that all too frequently leads to death.

Results of the Pig-Killing and Recent Protein Consumption Surveys

The results of both these surveys confirmed the finding of the food-intake studies that meat, and particularly domestic pork, form only a minor part of the Simbai diet. They also indicated that there was considerable regional variation in the availability of these protein sources. The results of the pig-killing survey are presented in Table 6.7. No Simbai Maring clan was holding a *kaiko*, or pig festival, during 1968 when the survey was made. Thus, all pigs were killed for purposes of affinal payments or to placate the ancestral spirits of persons who were seriously ill. Exceptions occurred at Fogaikumpf and Singanai where people claimed that sometimes they killed pigs just because they were hungry for pork. And in most places a few pigs were killed for local domestic celebrations, such as the return of plantation laborers. By 1974, this had become one of the major reasons for pig killing (Buchbinder, 1975). It therefore seems reasonable to assume that 1968 was a fairly typical year with respect to pig killing.

The total number of pigs killed by all the Simbai Maring clans included in this study in 1968 was 184. This yielded an average of 6.3 pounds of pork per person per year, or an average of 7887 calories and 478 grams of protein per person per year. Actually, the amount of pork available varies from one local group to another throughout the valley, with a high of 12 pounds per person at Gunt's and a low of 2.74 pounds at Gai. The pattern that emerged for pork consumption in 1968 was one of high consumption on the edges of Simbai Maring territory, particularly in the southeast, and of low consumption in the middle. The one exception to this pattern occurred at Tuguma, where pork consumption was higher than expected. This may have been because the Tuguma were so hard hit by the influenza epidemics that they were killing more pigs to appease angry ancestral spirits, and it might be that my presence in this community affected pig-killing behavior. However, this slight increase in the amount of animal protein consumed was not sufficient to protect the Tuguma from the lethal effects of the influenza epidemics.

The recent protein-consumption survey, in which people were asked to recall the meat they had eaten in the past week, indicated that little or no meat had been eaten in the northwestern part of Simbai Maring territory. Those who did eat meat in these local groups ate only very small game such as insects, birds, lizards, and rodents. Individual portions could not have been greater than an ounce at a time. Indeed, in many of these areas, people said that game was so scarce it was hardly worth their time to hunt, and many men had discarded their weapons.

TABLE 6.7

Results of Pig-Killing Survey

Location	Population	Number pigs killed	Total amount pork lbs.[a]	Pork per person—lbs.	Calories[b]	Protein[a] (gm)	Fat[a] (gm)	Calcium[a] (mg)
Fogaikumpf	113	10	700	6.2	7,762.4	469.96	638.6	279
Gunt's	297	51	3,570	12.0	15,024.0	909.6	1,203.0	540
Tsengamp	180	23	1,610	8.93	11,180.0	676.89	919.79	402
Singanai	197	17	1,190	6.0	7,512.0	454.8	618.0	270
Nimbra	·319	14	980	3.3	3,756.0	250.14	339.9	149
Gai	354	15	1,050	2.74	3,430.5	207.69	282.2	123
Tuguma	232	24	1,680	7.2	9,014.4	545.76	741.6	324.0
Tsembaga	209	16	1,120	5.3	6,635.6	401.74	545.9	239
Kinimbong	148	14	980	6.6	8,263.2	500.28	679.8	297.0
Total	2,049	184	12,800	6.3	7,887.6	477.54	648.9	284

[a] USDA (1963). 1687b—Composite of trimmed lean cuts, thin class, without bone and skin—81% lean, 19% fat.
[b] All calculated values based on average weight of pigs = 140 lbs., and edible portion = one-half total weight of pig.

In the southeastern part of Simbai Maring territory, the response was quite different. Here people reported a fairly consistent consumption of at least some animal food in the week prior to the survey. Frequently, it was in the form of small game, but this seemed to be fairly abundant. The groups on the edge of the forest reported having eaten quantities of large game, namely, cassowaries and feral pigs. People in these areas were very involved with hunting and found it to be a rewarding activity. They have access to an almost unlimited tract of primary forest, which stretches out to the southeast of their territory.

This impression of abundant game in the eastern part of Maring territory is confirmed by Clarke. He (1971, p. 90) noted that an average of 3 or 4 feral pigs were killed and eaten by the people in the Dwimba Basin during each month of his residence there, while 4 or 5 cassowaries were killed and eaten his year of residence there. He noted that the pigs were small, averaging only about 50 pounds, but this would yield over 1 pound of undressed pig per person per month. Cassowaries are about the same size as feral pigs and would provide a similar amount of meat. Clarke also estimated an additional consumption of about 10 ounces of additional animal flesh in the form of birds and marsupials per person per month. Thus, the total amount of edible wild animal flesh consumed by the forest-edge people would amount to about 12 ounces per person per month. This is equivalent to 1753 calories and 106 gm of protein.

In contrast, during my first 22 months at Tuguma, only 3 feral pigs were captured: Rappaport (1968, p. 78) reported a similar number during his stay with the adjacent Tsembaga. In this area, there are no wild cassowaries. Marsupials, eels, and birds were occasionally captured, but their numbers were small and probably yielded no more than an ounce of animal flesh per person per month.

Thus, among the Simbai Maring groups whose territory borders on the forest, game provides an average of about 3 gm of protein per person per day, while for those groups without access to large tracts of forest, the amount of protein provided by game is negligible.

SUMMARY AND CONCLUSIONS

I have presented data to demonstrate that the consequences of introduced infectious disease, following culture contact in a previously isolated New Guinea population, varied with the nutritional status of the various component local populations, such that those populations that were more adequately nourished experienced lower initial mortality and recovered more rapidly from the general population decline.

Those local populations that were located in the southeast on the edge of a vast forest had diets richer in both energy and protein than did those groups located further to the northwest whose land was more densely occupied. The southeastern groups had more land available to them and practiced longer periods of fallow between cropping than did the northwestern groups, and it is known that longer fallows return more fertility to the soil. This possible difference in soil fertility is reflected in the protein content of staple root crops grown in the two areas.

Food-intake studies indicated that the diet of the northwestern groups had a lower energy and protein content than did the diet of the southeastern groups. Further, while the nutrient content of the northwestern Simbai Maring groups marginally met the needs of adults, it was deficient for all other age groups. The southeastern Simbai Maring groups, in contrast, had a protein intake above the safe level for all age groups studied, and the energy content of their diet was low only for children under the age of 12. Anthropometric studies indicated that the difference in the diet between local groups was long standing, as there was a significant difference in both stature and weight in individuals of all ages.

It is thus suggested that the northwestern Simbai Maring local populations suffered higher mortality in the wake of introduced disease because of the effect of chronic malnutrition. The immune response of the individuals in the northwestern Simbai Maring groups was likely to be impaired. This impairment probably existed among children who were currently malnourished and also among adults who had experienced chronic malnutrition as children. The high mortality in epidemics of the 1960s affected all age and sex categories within the population

I have thus demonstrated the relationship of nutritional stress to postcontact population decline among previously isolated New Guinea population. In doing so, I have somewhat simplified the situation for ease of presentation. The degree of chronic PCM prevalent in the various local populations may not be the whole answer. It could be argued that because the northwestern groups were closer to the source of infection, they were more severely affected. However, it is well known that influenza spreads through a population with extreme rapidity. With the breakdown of local group-isolating mechanisms following pacification, there were no obstacles to its spread in the Simbai valley, and its point of entry into the population should thus make little difference in terms of its outcome. The presence of both iodine deficiency and malaria among the Maring also complicates the picture. But iodine deficiency was fairly recent among the Maring, and its distribution and effects parallel those of PCM. It is likely that the high prevalence of endemic goitrous cretinism encountered among the western Maring groups further lowered their ability to cope with the introduced stress of influenza. It certainly has an adverse effect on fertility and on infant survival (Buchbinder, 1976). Malaria is present throughout Simbai Maring territory, its prevalence is greater in the east, but endemic malaria tends to be a rather mild disease in well-nourished adults who have been exposed since birth. This acquired immunity breaks down under nutritional stress, and so it is likely that although malaria was less prevalent in the northwest, it was more lethal there, and that its significance as a health hazard increased in proportion to the level of malnutrition present in the community.

In an earlier work (Buchbinder, 1973), I argued that one might view the various Simbai Maring local populations as occupying various stages in a dynamic regional population regulation cycle. This postulated cycle consists of an initial pioneering stage, followed by population build-up, followed by resource depletion, followed by population decline, followed by resource replenishment, followed once more by population build-up. In this model, pioneering populations are characterized by their vigor and fecundity; as resources become depleted, both vigor and fecundity drop, and the population becomes more susceptible to infectious disease. High mortality from the combined effects of malnutrition and infectious disease lowers the population size and allows for environmental resource recovery, allowing the whole cycle to repeat itself. In terms of this model, the eastern Maring groups are the pioneers, and the western groups are the ones that have depleted their resources. Some evidence for the working of this model became apparent during my field work among the Maring in 1974. As mentioned earlier, by this time, the population decline had begun to level off for most groups and had, in fact, reversed itself in the southeast. What was particularly striking at that time was the increase in the amount of game and number of domestic pigs available among the northwestern groups. When asked about this, people said, "Of course, since there are so few people left, there is plenty of room and food for pigs and other animals, and so their numbers have increased." Indeed, more domestic pig and wild game of all sorts were consumed in July and August 1974 by the Tuguma than had been during my previous 3 years with them. In fact, the size of domestic pig herds had increased throughout the valley. In 1974, there were no obvious cases of malnutrition, and anthropometric studies revealed that children were both slightly taller and heavier for their age than they had been previously. (The difference in height and weight are consistent but small and not statistically significant.) This may signify that they will be able to cope with disease stress better than their parents' contemporaries had.

I have also suggested that it might be possible to predict the outcome of intergroup conflict on the basis of the health and nutritional status of the antagonists. One of the possible outcomes of Maring war is the routing of the defeated group from its territory. When this occurs, however, because of religious beliefs (Rappaport, 1968), a period of time of about a decade must intervene before the conquered land can be occupied by the victorious groups. This time interval would again allow for regeneration of environmental resources. Thus, it is possible that a density-dependent population-control mechanism might be operating to control population pressure over the entire Maring region and that this mechanism would allow for the build-up and decline of local populations. If this is the case, then the population decline of the 1960s might have simply represented one stage in a continuously repeating cycle.

However, in this chapter, I am most concerned with the effect of malnutrition on a population's ability to withstand disease stress. In particular, I wish to emphasize the positive feedback or amplification relationship between malnutrition and infectious disease at the local population level. As I have noted earlier, one of the more surprising results of my investigation of Maring diet was the amount of individual variation that was shown to exist among members of the same local group. This was not expected in an unstratified egalitarian society in which (with certain restrictions) food is freely shared and in which no one ever complains of being hungry.

Given this wide variation in individual intake, combined with a wide variation in group mean intake, with some groups showing very marginal means, it is obvious that a large proportion of the population of any group may in fact be malnourished and that the lower the mean intake, the larger the proportion of malnourished individuals in the group. Some of the observed variation in food intake was related to activity levels that, in turn, could be related to life-cycle stage. Young married adults were the most active and had the most adequate diets. All other individuals ate less, but their lower intake may well have been in balance with their lower requirements. However, it was noted that widows and widowers and others in mourning had particularly low intakes and that, in fact, some of these people did die from respiratory disease in the course of my study. Orphaned children had a high incidence of malnutrition and a very low survival rate. Thus, we have a situation in which a low average level of nutrition in a population results in some members who are severely malnourished and thus extremely susceptible to infectious disease. As the death rate from such diseases rises, more and more individuals are in a state of mourning and, while in this state, lower their food intake and increase their own susceptibility to disease leading to more and more deaths. It is also likely that individuals who are eating less because they are in mourning are also producing less food, thus lowering the availability of food for the rest of the community. In fact, Maring mortuary practices do forbid widows and other close female relatives of the deceased from entering gardens for several weeks after the death has occurred. I do not know what effect these prohibitions have on total food production, but it is not unreasonable to suspect that if there are large numbers of recent widows in a population, that its food production might fall. I have also observed that widowed and other bereaved men do little work, frequently for extended periods of time. It thus appears that malnutrition in the community not only leaves its members vulnerable to high mortality from infectious disease, but also that the high mortality increases the likelihood of malnutrition by removing not only the dead but also their close relatives from food production.

There is also evidence that in a chronically malnourished community, a certain proportion of adults will manifest both physical and psychological handicaps resulting from early severe malnutrition. The presence of these individuals in large numbers in a community might further reduce its food supply. Among the Maring, as well as among the other highland New Guinea societies, there are a certain number of men who never marry. Permanent bachelors among the Maring comprise over 6% of the male population over the age of 35 (C. Lowman, personal communication). These permanent bachelors are frequently stunted and somewhat dim-witted individuals, and it is likely that their consumption and production of food is low in proportion to their normal age mates. Among the Simbai Maring, there was a higher frequency of permanent bachelors in those groups that suffered the highest mortality in the 1960s and a lower frequency among those groups whose population was expanding. The increased frequency of bachelors in these already stressed groups may have put additional strain on already short food resources. Here, again, we see the positive feedback between malnutrition and food production.

One further consequence of the population decline of the 1960s

among the Maring must be mentioned. That which, for want of a
better term, I will call social disruption. The Maring were acutely
aware that their numbers were declining, and they were frightened by
this fact. The level of anxiety was, of course, greatest among the
groups that were declining most rapidly. Here sorcery accusations
were common, and there was frequent reluctance, particularly on the
part of young unmarried men to provide aid and assistance to a sick
parent or other relative. This behavior was severely condemned by
the community, but it continued to occur, and it is likely that a number
of people, particularly older people, died of neglect as well as of
influenza. Many people expressed a belief that there was something
wrong with the land of the most severely affected groups. With the
exception of a place called Singanai, which was a mixed border population of Maring and Gainj and had the highest death rate throughout
the study period, there were no mass migrations out of local groups as
a result of this belief. But young women were reluctant to marry into
high-mortality groups, and young men from the most depleted populations were leaving in large numbers for contract work on coastal
plantations. Frequently, as many as 50% of the men between the ages
of 20 and 45 were so engaged. We can only guess about the effect of
this high level of absenteeism on those who remained behind. Since
the introduction of the steel axe, the time required for men's share of
garden work has greatly diminished, and it is possible that large
numbers of men can be away at any time without affecting the food
supply of the community, but this is doubtful.

So it appears that at least among the Simbai Maring during the 1960s
that those local populations that suffered the greatest degree of
chronic malnutrition also suffered the greatest mortality from infectious disease, that this high mortality caused the greatest degree of
disruption of individual and of social behavior, and that the disturbed
behavior patterns aggravated both the malnutrition and the disease
fatality.

REFERENCES

Buchbinder, G. *Maring microadaptation: A study of demographic, nutritional, genotypic and phenotypic variation in a Highland New Guinea population.* Un-published Ph.D. dissertation, Columbia University, 1973.
Buchbinder, G. *Small body size among the Simbai Valley Maring.* Paper read at the American Association of Physical Anthropologists, 43rd Annual Meeting, Amherst, 1974.
Buchbinder, G. Endemic cretinism: A by-product of culture contact. In T. K. Fitzgerald

(Ed.), *Nutrition and anthropology in action*. Amsterdam: Van Gorcum Press, 1976. Pp. 106–116.

Buchbinder, G., & Clark, P. The Maring people of the Bismarck Ranges of New Guinea. *Human Biology in Oceania*, 1971, *1*, 121–133.

Clarke, W. C. *People and place*. Berkeley: University of California Press, 1971.

FAO/WHO Energy and protein requirements. Report of a joint FAO/WHO *Ad Hoc* Expert Committee, World Health Organization Technical Report Series No. 522, FAO Nutrition Meetings Report Series No. 52. World Health Organization, Geneva, 1973.

Hipsley, E. H., & Kirk, N. Studies of dietary intake and the expenditure of energy by New Guineans. South Pacific Commission, *Technical Paper* 147, Noumea, New Caledonia: South Pacific Commission.

Rappaport, R. *Pigs for the ancestors*. New Haven, Connecticut: Yale University Press, 1968.

U.S. Department of Agriculture. Handbook No. 8, *Composition of foods*. Washington, D.C., 1963.

Vayda, A. P. Phases of the process of war and peace among the Maring of New Guinea. *Oceania*, 1971, *42*, 1–24.

Venkatachalam, P. S. A study of the diet, nutrition and health of the people of the Chimbu area (New Guinea Highlands), territory of Papua and New Guinea. Department of Public Health. Monograph No. 4, 1962.

7

Social Structuring of Nutrition in Southern India[1]

EDWARD MONTGOMERY

Washington University—St. Louis

PROBLEM INTRODUCTION: NUTRITIONAL AND SOCIAL VARIATION

Few would consider variations in nutrition and nutritional status in human societies to be randomly distributed. Now it is generally accepted that nutritional variations are structured at all levels of analysis of societies, whether local, regional, national, or global. However, different explanations—with reference to either cultural, economic, or social determinants—have been proposed to account for observed variation for particular cases. Comparatively, the social dimension has been less fully explored. Certainly anthropological studies of food use and nutrition have paid it limited attention (Montgomery, forthcoming). Given this volume's concern with the relations among malnutrition, behavior, and social organization, it is appropriate in this chapter to

[1] The field research was supported by funds from NIH (Grant No. M.H. 13811-01), the Wellcome Research Unit, and Columbia University. Computerized analyses were generously supported by N.S.F.–B.S.S.G. funds through Washington University—St. Louis. Portions of the material in this chapter have been presented in lectures at Washington University—St. Louis, University of California—Davis, University of Texas School of Public Health—Houston, and Michigan State University.

investigate in detail the social structuring of nutrition. Here attention is focused on a population in rural southern India in which there are important nutritional and social variations. Elsewhere I have presented detailed quantitative evidence for this population that shows that the many significant economic variations within it (as measured in terms of a number of property, income, and expenditure variables) cannot be significantly related, positively or negatively, to the wide nutritional variations (Montgomery, unpublished ms). Hence this case is of interest not only for the need in this context to examine more closely the social variations but also because, as will become clear at one stage of the analysis, part of the results from this study contradicts the current view that differentials of nutritional status are simply and directly related to differences in social behavior or social position. This chapter has three aims: (1) indication of the need for more careful and detailed use of social variables in nutritional inquiries; (2) suggestion that consideration of a broad range of social relations is essential to thorough inquiry; and (3) provision of a partial solution to the apparent contradiction that arises in the analysis here.

METHODS

The anthropological and nutritional data presented in this chapter were obtained during a period of continuing research on the ecology of nutrition, health, and health care that was conducted in North Arcot District, Tamil Nadu (formerly Madras State), southern India, from December 1967 to May 1970. From April 1968 onward, particular attention was focused on the total population of the rural nucleated settlement Reddiur. This research site was situated about 165 km inland from the coastal city of Madras and was in the agriculturally productive Palar River valley. In this region, the population density then was about 275 persons per square kilometer (just over 700 per square mile). From the district's headquarters, the city of Vellore, to Reddiur was a distance of about 25 km. Certain details of the social, economic, and cultural life, demography, health, and nutrition of the people of Reddiur were studied as part of the research, and one major goal was the careful specification of all sources of nutrients, food energy, and health care of current significance for the population. Processes of food production, purchase, sale, and consumption were investigated for each family in the population, as were the various categories of home and local health-enhancing activities and medical practitioners that were used. (Relevant to the latter see Montgomery,

1974–1975; Montgomery, 1976b.) Study of the nutrient and energy-flow processes called for determining not only where and in what quantities various food items were grown, bought, earned, sold, and consumed but also those persons within and linked with the Reddiur population in food-related transactions. Previous anthropological studies indicated the importance of caste in commensal relations and food flows (Marriott, 1968; Mayer, 1956, 1960), and thus ranking of castes was one of a series of social variables that could be quantitatively measured as continuous or ordinal variables. Personal ranks (Hiebert, 1969) were not measured. As there was no shop or store within Reddiur in which food items could be bought, the people's uses of shops in a neighboring settlement, of a weekly market, and of the market in Vellore were included in the study. Data for all social variables reported here were obtained for all families and individuals in the population. The research was organized from within Reddiur where I maintained continuous residence during the study year June 1968–May 1969 and from Vellore during the next year.

The health and nutritional profile of the population was determined clinically, anthropometrically, biochemically, and through diet studies. Over the period December 1968 through March 1969, clinical examinations of a 50% sample ($N = 297$) were completed by an experienced southern Indian clinician, Dr. Gopala Krishna Khandige, and observations were recorded on a form (see Figure 7.1) appropriately modified to local conditions from those exemplified in the Interdepartmental Committee on Nutrition for National Defense (I.C.N.N.D.; 1963) and Jelliffe (1966) manuals. Nearly every member of the population through age 14 was part of this sample, and all older age, sex, and social groups were rather evenly represented in the remaining part. Just over one-quarter of all persons aged 15 or older were clinically examined. In conjunction with the clinical observations, anthropometric data were obtained for a 65% sample ($N = 380$) of the population, and the weights and heights were compared with the World Health Organization (WHO) and Indian Council of Medical Research (I.C.M.R.) Madras State standards for the appropriate age and sex categories (Jelliffe, 1966; Indian Council of Medical Research, 1972, Tables 25, 26, 29, 30). Stool specimens were obtained for 186 persons (32% sample), and part of the observations regarding locally important intestinal parasites have been reported (Jacob John, Montgomery, & Jayabal, 1971). Also, in March 1969, venous blood specimens (20 ml) were drawn from 134 Reddiur residents (23% sample) by a team of technicians from the Haematology Laboratory of the Wellcome Research Unit of the Christian Medical College Hospi-

IDENTIFICATION:

Name _____ M F Age___years___months S. No. _____

Father's Name_____ Address _____

Mother's age___	At	Total Preg-	Of Live-	Of Deaths
	breast	nancies	born	___died before 1 yr
Birth order___	or	___liveborn	___alive	___died 1–4 yrs
	Weaned	___stillborn	___died	___died 5+ years
		___abortions		

Weight___kg   Height___cm   Weight/Age___%

Mid
Left___cm
Arm circumference

CLINICAL EXAMINATION: date   examiner

General impressions: apathy / pallor / irritability / wasting / oedema

Chronic illness
and disability:

Diarrhoea,
G-I disorders:

Remarks:

Skin:	normal / pale / dry / scaly / follicular hyperkeratosis / scabies / tinea / ulcer / leprosy / other -
Head:	fontanelle - closed / open (size)
Hair:	normal / dry / thin / easily pluckable / depigmented
Eyes:	normal / pink-red / pale / muddy / Bitot's spots / vertical wrinkling / cornea - circum-C injection / quick-drying / dry w photophobia / keratomalacia / conjunctivitis / trachoma
Lips and Mouth:	normal / angular stomatitis / cheilosis / stomatitis / bleeding gums / pale tongue / filiform papillary atrophy - mild / moderate / severe
Teeth:	caries - mild / severe / malposition / debris or calculus
Glands:	thyroid enlargement / parotid enlargement
G-I:	splenomegaly / liver - hard / firm / soft
Musculo-skeletal:	epiphyseal enlargement / beading of ribs / craniotabes / pigeon chest / frontal & parietal bossing / knock-knee & bow legs / Harrison's sulcus
Other:	

Remarks on
nutritional
status:

                     marasmus / pre-kwashiorkor / kwashiorkor
probable
deficiencies: vit A / vit B / vit C / vit D / iron / other —

Figure 7.1 Clinical examination questionnaire.

tal (C.M.C.H.), Vellore, under the supervision of Drs. V. I. Mathan and Selwyn J. Baker. A few older children, some teen-agers, and mostly adults made up this sample, which was proportionately about twice the size usually obtained in blood surveys in southern India. The biochemical measurement of hemoglobin, hematocrit, serum B_{12}, serum folic acid, red blood cell folic acid, serum iron, and unsaturated iron-binding capacity was completed by Baker's laboratory in the Wellcome Unit. Determinations for total serum protein, serum albumin, plasma vitamin A, and serum vitamin C were completed by Dr. Barbara A. Underwood in the laboratories of the Nutrition Research Department, C.M.C.H., and the Institute of Human Nutrition, Columbia University. Also, during her collaboration, Dr. Underwood, with the assistance of nutritionists Regina S. Sundararaj and Sheila David Jones from C.M.C.H.'s Nutrition Research Department, completed random 1-day weighed dietary intake measurements in March 1969 for a sample of 25 Reddiur households (169 persons, 29% of the population). Previous work indicated the acceptability of random 1-day observations, given the low intrafamilial variability in food consumption from day to day in this region (Taskar, Swaminathan, & Shantha, 1967) and in Reddiur. Consumption unit and food-composition values then currently in use in nutrition work in India were consulted in the analysis of the weighed diets (Indian Council of Medical Research, 1966, p. 8 and Tables I, II, III). By one or more of these approaches to assessing nutritional status, almost all families (99 or 94%) in Reddiur were brought into the nutritional part of the study. Those six who were not were four single-person households (elderly widowers and widows), one elderly childless couple, and one disinterested four-person family. Computerized analyses of these various observations were done at the University Computing Facilities, Washington University, St. Louis.

FINDINGS

Reddiur, like most rural settlements in this region of southern India, is a dense aggregate of single-storied, whitewashed, tiled- or thatched-roofed houses packed along nearly parallel east–west and north–south streets. During the period of the nutritional investigations, 589 persons were its population, distributed among 105 families that lived in commensally separate households. Within a radius of 1.5 km about Reddiur were 6 other similar nucleated settlements. About them lay intensively cultivated family-owned fields on which crops of millets, rice, sugarcane, legumes, sorghum, mangoes, bananas, and coconuts were grown. In this region, electric-pump-raised irrigation water to supplement monsoon rainfall permitted millets, rice, and sugarcane to be grown year round. Farms 2–4 acres in size supported the average-sized family, and the modal-sized holding was then 2.6 acres. Eighty-nine of the 105 families owned some farmland, and amounts owned ranged from .23 to 41 acres. Residents of Reddiur were members of any one of 12 named endogamous caste populations, and the great majority of the cultivating families belonged to farmer castes, traditionally agriculturalist. In addition to the members from four farmer caste populations in Reddiur, families of accountant, artisan (carpenter-blacksmith), potter, herder, and two laborer castes lived in the settlement. The total membership of the population of each particular caste was distributed among dozens of villages, towns, and cities across the region (Montgomery, 1977). In general, life in Reddiur was predominantly locally oriented; everyone worked in the settlement (e.g., potters, artisans, housewives) or in the fields about it (e.g., farmers, herders, laborers) except for 4 men (a primary school teacher and 3 clerks or office workers who daily commuted to nearby settlements). Children attended either a local primary school or a neighboring settlement's high school and returned home for all meals. Family sizes were not large on the average; the mean size was 5.61 persons. Ever-married women had an average of 2.72 living children and had lost 1.04 children. As a whole, the population in 1969 was young: 14% of its members were aged less than 5 years, 40% were younger than 15 years, and 7% were 60 or older.

Food-relevant behavior in Reddiur was found to be rather precisely specifiable, and it can be described briefly. Raw food items were obtained through local crop production, through earnings as shares of leases or as wages, through ritual payments, and through purchases. Cooked foods were obtained either in meals in one's own home, as part of wages paid by one's employer, or as meals eaten when away from Reddiur. Nearly all meals were consumed locally; an average of fewer than 10 meals in a year per person were eaten away from Reddiur. These few meals away from home were eaten at weddings, funerals, or on visits to relatives, temples, and cities. Overwhelmingly, it was local consumption that was of nutritional significance. Three places were of importance for local meals: one's own home, one's employer's house, or one's own or one's employer's fields. The last was notable in the numerous instances when meals were taken to the fields for men and women engaged in agricultural activities. During all phases in acquiring foods, both raw and cooked, social links among members of the population or specifiable others were critical to the flows of nutrients and energy (Montgomery, 1972).

The social dimension was essential to several aspects of local food production. First, many families either gave out or received plots of farmland to other local families through annual lease agreements. In 1968—1969, nearly half (52) of the families had lease agreements with others, and the usual terms of the leases were that one-third of the crop was given to the landowner by the lessee. Such agreements enabled consolidation of widely dispersed plots and adjusted quantities of land cultivated to the farmers' capabilities or production aims. For a number of cultivators, part of their successes in production derived from skillful lease arrangements. Some thereby were able to increase significantly their production of food crops.

Next, social ties had consequence in the contributions of labor and various technological resources to the production of crops. Family size was one major variable that affected the area of land that could be cultivated and the kinds of crops that could be raised. Larger families tended to have more able men working regularly in cultivation, and they tended to cultivate larger acreages. (The usual categories of family types—nuclear, extended, etc.—are of limited relevance in this context in view of the evidence that the different forms are of relatively short duration (Montgomery, 1976a). Since the major crops (millets, rice, sugarcane) were labor intensive, and largely non-mechanized production techniques were used, the labor of the farmers and also of their wives was important for certain aspects of cropping, as was the assistance of local kinsmen. Kinsmen's labor was an essential component of the overall labor investment in cultivation for 80% of the farming families. Families varied markedly from one another in the numbers of houses locally in which they had kin and also in the total numbers of local kin. Those with large numbers of kin tended to cultivate larger holdings and to produce larger acreages of the staple food crops.

Third, friends and neighbors who were willing and able to help in cultivation—by providing labor, loaning or renting implements and draft animals, or making available irrigation water—were essential to many cultivators. Those with greater numbers of helper relationships tended to cultivate larger acreages. Finally, at crucial periods in the cropping sequences (e.g., transplanting, weeding, harvest), hired laborers were needed to complete productive work, and those farmers who hired greater numbers of daily wage laborers tended to produce greater acreages of the major food crops. Table 7.1 presents the distribution of observations for five of these social variables.

TABLE 7.1
Distributions of Five Social Variables

Family size	Frequency	Local families with kin	Frequency	Number of local kin	Frequency	Number of helpers	Frequency	Number of day laborers hired	Frequency
1	5	0	8	0	8	0	15	0	29
2	6	1	23	1	9	1	15	1–3	11
3	11	2	29	2	23	2	31	4–7	12
4	15	3	10	3	14	3	25	8–10	13
5	21	4	13	4	13	4	10	11–15	11
6	18	5	10	5	8	5	3	16–24	10
7	4	6	8	6	1	6	5	25–49	12
8	10	7	2	7	3	7	1	≥50	7
9	6	8	1	8	5				
10	3	9	1	9	4				
11	4			10	9				
15	2			11	3				
				12	3				
				14	1				
				16	1				
	105[a]		105[b]		105[c]		105[d]		105[e]

[a] Mean = 5.61, SD = 2.76.
[b] Mean = 2.78, SD = 1.98.
[c] Mean = 4.58, SD = 3.68.
[d] Mean = 2.32, SD = 1.58.
[e] Mean = 14.30, SD = 23.23.

As would be expected, those families cultivating greater acreages of the staple food crops needed to purchase lesser amounts or none for their own consumption. During the 1968–1969 study year, consumption needs for the following food crops were met out of family production (including lease earnings) by these numbers of the total 105 Reddiur families: rice, 27 families; finger millet, 29; red gram dhal, 35; black gram dhal, 13; groundnuts, 66; groundnut oil, 51; crude brown sugar, 62; and milk, 53. All other families, even those that produced or earned some quantities of these foods, purchased at least part of their consumption of these basics during the year. The quantities of staple foods obtained as payments for leases were significant for several families, but the very small amounts received as ritual payments by service caste households represented at best a few days of their annual consumption requirements. However, flows of cooked foods between families as part of wage payments had major nutritional significance for a number of persons in the population (Montgomery, 1972). Employees at daily wage labor received both a midday meal and a cash payment, and the meal usually was the same as that eaten by the employer's family. Day laborers were paid in meals of large balls of a cooked combination of millet flour and rice served along with a vegetable curry sauce. By tradition, men received 2 of the cooked cereal balls, and women, 1. Payment of day laborers in food has been reported for other parts of India, including West Bengal (Mukherjee, 1958, p. 83; Nicholas, 1963, p. 1191), south Gujarat (Breman, 1974, p. 196), Karimpur, Uttar Pradesh (Wadley, personal communication), Andhra Pradesh (Mahadevan, 1962, p. 44), and Pondicherry on the Madras coast (Datta, Kutty, & Gopalan, 1963, p. 149). In Reddiur, 27 families had 1 or more members working at least occasionally as day laborers. In some of the laborer caste families, the working adult members depended on wage meals an average of six days per week. The giving of cooked food frequently to laborers by employers did not, however, violate the commensal character of caste restrictions on co-dining, and it was learned that in general members of different castes would not eat in one another's homes. A clear composite rank of castes along a "high" to "low" dimension emerged from measures of caste ranking from 37 Reddiur adults. The composite rank is given in Table 7.2.

Purchased food items were obtained either locally, at small shops in the neighboring settlement southeast of Reddiur, at a weekly market at a settlement about 5 km distant, or from the large market in the city of Vellore. Rice, groundnuts and other legumes, and tamarind pulp were usually bought from local producers. The items usually bought from 1

TABLE 7.2

Castes and Caste Ranks

Name	Traditional occupation	Families ($N = 105$)	Composite rank position
Reddi (Yelnadu)	Agriculturalist	65[a]	1
Kannakka Pillai	Accountant	1	2
Mudaliar	Agriculturalist	2	3
Achari	Carpenter–blacksmith	3	4
Udayar	Potter	11	5
Mandiri	Herder	11[b]	6
Idiga Naidu	Palmwine producer	2	7
Goundar	Agriculturalist	0[c]	8
Vannan	Washerman	1	9
Adidravidar	Laborer	0[d]	10
Arundathiar	Laborer	9[b]	11

[a] Two residents are servants: one, Yelnadu Reddi, one, Pokanad Reddi.
[b] One resident is a servant.
[c] One resident is a servant, one is a tenant.
[d] Two residents are servants.

of the 3 small shops in the neighboring settlement (about 15 minutes' walk distant) were red gram, groundnut oil, onions, garlic, and chilies. Many families bought all their vegetables at the weekly market, and occasionally some bought meat (mutton, chicken) in small amounts there. During visits to Vellore city, some families bought finger millet, legumes other than groundnuts, and vegetables. Since almost none of the regularly consumed vegetables were raised locally, trips to the shops and markets were the main means by which most families got these items for their diets. Only very occasionally would some housewives buy vegetables from itinerant vendors who passed through the settlement (on bicycle or foot) with baskets of several kinds of vegetables. Table 7.3 presents the frequencies with which Reddiur residents made trips (other than to high school) to the neighboring settlement with shops and to the weekly and town marketplaces.

The various grains, legumes, vegetables, and condiments in use in Reddiur were integrated into one of two basic meals. One was patterned about cooked rice as the central item, and the other was based on cooked finger millet flour combined with broken grains of rice (preferably) or sorghum and shaped while still hot into balls about 10 cm in diameter. Sometimes pearl millet or maize were used as cheaper, less preferable substitutes for the rice. Sauces, made mainly

TABLE 7.3

Frequencies of Trips to Places with Shops and Markets

Ranges of frequencies of trips in a year	Persons going to neighboring settlement with shops	Persons going to weekly market settlement	Persons going to Vellore city
235–365	47	3	4
183–234	14	5	1
79–182	49	23	9
45–78	35	59	14
19–44	29	61	49
10–18	9	23	25
4–9	6	8	30
1–3	2	5	37

with red gram dhal and condiments, sometimes with one or another vegetable, were served as complements to the cereal preparations. Usually, cooked foods were prepared twice daily, for a midday meal and a night meal. Leftover millet balls or rice from the night meal were mixed with water, kept overnight, and drunk as a slightly fermented, unheated gruel around 7:00 or 8:00 the following morning. The distinction between families relying on the more prestigious rice-oriented meals and those depending on other cereals can be seen in Table 7.4, which presents some of the findings from the dietary study of 25 Reddiur families.

As can be seen in Table 7.4, these families were almost wholly vegetarian. In general, most families in the population were similarly vegetarian, although for economic rather than religious or ritual reasons. Most consumed meat (mutton or chicken) an average of four to six times a year on special festival occasions and then in quite small quantities. The major exception was laborer families, which fairly regularly consumed beef, as they were not bound by caste concerns to avoid its consumption. Laborer caste families from Reddiur would join other laborers of nearby settlements and as a group purchase aged bullocks (steers) no longer useful as draft animals and slaughter and share the beef. On an average, beef was consumed by laborer families approximately fortnightly and sometimes with greater frequency. Although many foreigners suppose that beef is not consumed within India, the practice of beef avoidance actually tends to be associated with the more Brahmanically oriented castes. In fact, beef consumption in India has been reported in previous nutritional studies (De-

TABLE 7.4

Foods in Weighed Diets of 25 Families[a]

Items	Families Consuming	Times Used during day 1	2	3	Calories	Protein	Fat	Carbohydrates	Calcium	Iron	Ionizable iron	Vitamin A	Riboflavin	Vitamin C	Thiamin	Niacin
Grains and grain foods																
Rice, parboiled	21	8	8	5	21	21	18	21	11	21	21	—	21	—	21	21
Rice, raw	6	1	4	1	6	6	3	6	3	5	6	—	5	—	5	6
Finger millet	15	8	6	1	15	15	15	15	15	15	15	13	15	—	14	14
Sorghum	8	4	3	1	8	8	7	8	3	6	8	8	8	—	8	8
Suji	1	—	—	1	1	1	—	1	1	1	1	1	1	—	1	—
Leftover rice in gruel	9	9	—	—	9	9	—	9	—	9	9	—	9	—	9	9
Leftover millet balls in gruel	1	1	—	—	1	1	1	1	1	1	1	—	1	—	1	1
Legumes and legume foods																
Red gram	22	18	3	1	10	21	4	4	9	9	20	18	22	—	19	9
Black gram	11	11	—	—	1	4	—	1	4	4	4	1	4	—	3	1
Bengal gram	4	3	1	—	—	1	—	—	—	—	1	—	—	—	—	—
Field bean	3	3	—	—	1	—	—	—	3	—	—	3	3	3	1	—
Horse gram	2	2	—	—	1	2	—	—	1	2	1	—	1	—	1	1
Green gram	2	2	—	—	1	2	1	1	1	1	2	2	2	—	2	—
Cow pea	1	1	—	—	1	1	—	—	1	—	1	—	1	—	1	1
Groundnut chutney	1	1	—	—	—	1	1	—	—	—	—	—	1	—	1	—
Leftover red gram sauce	2	2	—	—	1	2	—	—	1	1	2	2	2	—	2	1

Vegetables																
Onion	23	14	8	1	—	—	—	—	10	—	—	—	—	15	1	—
Tomato	9	7	2	—	—	—	—	—	5	—	—	9	6	9	4	—
Eggplant	7	7	—	—	—	1	1	—	3	1	5	6	6	7	—	3
Potato	5	5	—	—	—	—	—	—	—	—	—	1	—	4	—	—
Cabbage	3	3	—	—	—	—	—	—	—	—	—	3	—	3	—	—
Carrot	2	2	—	—	—	—	—	—	1	1	—	2	—	1	—	—
Radish, white	2	2	—	—	—	—	—	—	1	—	—	—	—	2	1	1
Greens	2	2	—	—	—	—	—	—	2	2	—	—	—	—	—	—
Beet	1	1	—	—	—	—	—	—	1	—	—	—	—	1	—	—
Drumstick	1	1	—	—	—	—	—	—	—	—	—	1	—	1	—	—
Knol-khol	1	1	—	—	—	—	—	—	—	—	—	—	1	1	—	—
Mango, green	1	1	—	—	—	—	—	—	—	—	—	—	—	1	—	—
Ridge gourd	1	1	—	—	—	—	—	—	—	—	—	—	—	1	—	—
Yam	1	1	—	—	1	—	—	1	1	—	—	1	—	—	—	—
Animal products																
Milk, water buffalo's	5	4	1	—	—	—	4	—	5	—	—	4	3	—	—	—
Milk, cow's	1	1	—	—	—	1	1	—	1	—	—	1	1	—	—	—
Milk, goat's	1	1	—	—	—	1	1	—	—	—	—	1	1	1	—	—
Buttermilk	4	4	—	—	—	—	2	—	3	—	—	—	—	—	—	—
Egg, hen's	1	1	—	—	—	1	1	—	—	1	—	1	1	—	1	—
Cooking oils																
Groundnut oil	24	4	17	3	8	—	24	—	—	—	—	—	—	—	—	—
Sesame seed oil	2	2	—	—	—	—	2	—	—	—	—	—	—	—	—	—
Condiments																
Garlic	22	8	11	3	—	—	—	—	—	—	—	—	—	7	—	—
Tamarind pulp	20	8	12	—	—	—	—	—	5	5	2	2	—	2	—	—
Chilies	19	13	6	—	—	1	1	—	1	—	—	7	2	14	2	1
Mustard seeds	17	9	7	1	—	—	2	—	3	—	—	—	—	—	—	—
Cumin seeds	12	10	1	1	—	—	—	—	2	—	—	2	—	—	—	—

TABLE 7.4 (Continued)

Foods in Weighed Diets of 25 Families[a]

Items	Families Consuming	Times used during day 1	2	3	Number of families with ≥5% day's intake this source — Calories	Protein	Fat	Carbohydrates	Calcium	Iron	Ionizable iron	Vitamin A	Riboflavin	Vitamin C	Thiamin	Niacin
Pepper	12	8	4	—	—	—	—	—	1	—	—	4	—	1	—	—
Turmeric	4	4	—	—	—	—	—	—	—	—	—	2	—	—	—	—
Coriander	2	2	—	—	—	—	—	—	—	—	—	2	—	—	—	—
Fenugreek seeds	1	1	—	—	—	—	—	—	—	—	—	—	—	—	—	—
Asafoetida	1	1	—	—	—	—	—	—	—	—	—	—	—	—	—	—
Coconut	2	2	—	—	2	2	2	—	2	2	—	—	—	—	1	—
Masala powder (prepared)	20	18	1	1	—	—	—	—	—	—	—	—	—	—	—	—
Vadagam (prepared spice)	5	4	1	—	—	—	—	1	1	—	1	—	—	—	—	—
Crude brown sugar	5	4	1	—	—	—	—	—	—	2	1	—	—	—	—	—
Curry leaves	13	9	4	—	—	—	—	—	—	—	—	6	—	—	—	—

Numbers of sources for nutrients/energy

	Calories	Protein	Fat	Carbohydrates	Calcium	Iron	Ionizable iron	Vitamin A	Riboflavin	Vitamin C	Thiamin	Niacin
Lowest total number of different food items which provide ≥5% of day's intake of nutrient/energy for one family:	1	2	1	1	1	1	2	2	3	1	2	1
Highest total number of different food items which provide ≥5% of day's intake of nutrient/energy for one family:	5	5	5	5	7	7	5	7	5	5	8	5
Average number of different food items which provide ≥5% of day's intake of nutrient/energy for 25 study families:	3.0	3.6	3.5	2.3	3.9	3.1	3.4	4.0	4.1	3.0	3.4	2.6

[a] Dashes indicate no...

vadas & Easwaran, 1967, p. 157; Pandit, Raghavachari, Subba Rao, & Krishnamurti, 1940, p. 558; Sundararaj, 1972, p. 89; Sundararaj, Begum, Jesudian, & Pereira, 1969, p. 253).

The amounts of nutrients and energy consumed by the 25 diet study families are shown in Table 7.5, expressed as mean values, standard deviations, and in relationship to the allowances recommended by the Nutrition Expert Group of I.C.M.R. (1968). The findings clearly indicate that some of the population of Reddiur experienced undernutrition in certain respects.

Before presenting the findings from the other approaches taken to assess the population's nutritional status, the practices of feeding infants should be mentioned briefly. In general, infants received first priority in families in feeding and were fed on demand. Infants were fed supplements to their breast-milk diet beginning at about age 6–10 months according to just over half of the mothers. Some mothers said they started supplementation when their babies got their first teeth, and others said they started as soon as the infant reached for cooked foods. Usually, small quantities of cooked rice or cooked millet flour–rice balls were early supplementary foods. Breast-feeding was continued until children were 2 years or older. Older women were proud of having breast-fed children for prolonged periods, and some

TABLE 7.5

Daily Intakes in Weighed Diets

Energy, nutrients	Daily intake per consumption unit, 25 households[a]		Nutrition expert group, India, recommended allowance	Families below recommended allowance	
	Mean	SD		(N)	(%)
Calories	1,992	440	2800	25	100
Protein, gm	45	11	55	19	76
Fat, gm	21	17	—	—	—
Carbohydrates, gm	407	97	—	—	—
Calcium, mg	560	338	400–500	9	36
Iron, total, mg	38	16	20	0	0
Iron, Ionizable, mg	7	2	—	—	—
Vitamin A, IU	731	746	5000	25	100
Riboflavin, mg	0.8	0.2	1.5	25	100
Vitamin C, mg	28	34	50	21	84
Thiamin, mg	1.5	0.5	1.4	11	44
Niacin, mg	16	5	19	17	68

[a] Composed of 169 individuals.

younger mothers were following the same practice. Some claimed to have continued breast-feeding until their children were 4 or 5 years old. That local infant-care practices generally served to maintain good nutritional health was indicated during the clinical assessments of the population.

In the clinical assessment, 297 persons were examined. The findings presented here have been classified according to clinical signs observed and in broad categories for clinical nutritional status, which indicate some probable deficiencies of energy and of particular nutrients. The clinical observations were summarized by the examining physician, with the following definitions of nutritional health levels:

1. Good = normal clinical picture with approximately standard weight and height
2. Fair = underweight or standard build with a definite clinical sign of one nutrient deficiency
3. Poor = definite clinical signs of one nutrient deficiency and underweight, definite clinical signs of two or more nutrient deficiencies, or advanced PCM (severe wasting, marasmus)

The frequencies with which particular signs were observed is shown in Table 7.6. No attempt has been made here to list the numerous combinations of signs seen.

The more clearly indicated deficiencies were those of energy and protein, vitamin A, riboflavin, and iron. These are the deficiencies seen in the state of Tamil Nadu as a whole (Devadas, 1972, p. 25). The overall assessment of the population in these respects is summarized in Table 7.7. More than twice as many (64 versus 30%) of the infants and young children through 24 months were in the "good" category when compared with the rest of the population, and for them a favorable comparison (18 versus 27%) was evident even in the "poor" category.

The anthropometric observations supported the clinical observations that a significant proportion of the population was underweight. The weight and height data as analyzed according to age-independent standards (Jelliffe, 1966, Annex 1, Tables 3, 10, 11, 15, and 16) revealed that 12% (of $N = 380$) had weights at the $\geq 100\%$ of standard level, 28% were in the 90–99% of standard range, 37% were in the 80–89% range, 18% were in the 70–79% range, and 5% were in the 60–69% range; 215 (57%) were below the 85th percentile. Local standards for India (Viweswara Rao & Singh, 1970; Indian Council of Medical Research, 1972) also were used to analyze the

TABLE 7.6

Clinical Observations

	N	Per-centage of sample		N	Per-centage of sample
Skin			Lips and Mouth		
Pale	30	10.1	Pale tongue	32	10.8
Dry	20	6.7	Angular stomatitis	39	13.1
Follicular			Cheilosis	2	0.7
hyperkeratosis	1	0.3	Filiform papillary		
Knuckle pigmentation	3	1.0	atrophy	10	3.4
Eyes			Other		
Pale	33	11.1	General pallor,		
Bitot's spots	5	1.7	mild anemia	27	9.1
Vertical wrinkling	10	3.4	Severe anemia	7	2.4
Muddy	17	5.7	Underweight, thin	107	36.0
			Underweight, severe;		
			wasting	15	5.1
			Marasmus	4	1.3

anthropometric data, and for 70 children aged 60 months or younger for whom month of birth was known, nearly a third had values on the weight-to-height squared index that were indicative of protein–calorie undernutrition. These data are presented in Table 7.8. This distribution is remarkably similar to that reported by Viweswara Rao and Singh in their study of 3,100 Hyderabad city preschool children, in which they found that 53%, 13%, and 34% of the indices were in the respective interpretive categories. That in the Reddiur sample 77% of all values <0.145 were those of children in the 25–60 months age group (or, proportionately, 44% of this group versus 16% of the younger) reinforces the view that children 0–24 months were generally better nourished.

The biochemical assessments of nutritional status further affirmed that protein, vitamin A, and iron were nutrients for which some members of the Reddiur population exhibited low or deficient levels. Table 7.9 presents the findings from 11 biochemical measurements made in the blood study. The parallels with the clinical, anthropometric, and dietary observations are striking. One exception is that the low levels of vitamin C shown biochemically were not manifest clinically. This exception is consistent with nutritional survey findings in the

TABLE 7.7

Clinical Nutritional Assessments[a]

Good	N	Fair	N	Poor	N
Normal clinical picture with approximately standard weight and height		Underweight	88	Underweight and anemic	31
		Anemic	16	Underweight and riboflavin deficiency	21
		Riboflavin deficiency	9	Underweight and vitamin A deficiency	7
	99	Vitamin A deficiency	6	Anemic and riboflavin deficiency	1
				Anemic and vitamin A deficiency	1
				Riboflavin deficiency and vitamin A deficiency	1
				Underweight and anemic and riboflavin deficiency	6
				Underweight and riboflavin deficiency and vitamin A deficiency	6
				Severe wasting or marasmus	5
Total	99 (33.3%)		119 (40.1%)		79 (26.6%)

[a] Overall: underweight, N = 164 (55.2%); anemic, N = 55 (18.5%); riboflavin deficiency, N = 44 (14.8%); vitamin A deficiency, N = 21 (7.1%).

TABLE 7.8

Weight-to-Height Squared × 100 Index Values[a]

Wt./Ht.² × 100 index levels	Suggested interpretation	Number	Percentage
≥.150	"Normals"	37	53%
.145–.149	"Earliest stages of growth retardation"	11	16%
< .145	"Indicative of protein-calorie malnutrition"	22	31%

[a] $N = 70$, Mean = 0.155, SD = 0.026.

state of Tamil Nadu as a whole, in which clinical signs of vitamin C deficiency have been seen most infrequently (Devadas, 1972, pp. 20–25).

RELATIONS BETWEEN NUTRITIONAL AND SOCIAL VARIATIONS

Given this broad view of variations in nutritional status found in the Reddiur population, it is appropriate, at this point, to test whether these variations can be related to the marked social differences that also characterize this population. It is widely considered that social position and social behavioral differences bear on nutritional status distinctions in a clear, direct way. Numerous examples can be cited in which investigators have considered social factors in India to be of significance in explaining observed undernutrition (Datta *et al.*, 1963; Devadas & Easwaran, 1967; Devadas, 1974; Gopalan, 1968, 1974; Grewal, Gopaldas, & Gadre, 1973; Indian Council of Medical Research, 1972, pp. 47–49; Mahadevan, 1962; Swaminathan, Apte, & Someswara Rao, 1960; Viweswara Rao & Gopalan, 1969). For the Reddiur population, the specific relationships between nutritional and social variables could be examined statistically to learn whether particular sets of variables might co-vary. Here the results of correlation analysis (Pearson's r and Spearman's r_s) are presented to show the relationships that became apparent in these analyses. In Table 7.10 are presented the correlations between 31 nutritional variables and 7 social variables. For all the social variables, values were determined for every family and used for all members of the family. (For example, each member of a particular-sized family has the same family size

TABLE 7.9
Biochemical Assessment of Nutritional Status in Reddiur

Determination	Observations			Percentage in category			Interpretive values utilized			
	N	Mean	SD	Deficient	Low	Acceptable	Deficient	Low	Acceptable	Reference[a]
Total serum protein, gm/100 ml	132	6.99	0.58	3	17	80	<6.0	6.0–6.4	≥6.5	1, p. 308
Serum albumin, gm/100 ml	61	3.48	0.71	16	43	41	<2.8	2.8–3.4	≥3.5	1, p. 308
Plasma vitamin A, μg/100 ml	127	28.87	10.45	1	19	80	<10	10–19	≥20	1, p. 222
Serum B_{12}, pg/ml	132	189	103	20	17	63	<100	100–149	≥150	1, p. 276
Serum folic acid, ng/ml	132	8.79	4.28	0	22	78	<3.0	3.0–5.9	≥6.0	1, p. 267
RBC folic acid, ng/ml	132	223	123	16	14	70	<140	140–159	≥160	1, p. 267
Serum vitamin C, mg/100 ml	132	0.20	0.15	55	18	27	<0.20	0.20–0.29	≥0.30	1, p. 230
Hemoglobin, gm/100 ml	134	10.83	2.44	36	31	33	a:<12 b & c:<10	12.0–13.9 10.0–10.9	≥14.0 ≥11.0	2, p. 235[b]
Hematocrit, %	134	37.1	6.2	13	38	49	a:<36 b:<30 c:<30	36–41 30–37 30–33	≥42 ≥38 ≥34	2, p. 235[b]
MCHC, gm/100 ml RBC	134	28.8	2.8	—	72	28	—	≤30	>30	3, p. 104
Serum iron, μg/100 ml	131	60.3	26.7	34	—	66	a:<60 b:<40 d:<50	—	≥60 ≥40 ≥50	1, p. 331[b]

[a] References: 1 = Sauberlich, Dowdy, & Skala, 1973; 2 = I.C.N.N.D., 1963; 3 = O'Neal, Johnson, & Schaefer, 1970.
[b] The age-sex groupings for these interpretive values are: a = males, ≥ 13 years; b = females, ≥ 13 years, c = children, 3–12 years; d = children, 6–12 years.

value.) Also included in Table 7.10 is one individual characteristic, age in years. None of the five anthropometric variables is correlated (positively or negatively) with the social variables at a level above .18, and none of the 11 biochemical variables shows a correlation exceeding .28. Similarly, for the 12 dietary intake variables, many of the correlations are extremely low, some virtually zero, and even for the single variable most clearly correlated with nutrient intakes, family size, the values are only in the .40–.60 range. The highest correlation in the table is just +0.60 ($p<.001$). Many of the positive correlations for any particular variable are offset by negative correlations in the same columns or rows elsewhere in the table. The lack of relation between age and serum vitamin A values identified by Underwood for this population (1974, p. 160) applies to the other nutritional variables as well. The overall remarkable lack of relationship between the nutritional and social variations is further evidenced in the rank correlations (r_s) for ordinal variables in Table 7.11. In short, these statistics demonstrate that when carefully examined, these nutritional and social variables are impressively unrelated. In the context of the position that social factors are implicated in malnutrition, this conclusion appears contradictory.

DISCUSSION

There are several ways by which one might seek to resolve this apparent contradiction. One would be to propose alternative social variables that would bring into consideration behaviors excluded in the above analysis or that would refine the above variables to increase their specificity. Another would be to use other statistical analytical techniques. A third way would be to suggest that resolution lies in some other (nonsocial and noneconomic) category of variables (e.g., demographic, such as sex; or cultural, such as food taboos). The resolution presented here utilizes aspects of all of these possibilities and in its essential form can be summarized briefly.

One critical feature of nutritional variation in Reddiur was that with a consistency approaching universality, it was manifest *within* families. The empirical evidence bearing on this point is decisive. In 95% of the families (84 of 88) in which 2 or more members were assessed biochemically, anthropometrically, or clinically, the particular assessments for different family members fell into contrasting categories or ranges. (E.g., 1 family member had the clinical status

TABLE 7.10

Correlations: 31 Nutritional and 7 Social Variables[a]

Nutritional Variables	Family size	Number of leases given	Number of leases received	Number of local families with kin	Number of local kin	Number of helpers	Number of laborers hired	Age in years
Weight for height, WHO standard	.12a*	.06	.11a*	.05	.04	.12a*	.16b*	-.04
Weight for age, WHO standard	-.01	-.04	.18	.15	.06	-.08	.04	.13
Height for age, WHO standard	-.16	.15	.18	.17	.10	.00	.06	.09
Weight for age, I.C.M.R. Madras standard	-.01	.06	.11	-.05	-.05	-.02	.07	-.02
Height for age, I.C.M.R. Madras standard	-.09	.07	.09	.09	.08	-.04	.03	-.01
Total serum protein	.05	.01	-.11	.01	-.05	-.12	.02	-.04
Serum albumin	.15	.00	.06	-.12	-.03	.09	.00	-.10
Plasma vitamin A	.04	.07	.04	.10	.17	.28b*	.22a*	.03
Serum B_{12}	.00	-.15	-.11	-.15	-.17	-.05	-.12	.10
Serum folic acid	-.03	-.03	.20a*	.11	.10	.11	.09	-.02
RBC folic acid	-.12	.04	-.10	.13	.15	.06	-.08	-.03
Serum vitamin C	-.06	.23b*	.08	.12	.15	.09	.05	-.22a*

Hemoglobin	.17a*	.01	−.01	.02	.05	.06	.11	−.03
Hematocrit	.17a*	−.01	.02	.02	.07	.04	.12	.02
MCHC	.12	.07	−.04	.00	.01	.07	.08	−.15
Serum iron	.07	.07	.03	.02	.00	.11	.11	.06
Calorie intake	.46c*	.15	.22a*	.03	.00	.04	.17a*	.14
Protein intake	.47c*	−.03	.15	−.13	−.20b*	−.06	.09	.07
Fat intake	−.18a*	.05	−.15	.47c*	.48c*	.21b*	−.12	.07
Carbohydrate intake	.53c*	.15	.28c*	−.12	−.16a*	−.03	.22b*	.13
Calcium intake	.45c*	−.31c*	.16a*	−.25c*	−.45c*	−.52c*	−.17a*	−.06
Total iron intake	.49c*	−.24c*	.16a*	−.39c*	−.55c*	−.50c*	−.14	−.04
Ionizable iron intake	.24	.25c	.08	.06	.07	.18a*	.19	.15
Vitamin A intake	.00	.00	.35c*	.39c*	.31c*	.11	−.16	.01
Riboflavin intake	.60c*	.01	.09	−.27c*	−.25c*	.08	.07	.01
Vitamin C intake	−.15	−.02	.52c*	.40c*	.28c*	−.02	−.07	.07
Phosphorous intake	.54c*	−.11	.24c*	−.17a*	−.30c*	−.25c*	−.07	.03
Phytin phosporous intake	.54c*	−.15	.21b*	−.38c*	−.53c*	−.43c*	−.04	−.02
Thiamin intake	.50c*	−.23b*	.11	−.46c*	−.56c*	−.38c*	−.15a*	−.04
Niacin intake	.29c*	.13	.16a*	−.11	−.04	.18a*	.13	.11
Clinical assessment levels	.03	.13a*	−.01	−.07	−.06	.06	.12a*	.03

[a] Rank correlations (r_s) for 31st nutritional variable, all others, Pearson's r.

* Levels of significance: a $\leq$ .05; b $\leq$ .01; c $\leq$ .001.

TABLE 7.11

Rank Correlations: 31 Nutritional and 4 Social Variables

Nutritional variables	Number of trips to settlement with shops	Number of trips to weekly market settlement	Number of trips to city of Vellore	Caste rank
Weight for height, WHO standard	.03	-.05	.08	-.05
Weight for age, WHO standard	—	—	—	-.03
Height for age, WHO standard	—	—	—	.12
Weight for age, I.C.M.R. Madras standard	-.01	-.05	-.15	.04
Height for age, I.C.M.R. Madras standard	.06	-.06	-.52a*	.05
Total serum protein	.03	.03	-.18	-.03
Serum albumin	-.44a*	-.24	-.04	-.04
Plasma vitamin A	-.14	-.21	.01	-.05
Serum B$_{12}$	-.04	-.02	.02	-.25b*
Serum folic acid	.14	.14	.16	.21b*
RBC folic acid	.08	-.08	-.01	.11
Serum vitamin C	.09	.26b*	-.10	.14a*
Hemoglobin	-.14	-.05	-.30a*	-.03

Hematocrit	−.07	−.02	−.27a*	−.01
MCHC	−.26a*	−.17	−.20	−.03
Serum iron	−.01	.04	−.24a*	.00
Calorie intake	.10	−.02	−.28a*	.19b*
Protein intake	.12	.12	−.25a*	−.05
Fat intake	−.04	−.24a*	−.16	.31c*
Carbohydrate intake	.08	−.04	−.31b*	.20b*
Calcium intake	.01	.36b*	.07	−.37c*
Total iron intake	−.05	.26a*	−.10	−.30c*
Ionizable iron intake	.05	−.22a*	−.38c*	.43c*
Vitamin A intake	.06	−.02	−.05	.03
Riboflavin intake	.08	.23a*	−.21a*	−.21b*
Vitamin C intake	.09	−.15	.01	.20b*
Phosphorous intake	.03	.16	−.22a*	−.16a*
Phytin phosphorous intake	−.07	.28a*	−.04	−.36c*
Thiamin intake	−.09	.29a*	−.05	−.32c*
Niacin intake	.02	−.07	−.28a*	.28c*
Clinical assessment levels	−.09	−.07	−.06	.07

* Levels of significance: a ≤ .05; b ≤ .01; c ≤ .001.

168 Edward Montgomery

"poor" and another was "fair" or "good".) At least 2 different types of assessment were made for 2 or more persons in 77 families; in 75 (97%) of these, contrasting levels among family members were evident. The clinical and biochemical contrasts among family members were particularly striking.

Another critical feature of nutritional variation in Reddiur is that only certain categories of individuals were in positions within families for which one can anticipate with some certainty their nutritional status vis-à-vis others in the family. The generally good nutritional status of infants and children in the first and second years of life was mentioned earlier. A second similar category was the group of young adolescents (aged from about 12 to 15) who were also usually better off nutritionally. Usually, these advantaged youth had nutritional values higher than those of either their fathers or mothers. The aged and disabled were a third category within which the nutritional contrasts among its members tended to be less disparate, but it differed from the previous 2 categories in that its members often were nutritionally disadvantaged. The great majority of the population, however, was in other than these 3 favored/disfavored categories. Parents also quite frequently contrasted nutritionally with their children in the less advantaged age range (2–12 years), but no clear trend of advantage of one group over the other can be indicated. Further, sex differences *were not* clearly shown (cf. Naik and Bardhan, 1974). Fathers in Reddiur seemed as likely as mothers to have nutritional values categorically lower (or higher) than those of their children in the 2–12 age range. In husband–wife comparisons, either spouse had about equal chance of being nutritionally better off than the other. The important sex-role differences favoring greater equality between women and men in southern India probably were implicated in these findings.

A combination of these two features can be considered to account for the low-order correlations found between the social and nutritional variations above. It also serves to indicate that these findings, which emerge from a population approach, do not necessarily contradict those concerning preschool children (Devadas & Easwaran, 1967; Gopalan, 1968, 1974; Grewal *et al.*, 1973; Viweswara Rao & Gopalan, 1974). Perhaps analyses for individuals in specific age ranges (e.g., 2–5 years) may demonstrate a greater significance of particular social variables as, for example, family size, which has been considered a determinant of preschool malnutrition in some instances (e.g., Viweswara Rao & Gopalan, 1969) but not others (e.g., Grewal *et al.*, 1973). However, a more important task for future investigations is the development of an improved understanding of the factors contributing to variations in the distribution of food within families.

ACKNOWLEDGMENTS

Appreciation is here expressed to Barbara A. Underwood, Gopala Krishna Khandige, Selwyn J. Baker, V. I. Mathan, Sheila David Jones, and Regina S. Sundararaj for their major contributions to this project. Thanks are also due to S. Lalitha Lakshmi, Joseph Jeyaraj Walser, J. Logan, K. Logan, and V. Sami for the essential and valuable assistance they provided in Reddiur.

REFERENCES

Breman, J. *Patronage and exploitation: Changing agrarian relations in south Gujarat, India.* Berkeley: University of California Press, 1974.

Datta, S. P., Kutty, V. K., & Gopalan, T. K. Diet and nutrition survey of Pondicherry Establishment, part I: Dietary survey. *Indian Journal of Medical Sciences,* 1963, *17,* 149–156.

Devadas, R. P. *Nutrition in Tamil Nadu.* Madras Institute of Development Studies Publication 3. Madras: Sangam Publishers, 1972.

Devadas, R. P. Social and economic dimensions of nutrition. *Proceedings of the Nutrition Society of India,* 1974, *17,* 66–72.

Devadas, R. P., & Easwaran, P. P. Influence of socio-economic factors on the nutritional status and food intake of preschool children in a rural community. *Indian Journal of Nutrition and Dietetics,* 1967, *4,* 156–161.

Gopalan, C. Special problems and preventive programmes (1) India. *Journal of Tropical Pediatrics,* 1968, *14,* 228–232.

Gopalan, C. Some aspects of nutrition in India. In Ashish Bose, P. B. Desai, Asok Mitra, & J. N. Sharma (Eds.), *Population in India's development 1947–2000.* Delhi: Vikas Publishing House, 1974. Pp. 101–108.

Grewal, T., Gopaldas, T., & Gadre, V. J. Etiology of malnutrition in rural Indian preschool children (Madhya Pradesh). *Journal of Tropical Pediatrics,* 1973, *19,* 265–270.

Hiebert, P. G. Caste and personal rank in an Indian village: An extension in techniques. *American Anthropologist,* 1969, *71,* 434–453.

Indian Council of Medical Research (I.C.M.R.). *The nutritive value of Indian foods and the planning of satisfactory diets* (6th ed.) Prepared by W. R. Aykroyd, C. Gopalan, & S. C. Balasubramanian. I.C.M.R. Special Report Series, No. 42. New Delhi: Indian Council of Medical Research, 1966.

Indian Council of Medical Research (I.C.M.R.) *Growth and physical development of Indian infants and children.* I.C.M.R. Technical Report Series, No. 18. New Delhi: Indian Council of Medical Research, 1972.

Interdepartmental Committee on Nutrition for National Defense (I.C.N.N.D.) *Manual for nutrition surveys* (2nd ed.) Washington, D. C.: U. S. Government Printing Office, 1963.

Jacob John, T., Montgomery, E., & Jayabal, P. The prevalence of intestinal parasitism and its relation to diarrhoea in children. *Indian Pediatrics,* 1971, *8,* 137–141.

Edward Montgomery

Jelliffe, D. B. *The assessment of the nutritional status of the community.* W. H. O. Monograph Series, No. 53. Geneva: World Health Organization, 1966.

Mahadevan, I. Social factors in some nutritional deficiency diseases. *Indian Journal of Social Work,* 1962, *23,* 41–51.

Marriott, McKim. Caste ranking and food transactions: A matrix analysis. In M. Singer & B.S. Cohn (Eds.), *Structure and change in Indian society.* Chicago: Aldine, 1968. Pp. 133–171.

Mayer, A. C. Some hierarchical aspects of caste. *Southwestern Journal of Anthropology,* 1956, *12,* 117–144.

Mayer, A. C. *Caste and kinship in Central India.* Berkeley: Univ. of California Press, 1960.

Montgomery, E. The significance of nutritional data in sociocultural research. In P. G. Tulpule & K. S. Jaya Rao (Eds.), *Proceedings of the First Asian Congress of Nutrition.* Hyderabad, India: Nutrition Society of India, National Institute of Nutrition, 1972. Pp. 851–852.

Montgomery, E. Trance mediumship therapy in southern India: A transcript of a session. *Ethnomedizin* (Hamburg), 1974–1975, *3,* 111–126.

Montgomery, E. A note on the relationship between natality and family form: A case study from southern India. In J. F. Marshall & S. Polgar (Eds.), *Culture, natality, and family planning.* Carolina Population Center Monograph 21. Chapel Hill: Univ. of North Carolina, Carolina Population Center, 1976. Pp. 50–58. (a)

Montgomery, E. Systems and the medical practitioners of a Tamil town. In C. Leslie (Ed.), *Asian medical systems.* Berkeley: Univ. of California Press, 1976. Pp. 272–284. (b)

Montgomery, E. Human ecology and the population concept: The Yelnadu Reddi population in India. *American Ethnologist,* 1977, *4,* 175–189.

Montgomery, E. Anthropological contributions to the study of food-related cultural variability. In S. Margen (Ed.), *Progress in human nutrition.* Vol. 2. Westport, Connecticut: AVI Publishing. Forthcoming.

Montgomery, E. Poverty and malnutrition: An anomalous case of few relationships. Unpublished manuscript.

Mukherjee, R. Six villages of Bengal: A socio-economic survey. *Journal of the Asiatic Society, Series Science,* 1958, *24,* 1–220.

Naik, J. P. & Bardhan, K. Nutritional problem of women in India: Some socio-economic aspects. *Proceedings of the Nutrition Society of India,* 1974, *17,* 61–65.

Nicholas, R. W. Ecology and village structure in deltaic West Bengal. *Economic Weekly* (Bombay), 1963, *15,* 1185–1196.

Nutrition Expert Group, Indian Council of Medical Research. *Recommended daily allowances of nutrients.* Hyderabad, India: Indian Council of Medical Research, National Institute of Nutrition, 1968.

O'Neal, R. M., Johnson, O. C., & Schaefer, A. E. Guidelines for classification and interpretation of group blood and urine data collected as part of the National Nutrition Survey. *Pediatric Research,* 1970, *4,* 103–106.

Pandit, C. G., Raghavachari, T. N. S., Subba Rao, D., & Krishnamurti, V. Endemic fluorosis in South India: A study of the factors involved in the production of mottled enamel in children and severe bone manifestations in adults. *Indian Journal of Medical Research,* 1940, *28,* 533–558.

Sauberlich, H. E., Dowdy, R. P., & Skala, J. H. Laboratory tests for the assessment of nutritional status. *Critical Reviews in Clinical Laboratory Science,* 1973, *4,* 215–340.

Sundararaj, R., Begum, A., Jesudian, G., & Pereira, S. M. Seasonal variation in the diets of pre-school children in a village (North Arcot District), part I: Intake of calories, protein and fat. *Indian Journal of Medical Research*, 1969, *57*, 249–259.

Sundararaj, R. Food intakes of rural preschool children (Tamil Nadu). *Indian Journal of Nutrition and Dietetics*, 1972, *9*, 88–90.

Swaminathan, M. C., Apte, S. V., & Someswara Rao, K. Nutrition of the people of Ankola Taluk, North Kanara. *Indian Journal of Medical Research*, 1960, *48*, 762–774.

Taskar, A. D., Swaminathan, M. C., & Shantha, M. Diet surveys by weighment method—a comparison of random day, three-day, and seven-day period. *Indian Journal of Medical Research*, 1967, *55*, 90–96.

Underwood, B. A. The determination of vitamin A and some aspects of its distribution, mobilization and transport in health and disease. *World Review of Nutrition and Dietetics*, 1974, *19*, 123–172.

Viweswara Rao, K., & Singh, D. An evaluation of the relationship between nutritional status and anthropometric measurements. *American Journal of Clinical Nutrition*, 1970, *23*, 83–93.

Viweswara Rao, K., & Gopalan, C. Nutrition and family size. *Indian Journal of Nutrition and Dietetics*, 1969, *6*, 258–266.

8

The Malthusian Proposition and Nutritional Stress: Differing Implications for Man and for Society

B. ABBOTT SEGRAVES

The University of Michigan

> First among the "iron laws" is that of Malthus: that if there are no checks on the growth of population except starvation and misery, then the population will grow until the people are miserable and starve. Given the major premise, there is no escape from the conclusion, and the condition of well over half the world's people is a shocking testimony to its truth. [Boulding, 1953, p. 77].

> The primary or fundamental check to the continued increase of man is the difficulty of gaining subsistence and living in comfort. We may infer that this is the case from what we see . . . [Darwin, 1871, Vol. I, p. 126].

MALNUTRITION: A GENERALIZING PERSPECTIVE

Following the particularly harsh winter of 1854, Charles Darwin noted that four-fifths of the local population of birds had not survived to nest that spring in his shrubberies or to visit his lawn. Remarking that we consider an epidemic that kills 10% of the human population as "frightful," Darwin estimated that the destruction of the birds that winter had reached at least 80% (1975, p. 185). This empirical notation to a general consideration of the limitations on natural increase in

173

animals should recall with force the statement made by Malthus some 25 years earlier:

Elevated as man is above all other animals by his intellectual faculties, it is not to be supposed that the physical laws to which he is subjected should be essentially different from those which are observed to prevail in other parts of animated nature [1970, p. 225].

While man may increase his numbers more slowly than Darwin's tomtit and certainly possesses means not given other animals of artificially increasing his means of subsistence, it is nevertheless the case that given the constants (Malthus' two postulata) of human reproduction and the necessity of food to human existence, the geometrical increase of population growth as compared with the arithmetical increase of the means of subsistence must imply a constant and powerful check on population (Boulding, 1955). Malthus in his *First Essay* (1798) and Darwin later (1871, Vol. II, pp. 369–370; 1975, pp. 175–176) pointed out that this check—the "misery" following upon the pressure of human numbers on the means of subsistence—must fall somewhere, and must of necessity be "severely" felt by "a large portion of mankind." While perhaps less dramatic than famine, pestilence, and war, malnutrition in its various forms is likewise among the significant "miseries" attendant upon our fecundity: the FAO (1974, p. 66) estimates over 400 million, as of 1970, including almost a quarter of the population of the underdeveloped (or nonindustrialized) nations except China, suffer nutritional inadequacy of varying degree.

The problem of population pressure on resources—and hence the matter of food availability, a central consideration in an ecology of malnutrition (Robson, 1972, Vol. I, p. 81)—is especially significant for man. For the human population in particular, there is a considerable time lag in the effects of self-crowding and also in the effects of resource-overuse (Bickel, 1956; Mackenroth, 1953; Odum, 1971, p. 514). Human population density, therefore, tends to "overshoot," to grow beyond its resources or baseline energy supply unless there are factors that sharply reduce the growth rate before the undesirable effects of crowding—the misery of which Malthus spoke—begin to be felt (Abelson, 1975, p. 501; Braudel, 1973, p. 3). As will be later indicated, such "factors" are not generally characteristic devices of post-Neolithic human populations. The successive major provisions of pristine high-energy environments (first by the food-producing and ultimately with the industrial "revolutions") notwithstanding, man continues to expand until inevitably his numbers once again exceed his means. And as the FAO estimate clearly indicates, this difference between numbers and means is expressed today, as in the past, in human misery.

From the Neolithic to the Industrial–Medical Revolution: Population Growth over Time

Aspects of Dietary Reconstruction

The reconstruction of adequate paleodemographic profiles is fraught with notorious difficulties (Angel, 1969; Brothwell, 1971; Dumond, 1975, p. 716; Goldstein, 1969, p. 480). The vital statistics of populations long dead, particularly pre- and protohistorical societies, is of necessity—due to the great relative durability of bone—confined primarily to inferences made on the basis of skeletal remains. Such studies have tended to be limited in number and scope, particularly as a sufficiently large "population" of skeletal material is rarely uncovered, especially of early man and of the long period preceding the Neolithic and the widespread appearance of sedentism. Even when large samples are available, the remains may be too fragmentary or in too poor a state of preservation for study. If recovery and preservation are generally possible, one still must ascertain how representative of a valid contemporaneous population or particular community the excavated material is. Data can be skewed due to the cultural factors that often bias burials: Neolithic and Bronze Age barrows may represent the internment of elites and an absence of the commoner class, for instance. It must also be noted that this concentration on skeletal material is itself especially problematic, particularly for the paleoepidemiologist and paleopathologist. While certain bone lesions may clearly be identified (Goldstein, 1969), the more numerous diseases—including those of severe malnutrition—that predominantly or solely affect the soft tissues are left unidentified. While such (soft) tissues are available from a very few desiccated or anaerobically preserved human remains from certain highly limited areas, the amount and quality of material is inadequate to provide useful, reliable data on the incidence of infectious diseases other than some metazoan and protozoan parasites (Black, 1975, p. 515). Furthermore, of course, such skeletal and dental indices of nutritional status as do exist present their own problems. For example, the development of extralocal hypoplastic or growth arrest lines in tooth enamel (Clement, 1963) is a variable response in those individuals suffering nutritional stress, and Harris lines of growth arrest in diaphysial bone can apparently be removed by remodeling.

In the attempt to reconstruct the nutritional status of past populations (including possible cases of dietary insufficiency), the problem of the representativeness of the cemetery sample is especially important (Brothwell, 1969, p. 534, 1972, p. 76). The standard biometric data on skeletal material, given the finding of significant physical differentiation within a population, could represent either (1) the intrusion of a distinct population or populations and variation within the sample as a result of this admixture or (2) change in the average physique as a result of local microevolution within the larger population, that is, the operation of differing selective pressures, such as the presence or absence of nutritional stress. This is an especially pertinent caution, as stature, derived from long bone lengths (Trotter & Glaser, 1958) and the depth index of the true pelvic inlet, is commonly used as a direct index of nutritional stress.

Perhaps the most serious single problem for the reconstruction of nutritional status of a population from skeletal remains is the previously mentioned frequent misrepresentation of infant and child (1–4, 5 years) deaths. As this vital statistic is a common barometer of significant dietary stress, that child samples are in many cases biased makes reliable inferences as to the mortality rates of that portion of the population most susceptible to the rigors of malnutrition extraordinarily difficult to render with any confidence. As Brothwell's (1972, p. 82, Table 24) data on the child—adult composition of certain early British samples suggest, child samples can be seriously underrepresented. They can also be overrepresented. Social distinction in burial practice along dimensions of age, sex, and rank—for example, infants interred apart from the rest of the population—is an especially critical variable, one that must be taken into account in order to construct a truly representative demographic assessment of any given community or population.

Information concerning the diets and health conditions of antiquity is not, of course, entirely limited to skeletal remains. The recovery and analysis of foodstuffs directly from human feces or "coprolites" is now recognized as a valuable aid in dietary reconstruction, particularly as it is now possible to successfully identify soft plant and animal tissues as well as seeds and bone fragments (Callen, 1969, p. 235; Bryant, 1974; Brothwell, 1969, p. 531; Heizer, 1969).

The Nutritional Status of Early Man

As Issac (1971, pp. 280–281) points out, in the reconstruction of Pleistocene diet, (1) the survival as paleoanthropological documents of only a part of the feces and food refuse of long-dead populations, and (2) the estimation of the number of hominids and the amount of time involved in refuse accumulation remain, as ever, the major archaeological problems. There are, however, further difficulties for this early period: the feeding habits of the average primate type—dispersed foraging—are hardly conducive to the formation of a clear depositional record. And if foodstuffs are transported for sharing at a central locale, bone refuse may be distorted by the predator danger inherent in its accumulation (Schaller & Lowther, 1969), by the fact that larger and heavier animals are perhaps less likely to be transported any great distance and the ever-present problem of dispersal and destruction by scavengers.

There are three additional—if somewhat less direct—lines of evidence for the diet of early man: (1) the morphology and wear patterns of hominid teeth (Brothwell, 1959); (2) subsistence-related functional attributes of artifacts; and (3) settlement patterns as they relate to paleoecology. Taking these three factors, as well as inferences gleaned from food refuse and excreta, into account, Issac (1971, pp. 279, 294) concludes that a flexible joint dependence on animal and plant foods would appear to have been fairly clearly established some 2 million years ago. (also cf. Poirier, 1973, pp. 55, 105). Keeping the above-noted problems in mind, the archaeological record would appear to support more readily a model of human evolution focused on broadly based subsistence patterns than one stressing intensive and voracious predation. Research concerning contemporary foraging populations (Lee & DeVore, 1968) generally concurs that an important feature of human development over time is the establishment of a partial division of labor between male hunters and female gatherers, an adaptive strategy unique to man. As Dunn (1968, p. 223) has stressed, even in arid environments dietary resources are diverse; normal exploitation of these resources by modern hunter–gatherers in relatively undisturbed environments appears to provide "at least the minimal" protein, carbohydrate, fat, mineral, and vitamin requirements. The expectation, then, for stable, well-adapted foraging populations, modern or prehistoric, is that *patent* malnutrition will be rare (cf. Stini, 1971).

Disease stress generally would appear to have been light for early man (see, e.g., Black, 1975). It is likewise agreed that both among modern foragers and for pre-Neolithic populations the birth rate is low, yielding a model for the Paleolithic in which natality is in approximate balance with mortality and the population is of a size well within the relevant regional carrying capacity (Dumond, 1975, pp. 714, 715; Hassan, 1973, p. 536). While early man had the advantage of a diverse resource base, the various components of his energy supply as a general rule would appear to have been often meager and sparsely distributed, necessitating a highly mobile exploitation carried out by small groups of often shifting composition (Sahlins, 1972). In other words, the technology and necessary adaptive strategy of early man set a relatively low ceiling on population growth. The primary mechanism ensuring this low growth rate would appear to be a considerable interval between live and viable births, generally thought to be a necessary accommodation to the demands and rigors of a mobile existence. The physiological stress of mobility considerably enhances the likelihood of spontaneous abortion, and deliberate spacing of births—for example postpartum restrictions on sexual intercourse, abortion, and infanticide[1]—is clearly documented for modern foraging populations. Further, Darwin's (1871, Vol. I, p. 127) suggestion that early man may have been "less prolific" due to "a lack of nutritious food" has recently received additional support. While it may be the case, as suggested earlier, that overt malnutrition is not characteristic of foraging populations, a diet only marginally adequate may delay resumption of the menstrual cycle after parturition, thus ensuring a spacing between births lengthy enough to prevent serious nutritional stress (Frisch & McArthur, 1974, p. 950; cf. Jelliffe, 1968, pp. 255–258). Coupled with a later onset of menarche, the resultant "incomplete" female childbearing period would clearly have served as a significant population check in the Paleolithic.

The "Agricultural Revolution" and Its Aftermath

With the transition to food production in the Neolithic and the resultant increase in productivity per unit area and hence in the carrying capacity of the land, the demographic profile for man alters radically, if not irrevocably. As Birdsell (1957) has documented for Australia, human populations, fecund enough to permit rapid growth in especially favorable circumstances, can expand greatly in size within a relatively short period (Dumond, 1975, p. 714; Hassan, 1973, p. 536). Factors that, in the Paleolithic, had encouraged a low birth rate were now no longer operative. On the most general level, of course, is the lifting of restraints on the size and density of local groups hitherto imposed by the basic (relative) scarcity and sparseness of available natural resources, a function of the low food-extractive

[1] Systematic infanticide, particularly of the female infant, is thought by some to have taken place among these early populations; Birdsell (1968) estimates that this practice terminated anywhere from 15 to 50% of the total number of live births.

efficiency of band-level technology (Hassan, 1975). The new technology—agriculture, intimately coupled with animal husbandry in the Old World and South America—redefined energy "availability": What had been often meager and variously distributed, both spatially and temporally, was now generally abundant and locally concentrated. With the artificial increase in the means of subsistence made possible by the domestication of plants and animals, man, for the first time in his history, was able, *as a general rule,* to steadily and regularly increase his numbers. Sedentary communities, small numbers of which may have appeared with the characteristically intensive collecting economies of the Mesolithic, now became firmly established,[2] and the need for mobility and its possible implications for family spacing was obviated. Perhaps most important for the human organism is the higher level of stored, easily mobilized energy that was made more generally available with the increase in resource productivity if, as Frisch and McArthur (1974, p. 949; Frisch, 1975) suggest, certain minimum levels are necessary for regular ovulation and menstrual cycles.

The increasing productivity of foodstuffs and concomitant expansion of population size and density are well documented for the period immediately following the Neolithic. A rapid increase in population is documented throughout the eastern Mediterranean with the establishment of farming towns and villages in the eighth and seventh millennia BC, from Jericho and Tell Mureybat west to Çatal Hüyük, Haçilar, Argissa, Nea Nikomedia, and Lerna, and south to Egypt (Angel, 1972; Barringer, 1966; Deevey, 1960). In many areas, this proliferation of settled communities and general population increase were given additional impetus by further agricultural innovations: Marked growth from the Neolithic to the Early Bronze Age in the number of settlements in regions of the southern Aegean, for example, was made possible by the addition of certain arboreal crops—notably the olive, the grape, and the fig, domesticated in the third millennium BC—to the more typical cereals and legumes of the eastern Mediterranean (Renfrew, 1972). Later and far to the west, in the period from the fifth to the second millennium in northern Italy, the exploitation of deer, pig, and woodland and aquatic plants becomes increasingly less significant relative to a more efficient economy based on caprines,

---

[2] Brothwell (1969, p. 534) suggests that thyroid malfunction, a localized phenomenon related to iodine-deficient soils in various areas of the world, may not have been significant prior to the predominantly post-Mesolithic advent of year-round, sedentary communities.

cattle, pigs, and cereals (Jarman, 1971). The Southeast Asian "Mesolithic," the Hoabinhian, sees the end of the broad spectrum exploitation of riverine, marine, and terrestrial flora and fauna: conservatively, rice *(Oryza sativa)* would appear, from its identification at Nok Nok Tha in central Thailand, to have been domesticated by perhaps 4000 BC (Flannery, 1973, p. 286; Gorman, 1971).

As population size, concentration, and hence, ultimately, pressure on available resources increased, the stress of infectious disease, and possibly malnutrition, increased. This increasing disease stress, in turn, helped to ensure over time a population increase certainly more gradual than "explosive" (Hassan, 1973, p. 538). Brothwell (1972, p. 86) estimates that the disease load was perhaps less heavy for early populations than in many of the less developed countries today. Black (1975, p. 518) concurs, arguing that diseases infectious only in the acute phase require a larger group for their perpetuation or maintenance than existed in any coherent community in Neolithic times.

However, it must be noted that the problem of increasing disease stress following the transition to agriculture is more complex than this general account alone would indicate. While animal husbandry developed concomitantly with plant cultivation in the Old World, in the New World (with the exception of the llama and alpaca in South America) domesticated animals were of relatively minor significance. As the absence of the stress of infectious disease in the archaic states of the New World documents, these animal populations constituted a major vector of disease for the human population with which they were, for the most part, in daily and intimate contact. While nutritional and metabolic problems certainly are not thereby precluded for the New World, this geographical area must be excluded in any general discussion of the increasing incidence of infectious disease attendant upon increasing social complexity and community size. For the Old World, however, such a correlation (between population concentration and infectious disease) is abundantly evident. In ancient Britain, for example, osteological evidence indicates that tuberculosis was probably not a significant health problem until Roman times or later (Brothwell, 1972, p. 86). The crowded conditions generally associated with urban life have long been recognized as conducive to the generation, spread, and maintenance of infectious disease, providing, as Black has suggested, the requisite concentration of human numbers to ensure a quickly ramifying transmission throughout the population (cf. Darwin, 1975, p. 190). The notorious urban problems of waste disposal and the provision of a clean and adequate water supply are well documented (Barth, 1961, p. 120; Caillé, 1949, p. 558; Salusbury,

1948, p. 77; Sjoberg, 1960, pp. 93–95), as is the general association between (Old World) cities and the most fierce ravages of epidemic disease (Angel, 1975, p. 174; Herlihy, 1958, pp. 47 ff.; Mols, 1955, p. 39).

It is clear that with the evolution of highly complex societies, the dangers inherent in agricultural specialization become increasingly more significant. The agriculturalist highly dependent on one or more staple crop is clearly at greater risk from food-supply failure and famine than is the forager (Barnicot, 1969, p. 525; Dunn, 1968, p. 223). Perhaps most significant, dietary overspecialization may imply a shortage of vital food constituents and hence nutritional diseases, as Yudkin (1969, p. 549), Barnicot (1969, p. 525) and Brothwell (1969, pp. 532–533) have suggested. However, it must be remembered that relatively small-scale traditional agricultural societies generally possess the means of ameliorating the possibly harsh effects of unanticipated environmental destabilizations, by socially and often ritually based redistributive networks and the cultivation of various wild "famine foods," for instance.[3] Furthermore, most prehistoric and early historical societies of which we are aware cultivated not one crop but several, combinations—like the familiar maize, beans, and squash—that generally provided a balanced food supply, each of the various items complementing one another. This is hardly surprising: Those societies or communities that did not, over time, develop such basically adequate energy sources would ultimately have been selected against and should not have long survived. As I shall discuss in somewhat more detail later, overemphasis on a single and sometimes nutritionally deficient staple, while certainly not possible prior to domestication, is rather more directly the result of the vicissitudes of a world market and the price of the economics of colonialism.

An increase in disease stress would appear, then, to have slowed somewhat the rate of population growth made possible by the agricultural "revolution." However, even if the rate of increase in the Neolithic was as low as .1% (Carneiro & Hilse, 1966), the cumulative result was to lead inexorably to a considerable increase in population density. The more notable fluctuations in this overall growth trend provide illustration of the often harsh checks periodically attendant upon the pressure of population on resources. The prolonged popula-

---

[3] Some 1800 famines have been recorded for China in the period between 100 BC and AD 1910; as early as the first century BC, it would appear that the water darnel, tolerant to both drought and flood, was intentionally encouraged by agriculturalists as a critical provision in times of crop damage or failure (Shêng-Han, 1965).

tion rise that took place in Western Europe between approximately
AD 1100 and 1350 was followed by an especially sharp recession
between 1350 and 1450. The Black Death in the mid-fourteenth century is said to have eliminated between one-quarter to one-third of the
population. While admittedly a drastic remedy for the burden of too
many on the land, this "cutting back" did, for a time, bring clear
benefits for those who survived. Inherited property was to become
concentrated in considerably fewer hands as a result of the "Great
Dying." Only the best land was cultivated, and the standard of living
and real earnings of the survivors rose. Even in periods of general
population growth, there were, of course, short-term "set backs."
Characteristically, these were almost immediately compensated for.
In 1581, 790 died (presumably from "plague"), 10 times the normal
mortality figure, in Salzawedel in the old Brandenburg marches; marriages fell from an average of 30 to 10. In 1582, despite the reduced
population, 30 marriages were celebrated, followed by numerous
compensatory births (Braudel, 1973, p. 37). Emigration and civil and
religious disorder complemented periodic outbreaks of virulent
epidemic following upon the European population rise of 1450–1650.
The French historian Braudel (1973, pp. 23–24) provides a vivid
picture of "recession." In 1600 Brantôme warned that France was
"full as an egg"; emigration to Spain, which had begun in the sixteenth century, increased in the seventeenth. By 1669, it was calculated that some 200,000 French were to be found in the Iberian
peninsula. Religious exile was more haphazard and certainly more
harsh. The first systematic prosecution of the Protestants began in
1540; it was not to end until 1752–1753, at which time the last great
emigration movement took place after the bloody repressions of Lan-
guedoc.
   A final great upsurge in the population of Europe began about 1760;
within only a century, the population had doubled, rising from approximately 140 million in 1750 to almost 300 million in 1850. During all
of the preceding four centuries of the *ancien régime,* from 1400 to
1800, *world* population had but doubled. This tremendous increase in
the growth rate that Langer (1972, 1963) has documented for the
beginning of the nineteenth century in Western Europe was never
again to slow for any appreciable period or place to pre-nineteenth
century levels.
   While it has been common to attribute the beginnings of this population increase in the West to medical improvements (Marshall,
Brown, & Goodrich, 1971; McKeown, 1965, pp. 21–38), it has been
more recently pointed out (Brown & Wray, 1974, p. 4; McKeown &

Brown, 1968, pp. 17–24) that the eighteenth-century physician—vaccination against smallpox notwithstanding—had little technology to offer his patients. There appears to be a much clearer relationship between population growth and certain fundamental changes in the resource base. Concurrent with the European population explosion was the introduction of important new field crops, notably maize and, most particularly, potatoes (Fussell, 1927; Handley, 1953, Chapter 8). The establishment and exploitation of these crops resulted in an increase of 25–35% in the food supply; significantly, it was a supply available even to the lowest social classes (Langer, 1963). Whether it is the case that this permitted an enhanced fertility or ensured a decline in mortality rates, the result was undeniably a sudden and marked expansion in human numbers. Changes in the resource base and concomitant population growth were not confined to Europe. China's big demographic increase began late in the sixteenth century with the occupation of Formosa. During this period, crops introduced by the Portuguese (groundnuts, sweet potatoes, and above all, maize) spread widely, and colonization proceeded apace (Brown & Wray, 1974, p. 7). From a population of approximately 120 million in 1680, China had grown by 1740 (and the end of the colonization period) to some 165 million. After this time, the portion of land reserved to each individual gradually diminished as the population continued to expand, from 246 million by 1770 to 430 million in 1850 (Braudel, 1973, p. 14).

Limitations on population increase did not, however, cease to operate throughout the eighteenth and much of the nineteenth centuries. While traditionally it is more common to stress the positive checks on population growth, the aspects of mortality that seem the predominant feature in the preindustrial period (Cipolla, 1962, Chapter 4; Hawley, 1950, p. 150; Ho, 1959, p. 256; Thompson, 1959, p. 17), there were clearly controls on fertility or reproductivity as well (see Dumond, 1965). In the eighteenth century, a limitation on population growth was set by the legal restrictions imposed on marriage by a number of European states, the German principalities in particular. Governments were constantly devising means whereby the poor would be prevented from multiplying unduly. Langer (1972, p. 5) reports a series of decrees from Württemberg, instituted in 1712, which required official approval of every marriage. Each prospective husband had to show proof of his ability to support a family; this requirement effectively denied many the right to marry. It is interesting to note that in 1871 Darwin (Vol. 2, p. 385) strongly advocated that all those who "cannot avoid abject poverty for their children" ought to refrain from marriage, as poverty otherwise will "tend to its own increase." He further identifies celibacy through restraints on marriage as the primary check on population pressure in "civilized nations" (Vol. 1, p. 127).

"Disguised infanticide" was a further limiting device prevalent throughout Western Europe in the late eighteenth and early nineteenth centuries (Darwin, 1871, Vol. 1, p. 129; von Öttingen, 1882, pp. 236ff.). Langer (1972, pp. 6–8) provides vivid documentation of this widespread practice as it was systematically carried out in England and France. The London Foundling Hospital, which after open admissions in 1756 was to accept some 15,000 children over the next 4 years, was called by one of its governors a "slaughterhouse of infants" because the mortality there was nearly equal to its admissions. There were always, of course, the more common, direct physical means of ridding oneself of an unwanted child. Legal sanctions against it were light and ineffectual: The physician W. B. Ryan wrote in 1862 that not only is infanticide not considered by the general public "in the same light" as other murders, but there is no other crime that "meets with so much sympathy." And infanticide was equally prevalent on the continent. Between 1824 and 1833, a single decade, 336,297 infants were consigned to the French hospices, there to meet the same fate as their opposite numbers in England. It would appear that late in the eighteenth century and early in the nineteenth, fully 80% of the foundlings died within a year after birth.

The "Demographic Transition"

The strength of the population trend that began in Europe in the late eighteenth century is notable in light of its persistence despite the operation of the limiting measures discussed above. The industrial and the medical "revolutions" ensured, if not guaranteed, the tremendous growth of world population that characterizes the modern period: the quantum jump in the productive power of society considerably increased the population "ceiling," and the specific health technology developed not long thereafter ensured at the same time a general decline in morbidity and mortality. The removal of a considerable portion of the disease load and its ravages—undoubtedly responsible in part for the slower rate of growth following the transition to food production—clearly allowed a more rapid rate of increase. While those countries that participated directly in the "revolutions" soon reached a relatively low and somewhat stable rate of growth with the "transition" to low rates of mortality and ultimately of low fertility (Dumond, 1975, p. 719; Wrigley, 1969, p. 54), in the nonindustrialized or so-called "developing" countries, mortality has declined at a greater rate than has fertility. The birth rate in the nonindustrialized countries is now approximately one and one-half times that of the industrialized West, and the net result is an overly pronounced and continuing expansion of population in the less developed world (Brown & Wray, 1974; Echols, 1976, pp. 165, 169; Pearson, 1968, p. 10).

While it is clear that the general downturn in the mortality curve is very real, it does appear that, for a certain considerable portion of the world's population, it nonetheless remains a significant stress. That is to say, within a specific environment—that of the lowest socioeconomic stratum—childhood mortality, in particular, does constitute an effective and continuing stress (Darwin, 1871, Vol. 1, p. 127; Scrimshaw & Béhar, 1961, p. 2039). The persistently high growth rate characteristic of the nonindustrialized countries, those countries marked by a lower "standard of living" relative to the industrialized "developed" countries, may, in part, reflect the outcome of a pronounced compensation within the affected portion of the population for this higher mortality rate. It has recently been demonstrated that females of low socioeconomic status enjoy a more complete childbearing period (Frisancho, Klayman, & Matos, 1976, also cf. Brown & Wray, 1974, pp. 8–9; McDermott, 1966). This compensatory mechanism ensures, by a greater number of live births, that an equivalent number of children from a marginal environment will survive the first crucial 5 years of life, as will those from an adequate, less regularly "fatal" environment.

The Implication of Differential Access to Strategic Resources

The Population at Risk

In a recent number of the journal of the American Association for the Advancement of Science, devoted entirely to food and nutrition, the lead article (Sanderson, 1975) notes bluntly that the growth of world population has exceeded the most pessimistic expectations. Sanderson's (1975, p. 503) assessment of the problem is echoed by other contributors (Poleman, 1975, p. 515; Walters, 1975, p. 525; and cf. Heiser, 1973, p. 203). World grain production (which accounts for the majority of food energy produced), growing during the past 20 years at approximately the same rate (70 or 2.8% annually) in both the developing and developed countries, clearly exceeded the 2% annual growth in world population and theoretically permitted an annual improvement in per capita consumption of about 1%. However, the

exploitation of this enhancement of the resource base was—and is—
severely biased by its differential availability. In the developed industrialized countries, population growth was fairly stable throughout the
1950s at 1.3%/year; during the 1960s, it declined to its present level of
.9%. In these countries, per capita food production thus rose at approximately 1.5%/year annually. But in the developing countries, these
gains in productivity were almost wholly neutralized by an increase in
annual population growth from 1.9% in 1950 to 2.5% by 1964, a level
at which it has remained since. Rapid population growth in the developing countries has thus limited per capita food production to less
than .4% annually. Furthermore, some underdeveloped countries, and
some groups within many of these countries, experienced no improvement in per capita consumption at all. As 86% of the world's
population growth is confined to these areas in which perhaps a third
of the population lives on the very margins of subsistence, the probability of nutritional stress is unavoidably significant. However, as
Sanderson points out, the problem is not new.

That a certain proportion of the population seems always to suffer
more acutely than the rest was, in fact, addressed in the nineteenth
century by Darwin (1975, pp. 185–186). He noted that within any
given population differential death rates are to be anticipated, following from the high rate of natural increase characteristic of all living
beings. The means of support being ever (ultimately) finite, some
proportion of the population will necessarily be pressed to the "extreme confines of their natural range," there "to perish in larger
numbers than elsewhere." Ever since the advent of sufficiently large
and complex societies some five millennia before the present, man has
been a part of a highly structured system predicated on a differential
access to strategic resources. That portion of the population with the
most limited access will by definition suffer the greatest "lack
stress"—inadequate rates of input of certain essential sorts of matter-
energy (Miller, 1965b, pp. 364–365). That is to say, lack stress, of
which malnutrition is a particularly striking example, is a function of
social stratification.

Braudel (1973, pp. 39, 40, 42, 89–91) has carefully detailed the table
of the European poor as it was during the four centuries of the old order, the *ancien régime*. The tables of the rich—those always with the
greatest access to essential energy resources—were clearly not only
more replete but more varied in terms of quality than those of the
poor. In the grand house of Spinola in Genoa in the early fifteenth
century, cereals represented only 52% of the total caloric intake; at the

same date, cereals accounted for 81% of the diet of the poor at the Hospital for Incurables of that city. It is estimated that the Spinolas consumed twice as much meat and fish and three times as much dairy produce and fats as did the inmates of the hospital. As the French historian puts it, for the poor eating consisted of a lifetime of consuming "bread, more bread, and still more bread and gruels." Bread was the food not of the towns but of the rural peasantry and the lowest stratum of the working class. According to Le Grand d'Aussy in 1782, a peasant or laborer in France ate some two to three pounds of bread a day. The reason for the dietary predominance of bread was, of course, the fact that it was clearly the cheapest food readily available. Furthermore, the bread of which Braudel speaks is not a freshly baked, fragrant loaf but a hard and "mouldy" adjunct to gruel and sops. In some regions, it was commonly cut with an axe, hardly surprising, as it was generally only cooked once every month or two; in the Tyrol it was baked—and made to last between times—only two or three times a year. As the *Dictionnaire de Trévoux* noted bluntly in 1771, "The peasants are usually so stupid because they only live on coarse foods."

This, however, was the normal diet characteristic of generally unstressed agricultural conditions; in the all too frequent times of famine, the resources of the poor nearly vanished altogether. The towns, site of corn exchanges, enjoyed reserves of food and purchases from abroad—altogether, considerable insurance against the unanticipated. It was the countryside that experienced the greater suffering when famine struck, for the majority of the rural folk of Western Europe characteristically lived in a state of marked dependence on the merchants and nobles of the towns and great estates and had scarcely any reserves of their own. In Venice and Amiens in the sixteenth century, the rural poor are described as crowding together in the towns when famine threatened, begging in the streets, or, more often, dying in the public squares. In Blésois in 1662, the poor attempted to survive a period of famine on a diet of "cabbage runts," taken with bran soaked in cod water. A chronicler of the times reported that people ate wild plants at random, the grass of the meadows, or, failing that, human flesh.

Social stratification and the restriction of a considerable proportion of the population to a marginal, resource-deficient environment did not, of course, alter with the demise of the old order; the advent of the modern period with the industrial revolution has not seen a magical transformation of the poor nor a decline in their suffering—only, perhaps, the emergence of a most distinct differential geography of poverty. The tables of the poor of the world are still bare: in India today, the poorest one-third of the population normally receives 20–30% less food than the national average (Gavan & Dixon, 1975, p. 548). Much of the literature concerned with nutritional inadequacies reflects an increasingly acute awareness of the environmental specificity of this important lack stress (Cabak & Najdanvic, 1965; Dwyer & Mayer, 1975, p. 568; Gopalan, 1970; Graham & Morales, 1963; Robson, 1972, Vol. 1, p. 71; Walters, 1975, pp. 525, 530). Cravioto and DeLicardie (1968, p. 253) have asserted that an association between any damage to physical or mental growth following upon malnutrition will inevitably be associated with social status; the underprivileged segments of the population not only suffer increased exposure to nutritional stress but also tend to have poorer housing, lower levels of formal education, and a higher incidence of infectious disease—in short, a grossly deficient environment in terms of a whole interlocking complex of variables. Both Greene (1973, p. 132; this volume) and Stanbury (this volume) have noted the marked association of a specific deficiency, that of endemic goiter, with a highly limited access to basic resources. The Andean Indian population studied by Greene suffers a "very constricted resource base," confined to "the most marginal and inhospitable lands." Stanbury stresses the more general nature of the association: This specific deficiency disease is commonly coextensive with borderline or even overt malnutrition, lack of dietary variety, inadequate clothing and housing, frequent infections and parasitism, and limited educational opportunities.

As I shall later discuss in greater detail, physical growth and development, traditionally a major index of nutritional stress, varies directly with socioeconomic status (Cravioto & DeLicardie, 1968, p. 253; Dairy Council Digest, 1974; Frankova, 1968, pp. 321–322; Guzman, 1968, p. 52; Keppel, 1968, p. 6; Lechtig, Delgado, & Lasky, 1975a, pp. 434–436; Rafalski & Mackiewicz, 1968, pp. 77–78; Robson, 1972, Vol. 2, pp. 416, 418, 420–421; Scrimshaw & Gordon, 1968, pp. 54, 90). The environment characterized by generalized lack stress also has a profound impact on learning and mental development, so profound, in fact, that it has been impossible to isolate and hence adequately assess the effects of nutritional stress alone on this aspect of human development (Richardson, 1968, p. 355; Scrimshaw & Gordon, 1968, pp. 71, 310, 384–385). Malnutrition is generally attended by economic deprivation, illiteracy, diminished social stimulation, often less well integrated family units (particularly among the urban poor), "suboptimal parenting," and an increased incidence of infectious disease and hospitalization, all of which tend to retard experience and stimulation at a critical stage in the course of cognitive development (Dairy Council Digest, 1973, p. 31; Thomson & Pollitt, this volume). These critical relationships in mind, a number of researchers have advocated or outlined a basic ecological approach to the problem of nutritional stress, a research design focusing on interactions between the human population and its effective environment (e.g., Canosa, 1968; Jelliffe, 1966, p. 106; Robson, 1972, Vols. I and II).

Infection: an additional environment-specific stress. Brown and Wray (1974, p. 4) strongly suggest that the developing countries have not, perhaps, felt the really comprehensive impact of modern health technology, estimating that an average of less than 10% of these populations enjoy adequate sanitation, safe water, or have access to health-care faculties. In other words, the population most liable to the rigors of nutritional deficiency is also the population most vulnerable to infectious disease. This association is not random but *systematic*, for it is the case that the interaction between malnutrition and infection is regularly synergistic, a compound stress specific to the deprived environment. Scrimshaw, Taylor, and Gordon (1968, pp. 11, 16, 262) provide a definition of this synergistic relationship: The presence together of malnutrition and infection results in an interaction more serious than would result from the effects taken together of the two working alone. In other words, a ramifying positive feedback operates between the two, leading often to a fatal resolution (Beisel, 1975, p. 573; Hansen, Wittman, Moodie, & Fellingham, 1968, p. 438; Latham, 1975, pp. 561, 564; Pearson, 1968, p. 10; Robson, 1972, Vol. 1, p. 13; Scrimshaw & Gordon, 1968, pp. 13, 16–17).

A brief glance once again at preindustrial Europe will serve to illustrate the enhanced disposition to infectious disease characteristic of members of the lowest socioeconomic stratum. The poor were always, of course, the first to suffer the effects of epidemics. What Braudel (1973, p. 38) terms "social massacres" occurred innumerable times between the fifteenth and the nineteenth centuries: In 1498, at Crépy near Senlis, a third of the town was said to be begging in the countryside; old people were dying each day "in squalor." But even had the poor been in good nutritional health—as they certainly were not—they would nonetheless still have suffered the most brutal effects of diseases like the plague. As Sartre noted in *La Peste*, the plague served to clearly define distinctions of social class, striking at the poor and sparing the rich. When this dread disease struck, the rich immediately took to their country homes, while the poor remained "penned up" in the contaminated towns, where the state isolated them and "kept them under observation [Braudel, 1973, p. 48]"; like the canary carried into the mine, the eventual decline in their death rate undoubtedly served as the sign that the urban elites could once again return to their shops and town houses.

Infection has an adverse effect on nutritional status that is both clear and measurable. As Scrimshaw (1973) has detailed, infection generally reduces food intake, while it increases metabolic losses, and if the gastrointestinal tract is involved, sometimes also affects the absorption of nutrients; further, increased nutrients are generally required during the recovery phase (Jelliffe, 1966, p. 112; Latham, 1975, p. 561). While the well nourished, with available body reserves and normal dietary intake, are unlikely to develop overt malnutrition unless infection is unusually prolonged, for the already poorly nourished an infection is of far greater consequence. The stress of infection in this latter case will often precipitate the appearance of a frank nutritional pathology such as kwashiorkor (Jelliffe, 1966, p. 106; Scrimshaw & Béhar, 1961, p. 2046). The poor of the 14th century, given the exceedingly restricted general level of dietary intake noted in the preceding subsection, would thus be very likely to exhibit the more overt signs of nutritional stress following one or another of the periodic epidemics that swept the continent—that is, if they survived the epidemic at all. As nutritional deficiencies generally increase the deleterious effects of infectious disease, lowering the capacity of the organism to resist by interfering with its normal mechanisms to bar the proliferation or progress of infectious agents (Eichenwald, 1968, p. 434; Kunitz & Euler, 1972, p. 39; Latham, 1975, p. 563; Scrimshaw et al., 1968, pp. 13, 142, 263), it is of course unlikely that many would have survived. While it is clearly established that the malnourished child is more susceptible to infection, more frequently suffers infection, and is less likely to combat it and survive, the mechanisms involved are apparently still somewhat unclear (Latham, 1975, pp. 561, 563; Scrimshaw & Béhar, 1961, pp. 2039, 2046; Robson, 1972, Vol. 1, p. 110; T. Smith, 1934, pp. 2ff.). The syndrome known as "weanling diarrhoea," caused by a vicious interaction of alimentary bacterial infection and protein–calorie malnutrition, (PCM) is thought to be a major contributing factor to the higher child mortality rates of the deprived segment of the population (Béhar, 1968, pp. 35–36; Jelliffe, 1966, p. 105; Robson, 1972, Vol. 1, p. 104; Scrimshaw et al., 1968, pp. 216, 217, 220–221).

The "developing" country: The stratified hierarchy of nation-states. "Social stratification" is generally understood to refer to the relative ranking of population elements within a given society. At a higher level of ordering, however, societies can be ranked relative to one another. This is important, for just as a proportion of the population within a given society—that with the most limited access to strategic resources—can be expected to suffer significant lack stress, so also will a proportion of the world's societies—those countries with the most limited access to the world's vital resources. The marked prevalence in the "developing" countries of both malnutrition and infectious disease, especially during the first 5–7 years of life, has been variously noted in the literature; Scrimshaw et al. (1968, p. 265) estimate its near universality in this setting (also see, Lasky et al., 1975; Lechtig et al., 1975a, p. 434; Lechtig, Delgado, & Lasky, 1975b, p. 553; Pearson, 1968, p. 10; Robson, 1972, Vol. 1, p. 110).

The historical consolidations of an expanding colonialism are to a large extent responsible for the differential access evidenced today in the common dichotomy between the so-called "developed" and the "developing" or "less-" or "underdeveloped" countries. As Ford (1974, pp. 888–889) has pointed out, regional and sometimes national "monoculture," agricultural systems of extreme specialization generally heavily dependent on the markets and manufactories of distant, highly complex industrialized countries, has rendered entire populations highly vulnerable to destabilizing forces over which they have no real control. Mill's predictions to the contrary, international trade—and the cyclical fluctuations in world market prices that attend it—has been more of a deterrent than an aid to balanced economic development. With little or no economic diversification even, often, in the agricultural sector, exports excessively concentrated in one or a few commodities, the "developing" countries can ill afford a sudden shift downward in the demand for their products (Higgins, 1968, pp. 267–268). Serious nutritional stress can often prove the outcome of the ultimately "false" economy of sacrificing a more traditional diet for the generally imported, less expensive, high yielding, and nutritionally inferior crops (Ford, 1974, p. 889).

The case of Indonesia as described by Geertz (1963) and Higgins (1968, pp. 679–705) is perhaps one of the best-known and well-documented examples of the process of "underdevelopment," a process in which one country becomes over time the dependent subsystem (the "producer") of a (generally distant) mercantile economy (the "ingester"). In the outward dispersion of productive processes, an important area of system control and coordination is preempted by the colonizing superstructure. The ramifications of this are profound. The integration and stabilization of an increasingly overburdened productive system necessarily imply a significant measure of internal regulation, but this would not have suited the interests of the larger system of which Indonesia had become a part. Resolution of the "dual" economy (Higgins, 1968, p. 87), perhaps in the financing of an industrial or indigenous commercial sector underwritten by the expanding productivity of the peasant sector, might otherwise have resulted. On the most basic level, and more pertinent to our concerns here, however, is the general intensification of various lack stresses that results from the dependency of one system on another that is characteristic of widespread commercial "cash" cropping for foreign markets. The delta of lower Burma in the early nineteenth century provides a further case in point. Although the area under cultivation, and hence production, grew rapidly, the Burmese cultivators shared little, if at all, in the benefits and prosperity this brought to the colonizing elites (Pfanner, 1969, p. 47). The familiar Cornell project in Vicos, Peru, illustrates the seriousness of the problem for the producers, the poorest members of a poor land. The produce of the fields of the Andean manor at Vicos, after providing subsistence for the owner's family, were destined primarily for external sale. The plots of the serfs yielded so little that they generally had to seek wage labor outside the estate in order to feed their families (Holmberg & Dobyns, 1969, pp. 394–395).

Increasing Size, Differentiation, and Integration: The Inexorable Procedure of System Evolution

It is certainly probable that the effects of the stress of malnutrition, particularly in synergistic combination with infectious disease, can to some extent confirm static membership in the lowest level of the socioeconomic hierarchy. As shall be discussed later, while the extent and permanence of damage due to this particular lack stress is notably difficult to estimate (Thomson & Pollitt, this volume), in those instances in which it is significant, malnutrition could be expected to inhibit or perhaps in some few cases even proscribe vertical mobility (Greene, 1973, p. 132; Robson, 1972, Vol. 1, p. 29). However, it is important to understand that in the elucidation of the structure and operation of the social system, biological or psychological characteristics of the human organism function as *constants* rather than as meaningful dimensions of variation. In other words, the behavioral characteristics of the malnourished population—even those in which is found damage so marked as to provoke some degree of neurological deficit—are not germane to our understanding of the generation or persistence of social stratification or the centralization of power, as the logical extension of a reductionist thesis must inevitably imply (d'Aquili & Mihalik, this volume). Those populations pressed to the extreme margins of their natural range will exhibit, in varying degree but nevertheless without exception, the consequences of the numerous deprivations attendant upon a highly restricted access to basic resources. But consequences should not be confused with "cause": The generation and evolution of social stratification or differential access to resources proceeds quite independently of any particular lack stress (such as malnutrition) that it might occasion.

The generation of social stratification   As system size increases, structural differentiation increases and integration progresses. This is the basic process of growth and evolution common to all veridical or "living" systems (von Bertalanffy, 1962, p. 16; Hall & Fagen, 1956; Spencer, 1967, pp. 14–16). The organization of systems through progressive differentiation and increasing complexity, a change in the direction of increasing division into subsystems and sub-subsystems or differentiation of functions, is a macroscopic system property amenable to measurement (on the most fundamental level, in terms of decreasing entropy). Social stratification is a type of structural differentiation (Blau, 1970) and as such is an increasing function of system size. In other words, as the size of human societies increases, structural differentiation increases.[4] Status barriers, points in the status hierarchy beyond which it is not possible for a population element to be upwardly mobile without leaving (and possibly reentering) the system,[5] likewise increase with size. As Spencer (1967, p. 79) noted, progression in system size, complexity, and integration is attended by a decreased ability to move from group to group and from place to place within the group.

As societies increase in size beyond a certain point, population density (number of people per unit area) rises. Small, mobile groups (e.g., those societies common prior to the Neolithic, modern band-organized foragers, some pastoral groups) could often readily fission and establish themselves in new areas; as settled communities based on plant cultivation proliferated, fissioning was no longer a viable means of assuring a sufficient energy supply. As human societies grew in size, a restructuring or reorganization occurred, a reorganization taking the form of social ranking or "stratification." Social stratification effectively regulates a population vis-à-vis the available natural resources or major factors of production (land, labor, capital). That this

[4] The relationship is assumed to be curvilinear, certainly, rather than linear.

[5] For instance, a population element might be able to cross a status barrier by leaving the system and returning with a new set of credentials, for example, further education.

establishment of a dominance hierarchy functions as a mechanism for the regulation of the size of the population has been demonstrated by research on all levels of living systems. It is well known that a clear "pecking order" in animals emerges under extremely constricted conditions (Schjelderup-Ebbe, 1921). The green sunfish (*Lepomis cyanellus*) is a case in point. If the sunfish are crowded, territories will be established by the males, the dominant males getting the choicer territories and the lowest-ranking males getting the poorer territories or no territory at all (Greenburg, 1947). Thus, as population density and hence pressure on resources increases, a certain proportion of the population is necessarily forced to attempt to subsist on very little; many members of this deprived category, of course, die, a stark but surely effective means of controlling the size of the group overall. As Darwin observed of the tomtits in his garden, the misery of which Malthus so eloquently spoke clearly waits upon all creatures.

Randsborg (1975, p. 159, Fig. 11) has demonstrated the relationship of status differentiation to population density for Early Bronze Age Denmark. He found a very strong correlation between population density and male degree of social stratification, inequality being more pronounced the denser the settlements. Competition attendant upon resource scarcity and the differential success resulting from such competition have been cited by a number of anthropologists and sociologists as the critical factors in the evolution of class stratification (Carneiro, 1961, pp. 60–61; Harner, 1970, 1975; Spencer, 1852, p. 501; Sumner & Keller, 1927, pp. 4–5; Tylor, 1889, p. 267; White, 1959, p. 352).

The generation of political centralization. While it is undoubtedly the case that such behavioral limitations as may persist in a severely malnourished sector of the population will facilitate the power—and hence control (Miller, 1965a, p. 229)—of the central governing authorities over that sector (Greene, 1973, p. 132), the degree of political centralization per se is independent of any environmental stress, such as malnutrition, specific to a particular system component. On the most general level, political centralization, as social stratification, is a direct function of system size. As Hall and Fagen (1956, p. 86) have noted, as a system evolves in size and complexity, a progressive centralization occurs, one part of the system emerging as a "central and controlling" agency. To paraphrase Montesquieu, the nature of the system changes to the extent that the system constricts or extends its limits (1748, p. 199; Durkheim, 1933, p. 223; Spencer, 1967, pp. 79, 162).

This is necessarily the case, for as system size increases, the rate of interaction increases, and the system becomes more fragile. A large system is inherently more "point vulnerable"; having more points of articulation, it thus has more points at which it can become disarticulated. A unitary control structure, the form of control structure characterized by a minority elite, minimizes point vulnerability (Mayhew, 1973; cf. Durkheim, 1933, pp. 365–367). In other words, the pressure to minimize this system vulnerability generates an oligarchy, a political structure in which a minority of the population controls the system (Michels, 1910; Pareto, 1916); the relative size of this ruling elite or administrative component is thus a decreasing function of the size of the system it governs (Mosca, 1896).

THE HUMAN POPULATION AS ANALYTICAL LEVEL

As Brace and Livingstone (1975, pp. 109–110) have stressed, differentiation between individual and populational phenomena is a critical prerequisite for the recognition of significant aspects of human variation. While birth rates, morbidity rates, and mortality rates are the result of individual performances, their variability among human populations is not primarily due to individual differences. The physiological or neurological status of any individual or individuals is merely a reflection or special case of the status of the population of which he is a member (or they are members), and this in turn reflects interaction (of the population) with the (relevant) environment (King, 1971, p. 89; Simpson, 1971, pp. 7–8). Thus it is that Robson (1972, Vol. 1, pp. 1–2, 4, 72) has concluded that the problem of malnutrition is addressed to the extent that it is viewed as a community problem rather than a clinical problem, a result of the coincident pressure of multiple environment-specific stresses. Gordon (1968, pp. 535–536) concurs, outlining what he terms an ecological approach to epidemiological investigation. Man is studied not as a "series of organ systems" nor as a collection of individuals but as a population unit or common aggregate within a given environment.

The general nature of the environment to which malnutrition is specific was identified earlier. The implications for the human population of this particular lack stress are here briefly examined. As man and society comprise distinct levels of observation or analysis, the implications of malnutrition for social-system operation will be considered separately later.

The Nature of the Data

It is unhappily the case, substantial research efforts and accumulation of knowledge relating to nutrition notwithstanding, that the "true nature and extent" of malnutrition throughout the world remains largely unknown (Robson, 1972, Vol. 1, p. 3; Goldsmith, 1969, p. 694; Thomson, 1968, p. 25). The factors accounting for this are multiple. As Hansen et al., 1968, pp. 445, 453) have pointed out, and as Jelliffe (1966, pp. 10, 11, 42) has detailed, the useful physical signs are relatively few and often nonspecific. Almost all of the signs of malnutrition usually recorded lack nutrient specificity, and nonnutritional stresses of the generally deprived environment can often result in an identical outcome. As noted earlier, it is thus often difficult if not almost impossible to assess the precise role of nutrition, only one component of a whole interlocking—and interacting—configuration of deprivation. Both Pearson (1968, p. 10) and Thomson (1968, p. 25) judge that the problem of isolating malnutrition-related effects from various other "contaminating" factors in the environment has resulted in large part from the paucity of field studies and the derivation of the bulk of the data from hospitals and clinics. And productive field studies are themselves severely limited by the general inadequacy of measurement techniques (Scrimshaw & Gordon, 1968, pp. 13, 461; Riecken, 1968, p. 529). Criteria commonly accepted in identifying and measuring nutritional status, and the relationship between actual food intake and health, lack reliability and specificity. The definition of malnutrition can be based on clinical, anthropometric, biochemical, or dietary—and of late even psychological—criteria; to choose between them is to some extent a subjective matter fraught with uncertainty, as Dwyer and Mayer (1975, p. 568) have stressed. Furthermore, Dwyer and Mayer point out that the standards for all of these criteria are arbitrary, small variations in cutoff points resulting in markedly distinct estimates of the prevalence of malnutrition. The standards for caloric and general nutrient requirements, such as those proposed by the FAO and the U. S. National Research Council, have been increasingly discarded as a tool in the direct assessment of nutritional status, as they make no allowances for the possible environment-specific variations in human needs and adaptations (Jelliffe, 1966, p. 117; Robson, 1972, Vol. II, p. 346).

Poleman (1975, pp. 515–516) provides a striking illustration of this problem in the calculation of apparent per capita diurnal energy and protein availabilities in Sri Lanka by income class from 1969 to 1970. A rather weak tendency for the starchy staple ratio to fall as income rises was observed among the 4 topmost income classes, some 20% of the total population. Between the lowest (43% of the population) and the next lowest class (37%), the only change was quantitative: while diet composition remained equivalent, a difference in apparent per capita daily availabilities of 200 kilocalories and 10 gm of protein was noted. As the FAO estimates average energy needs in South Asia at approximately 1900 kilocalories a day and takes protein adequacy as a function of energy adequacy, and if the standard factor of 15% can be understood to account for the wastage between purchase and actual consumption, the 200-kilocalorie gap could mean either of 2 things: (1) enforced reduced activity or actual physical deterioration (or both) among the poor or (2) caloric adequacy among that element of society "too poor to waste anything" and that, due to the local high unemployment rate, leads a less active life, thus requiring less energy. In other words, proceeding from different assumptions, it is possible to offer statistical proof that 43% of the Ceylonese suffer significant PCM or that none do. The significant fact that the same data can readily be interpreted in two distinct ways will be discussed in more detail in the following section, when variation in body size is considered.

Many of these general problems have proved particularly acute in attempting to assess the hypothesized impact of malnutrition on learning and behavior. As Thomson and Pollitt have noted in their review of studies concerning the behavior of children who have suffered marasmus or kwashiorkor—the concentration of studies on acute or severe forms of malnutrition itself a problem (Béhar, 1968, p. 30; Scrimshaw & Gordon, 1968, p. 42; Dairy Council Digest 1973, p. 32)—the information available is of an overwhelmingly anecdotal nature and based almost entirely on clinical impressions. The measurement of mental development and/or ability is especially problematic (Birch, 1968, p. 505). Techniques in this area are not yet generally well developed; the meaning of the tests is often uncertain, and the results often defy replication (Pearson, 1968, p. 10; Riecken, 1968, p. 505; Scrimshaw & Béhar, 1961, p. 2043). As Scrimshaw and Gordon (1968, p. 13) have pointed out, problems of methodological inadequacy are especially great in the evaluation of children at the young age at which nutritional damage is most likely to occur and to be most severe. But perhaps the most serious difficulty with the tests generally used to measure mental development and performance is the question of their cross-cultural validity (Robson, 1972, Vol. I, p. 64). It has been suggested that even tests based on pictures or abstract shapes might certainly be as susceptible to cultural "skewing" as tests in a verbal medium (Vernon, 1968, pp. 489, 494–495). Richardson (1968, p. 358) adds that most of the tests now in use were devised to measure the sorts of skills necessary in classroom performance; these skills may not be appropriate in societies in which differing skills and social roles are valued. Certain basic characteristics of the test situation itself, such as working by oneself, finishing a given task within a proscribed and limited time period, and the notion of the "valuable" goad of competition can subtly bias the test results of a considerable number of non-Western groups.

The environment to which malnutrition is specific, the generally deprived context of the lower socioeconomic stratum, is by definition an environment relatively lacking in the opportunities and incentives for the development of mental or intellectual skills. Demand for performance is relatively more limited; furthermore, valuable interactions with the environment and learning time in general is often abbreviated due to the increased incidence of infectious disease among the poor. In other words, "strictly experiential factors" can have an even greater effect on test performance and may completely "mask" the possible nutritional factors (Brace & Livingstone, 1975, p. 112; Robson, 1972, Vol. I, p. 65). Thus, it is not surprising that Birch, after reviewing these formidable problems of interpretation concerning the association between malnutrition and mental development, advances the "third verdict" of *not proven:* The evidence is suggestive rather than definitive (1968, p. 503).

These cautions in mind, the general significance of the lack stress of malnutrition for the human population will be considered.

Adaptation to Lack Stress

Reduction in body size or "growth failure" is commonly considered one of the major indices of nutritional stress (Béhar, 1968, pp. 30, 37; Robson, 1972, Vol. 2, p. 417; Scrimshaw & Béhar, 1961, p. 2040; Scrimshaw & Gordon, 1968, p. 42). As has been indicated previously, malnutrition is very difficult to measure except in its extreme manifestations (the overt pathologies, such as marasmus and kwashiorkor); smaller body size is generally taken as a reliable indicator of dietary deficiency in the absence of other clinical signs.

That a child's height is influenced by a number of nonnutritional variables is clearly recognized (Robson, 1972, Vol. 2, p. 417; Richardson, 1968, pp. 357–358). The generally deprived and relatively more infection-ridden environment of the lowest socioeconomic levels of society with which a reduced body size is strongly associated is, of course, the critical and subsumptive conditioning factor (Tanner, 1964). One further point in particular would appear to indicate the value of a closer examination of the nature of the relationship of body size to malnutrition. Quite aside from the normal variation in body size within any given population or subpopulation, it is the case that the optimal or certainly baseline anthropometric values or standards of normal growth are not known with certainty for any community, as the limits of normality are, in fact, arbitrary, specific to general research objectives (Jelliffe, 1966, p. 53; Robson, 1972, Vol. 2, p. 425). The variation of body size with socioeconomic level is thus suggestive of the possibility of correspondingly variable ranges of functional normality in body size by social class. That is to say, the reduced body size characteristic of the poor may represent not a pathological resoonse to the stress of deprivation but an *adaptation* to such stress, as the smaller organism has reduced energy requirements (Frisancho, Garn, & Ascoli, 1970; Frisancho, Sanchez, Pallardel, & Yanez, 1973). Before considering this hypothesis in more detail, it is important to consider first the general theoretical basis for such an argument.

The Maintenance of System Equilibrium under Stress

The greater proportion of the human population falls between the extremes of an excess of calories and protein on the one hand and clinical pathologies on the other, indicating a generalized adjustment to nutritive intake. The range of normal, a-pathological variation is thus broad, ranging from some 3500 calories/day in the United States to under 1000 calories/day among the Masai; nutritionally related clinical pathology is in both cases absent. This is clearly illustrated by the fact that perhaps the most persistent feature of human reproduction, a notoriously high risk category, is its resistance, not its vulnerability to apparently adverse nutritional conditions (Dairy Council Digest, 1974, p. 20; C. A. Smith, 1947; Stein, Susser, Saenger, and Marolla, 1975, pp. 3, 236; Thomson, 1968, p. 23).

That a considerable range of nonpathological adjustment to protein and calorie intake is the rule rather than the exception is predicted by certain general characteristics of system structure and operation. For each of the many variables in a living system—or system component, as we are concerned with a certain portion of the population, the lower socioeconomic stratum—there is a range of stability. An input of matter-energy, which by lack of some characteristic, forces the variables beyond the range of stability,[6] constitutes a stress and is produc-

[6] Certainly stresses can also be produced by outputs, of information as well as

tive of a strain or strains within the system or, in this case, system part. Depending on the intensity of the stress and the resources of the system or pertinent system component, strains may or may not be capable of being reduced. In the following section, the failure of stress reduction is briefly discussed. However, all living systems possess remarkably effective means of responding to and mitigating stress and hence preventing serious strain. The system under stress will move in that direction that tends to minimize the stress. A compensatory force, exerted opposite to the stress, will develop that dampens its effects. Furthermore, this compensatory force is generally accompanied by changes in other subsidiary variables not directly affected by the disturbance. In this general fashion, systems tend to maintain a steady state or equilibrium (Le Chatelier, 1888; adapted for open systems by Prigogine, 1955; also cf. Ashby, 1954, pp. 153–158, 210–211). As Kempf (1958, pp. 894–895) has noted, every level of organization—from atomic through crystalline and enzymatic to cellular, organic, and societal—has component processes that function to maintain system equilibrium in the presence of stress. If they did not, they would not continue to exist (Cannon, 1939, pp. 287, 293; Weiss, 1959, p. 8).

These adjustment processes that maintain system equilibrium are collectively termed *negative feedback*. Negative feedback decreases the deviation of system output from a steady state, effectively canceling the initial deviation or error in performance. A living system is self-regulating because input not only affects output, but *output often adjusts input*. That is to say, the operation of the system or system component is controlled on the basis of *actual* rather than expected performance (Rosenbleuth, Wiener, & Bigelow, 1943, p. 19). On this more general level, nutritional inadequacy clearly constitutes a case of energy insufficiency or lack stress, the input rate falling below the standard range (Miller, 1965a, p. 225). There are several different types of negative feedback discussed by Miller (1965a, p. 229), certain of which are pertinent to two somewhat distinct forms of dietary stress. The specific stress of iodine deficiency resulting in goiter and cretinism (Greene; Stanbury, this volume) can generally be readily eliminated by a "passive adaptation" dependent on "external feedback": by means of a feedback loop passing outside the boundary of the affected system or system component, it is possible to alter the problematic environmental variable without changing system vari-

---

energy; furthermore, the output or input can be excessive in some sense rather than insufficient. As malnutrition constitutes a case of insufficiency in certain matter-energy inputs, stress is considered here solely in these terms.

ables. In other words, the addition from some external source of iodized salt or an equivalent supplement to the diet of the affected population will generally eliminate the stress altogether (Buchbinder, this volume).

In the absence of inputs of massive amounts of high-quality foods, it is most probable that the response of the affected part of the system to generalized nutritional stress will involve an "input signal adaptation," an adaptation to changes in the characteristics of the input signal by the alteration of system variables. That is, the system or system component (the poor), subjected over time to a reduced energy input (general nutritional inadequacy), will itself ultimately alter. The generally invariable correlation of reduced body size with the nutritionally deprived population strongly suggests that this alteration involves an adjustment of nutritional demand to nutritional availability, as the smaller organism has correspondingly reduced energy needs. Such self-adjustment for a minimum of a certain variable—in this case calories and protein—is known as "extremum adaptation."

Small Body Size: A Case of "Extremum" Adaptation

As noted above, there is a direct relationship between body size and nutritional resources; they vary together. This is strongly suggestive of a significant instance of human adaptation, an adjustment to chronic dietary stress or long-term restricted caloric intake by the deprived segment of the population. The larger the body mass, the greater the caloric or general dietary requirements for growth and maintenance of that mass. While greater energy reserves are important, certainly, in instances of acute nutritional stress, the larger organism is at greater risk than the smaller if the stress is chronic. A small body quite simply requires less food (Garrow & Pike, 1967). Reduction in growth rate as an adaptation to consistently restricted caloric intake is a remarkably clear example of system cybernetics or self-regulation, of "output adjusting input."

This hypothesis, so strongly suggested by general theories of system behavior, has been closely—and, it would appear, fruitfully—examined by Frisancho and co-workers (Frisancho et al., 1970; Frisancho et al., 1973). The nutritional limitations generally associated with poor socioeconomic conditions constitutes an environmental stress that very definitely influences body size during growth and at maturity. While retardation in skeletal maturation during childhood is significantly greater than during adolescence, growth in body size shows a progressive delay from infancy through adolescence. As similar results obtain for both Central American and Asiatic populations, it is not likely that this phenomenon is "race" or population-specific (Frisancho *et al.*, 1970, p. 333). Frisancho *et al.*'s 1973 study in a south Peru *barriada* found evidence of a significant association between high offspring survival rates and small parental body size. This finding suggests that small body size is both a reflection of the influence of and an adaptive response to poor socioeconomic conditions and malnutrition, due, it is presumed, to the lower caloric or nutritional requirements for growth and maintenance noted earlier (Frisancho *et al.*, 1973, p. 260). Others have postulated for reduced body size in deprived circumstances a similar thesis of adaptive significance (Allen, 1968b; Garn, Nagy, Paznanski, & McCann, 1972; Graham & Adrianzen, 1971; Guzman, 1968, p. 43; Malcom, 1969, 1970).

Measurable human variation is coincident with the differing environment-specific selective forces to which man is subject. The stress of malnutrition, associated with the generally deprived environment of the lowest socioeconomic stratum, appears to be a most potent force of natural selection: With the exception of pregnant and lactating women, nutritional deprivation has its most marked deleterious effect, in terms both of morbidity and mortality, on the young, adults being the least vulnerable (Dairy Council Digest, 1974, pp. 19–20; Hansen *et al.*, 1968, p. 439; Jelliffe, 1966, pp. 97, 102, 176, 178–179; Newberne, 1975, p. 576; Robson, 1972, Vol. I, pp. 29, 64; Scrimshaw & Gordon, 1968, p. 250; Scrimshaw *et al.*, 1968, p. 265; Wills & Waterlow, 1958, p. 167). The work of Frisancho and others here reviewed strongly suggests that those with slow growth rates are favored by this evolutionary mechanism, for where nutritional resources are limited, the rapidly growing child, due to relatively greater nutritional requirements, will predictably be selected against (Frisancho *et al.*, 1970, p. 334; Widdowson, 1968; Brues, 1959). As Allen (1968a, pp. 102, 103) has noted, optimal nutrition—what Graham (1968, pp. 86–87) calls "ideal controlled undernutrition"—is not necessarily maximal nutrition. If, in fact, a physiological tolerance (such as that possibly conferred by reduced body size) for relatively more limited nourishment can reasonably be assumed to have developed over time in some proportion of the human population, then impairment of this population should not be anticipated (Brothwell, 1969, p. 542; Gruenwald, 1968; Thomson, 1968, pp. 22, 26). Clearly, pathological levels of malnutrition cannot continue to be assumed in the absence of clinical indicators other than that of a reduced body size and/or the dietary requirements of the nonstressed population.

While living systems characteristically initiate adjustment processes when threatened by potential strains, thus avoiding significant destabilization, this internal regulation is not without its costs (Miller, 1965a, p. 234). One possible cost of reduction in body size has recently been reported by Spurr, Barac-Nieto, and Maksud (1975). Among a group of Columbian sugarcane cutters, all judged to be in adequate nutritional condition, it was found that those who produced least weighed less and were shorter than those cutters who were the most productive; the taller, heavier men, enjoying a higher efficiency of cane cutting, were the better producers. A similar tendency is seen in data from East Africa (Davies, 1973).

Malthusian "Misery": The Failure of Adaptation

If a certain measure of adaptive response to nutritional stress can be presumed—and this would appear to be a valid assumption on both theoretical and empirical or analytical grounds—the common notion of significant numbers of inapparent or subclinical cases of dietary stress (the "iceberg" analogy [Brock, 1966, p. 890; Dairy Council Digest, 1973, p. 32; Gordon, 1968, p. 538; Jelliffe, 1966, pp. 188–189; Robson, 1972, Vol. 1, pp. 30–31; Scrimshaw & Gordon, 1968, pp. 19, 29]) should perhaps be modified somewhat. The existence of a "continuum" or "gradient" from sick to well is of course inarguable; the "sick" or significantly stressed, however, constitute the extreme end of the continuum, while the remainder, likewise members of the deprived socioeconomic environment to which low dietary input is specific, manage with varying degrees of success to avoid frank strain by means of numerous "adjustments" undoubtedly long characteristic of their circumstances. The adjustments—possibly, for instance, some reduction in activity, a maximization of food with more of it being utilized and less excreted—carry their own costs, as has been indicated; nevertheless, they enable a great many of those who commonly experience a generally low dietary intake to maintain a rough equilibrium vis-à-vis their environment.

Disequilibration, or a failure of adaptation, can occur if strains are of sufficient intensity, particularly as the resources of the affected population, the poor, are already at a relative minimum. A certain proportion of the population of the environment to which nutritional inadequacy is specific will manifest pathological strain. This affected "subpopulation" constitutes (on the most general level) that part of the population as a whole necessarily pressed, by weight of numbers, to the extreme limits of its range, there, as noted earlier, "to perish in larger numbers than elsewhere [Darwin, 1975, pp. 185–186]." It is that part of the population with the most markedly restricted access to basic energy resources that will, by definition, suffer the most significant consequences of nutritional deprivation. Iodine deficiency is most interesting in this regard (Greene, 1973, and this volume; Stanbury, this volume). Populations affected with goiter and cretinism (and their numbers are apparently not insignificant) live in regions of the world in which the soil that feeds them, due to the vagaries of geological or climatic events, is deficient in this critical mineral. These generally discrete and discontinuous areas are clearly *highly* marginal zones from the standpoint of the support of human life, providing important illustration of the rigors of a restricted access to basic resources, a restriction generated ultimately by the worldwide expansion of human numbers, an expansion great enough to have pressed into even these most deprived of environments.

While in accord with the Malthusian proposition the mortality rate of the pathologically affected malnourished population is certainly enhanced, the extent and significance of permanent impairment to that portion of the affected group that survives is unclear. Kwashiorkor is commonly severe and acute, suffered only for a few weeks (Scrimshaw & Gordon, 1968, p. 29). Thomson and Pollitt conclude that the available evidence would indicate that it may, but generally does not, leave any measurable deficit in behavior (Robson, 1972, Vol. 1, p. 64). Marasmus, however, occurs during a period of rapid brain growth, and being severe and chronic, Thomson and Pollitt feel it results in a significant decline in child–environment interaction. Thus, they have determined that a deficit in mental function may well result. Their review of the literature does not yield any determination concerning the possibility of deleterious aftereffects resulting from severe and acute episodes of malnutrition in the first year or severe and chronic problems later.

THE SOCIOCULTURAL SYSTEM AS ANALYTICAL LEVEL

The implications of malnutrition or dietary stress for social-system operation are necessarily distinct from its implications for man. As this statement will undoubtedly seem incomprehensible to some, possibly reprehensible to others, I shall briefly outline the basis for such an assertion. Nor should this be considered a trivial or perhaps self-indulgent digression: Science assumes certain logical prerequisites;

they are violated at the cost of a failure to achieve rigorous comprehension of the problem under examination.

A Comment on Reductionism and Logical Rigor

With a shift in *level* of analysis, a concomitant shift is observed in the relevant *unit* of analysis, as it is logically impossible to explain a phenomena on one analytical level by means of the analytical unit of another. In other words, if our objective is the understanding of some aspect of sociocultural organization or change (sociocultural behavior), then the biological or psychological characteristics of the human organism—while wholly pertinent to comprehending human behavior—will not function as explanatory variables but as constants or "givens."

The universe comprises a hierarchy of systems; that is to say, each higher level of system is composed of systems at lower levels. The criteria on which such distinctions are based stem directly from empirical observation of the whole range of living systems. As Miller (1965a, pp. 213, 216) has pointed out, these observations have led to a consensus among members of the scientific community that there exist certain fundamental forms of organization ("systems") of living matter-energy. All systems at each general level share certain common characteristics that differentiate them from systems at other levels. And as a measure of the sum of a system's parts is greater than the sum of that measure of its parts, the more complex systems at higher levels manifest characteristics, greater than the sum of the characteristics of the parts, not observed at lower levels.

Thus culture, or the social system, is not, as has been adduced (d'Aquili & Mihalik, this volume), the summed behavior of an aggregate of human organisms. It is a wholly distinct level of organization, a systematized structuring of activity, a patterned regularity that is generated by human interaction over time (Boulding, 1968, p. 8). It has been mathematically demonstrated that if human beings engage in sustained communication over time, a set of relations (a system or organization, a "culture" or "society") will emerge, the properties of which cannot be reduced to and/or explained in terms of the properties of the aggregate or the individuals composing this aggregate on which the system is defined (Ashby, 1964; q.e.d. Krippendorff, 1971; also Cf. Durkheim, 1895, p. 103). The scientific analysis and evaluation of veridical or living systems does not concern itself with the "hardware" that makes up a system but with the operation of the system as a whole, its internal relations and its behavior in a particular environment (Hall & Fagen, 1956, p. 28). In Ashby's (1968, p. 111) terms, the nature of materiality is a gross irrelevancy; it could be "angels" or "ectoplasm," he asserts, for as long as critical interdependencies operate in some regular fashion between them, then organization—a system—is defined.

Thus, insofar as human behavior and social or cultural behavior comprise two very distinct analytical levels, it follows that what constitutes significant stress for the human organism or a particular segment of the human population may *not*, in fact, constitute significant stress for the sociocultural system.

Significant Lack Stress: Energy Depletion

Energy depletion of sufficiently critical level to have a measurable impact on the operation of the sociocultural system must considerably exceed the relatively constant and predictable levels of nutritional stress long associated with poor socioeconomic conditions; even if this stress, chronic or acute, is severe, it remains basically environment specific. Significant energy depletion for sociocultural system requires, in fact, a scourge, a devastation of extraordinary magnitude that in some way disrupts normal social function system-wide. It requires, in fact, something very like "the Plague." Historically, this was an event of sudden onset that radically depleted the social system of critical manpower within a relatively short period of time, further disorganizing system coordination or normal information flow in the suspension of governance it so often precipitated. A momentary digression on the "Great Dying" and related epidemics should serve to exemplify the very distinct nature of "lack stress" on this (sociocultural) level.

Whether the apparently older "bubonic" plague, or the so-called "Black Death" or pulmonary plague which apparently arrived in central Europe by the eleventh century at the latest, the "Plague" could reasonably be hypothesized to have constituted a serious energy drain for those societies that it so frequently overwhelmed. The plague of 545, which persisted intermittently for the following two decades, is said to have resulted in a population decrease in Western Europe of 40% or more (Russell, 1968). That the collapse of the Roman Empire in the *Pars Occidentalis* could well have been hastened by this great decline in manpower is not improbable: The armies necessary to carry out imperial orders and maintain imperial control would have been severely depleted. The "pandemic" of 1348–1350, the "Black

Death," saw the demise of a quarter of the population of Europe; it was followed by a long series of recurrent outbreaks all over Europe at intervals of approximately a decade or so (Langer, 1964). Furthermore, these epidemics were frequently accompanied by severe outbreaks of diseases such as typhus and the so-called "English Sweat," a most deadly form of influenza (Ackerknecht, 1965). The social disorganization attendant upon the "Great Dying," as the Germans called it, was equally severe.

Even if they fell short of the chroniclers' often exaggerated figures, the losses were nonetheless heavy with each new outbreak. Braudel's (1973, pp. 48–50) reliable account gives some idea of the frequency and severity of the plague. Besançon reported plague 40 times between the years 1439 and 1640; Dôle suffered its ravages in 1565, 1586, 1629, 1632, and again in 1637. In the sixteenth century, the whole of Limousin was subjected to the plague on 10 occasions and Orleans on some 22. Seville was hit between 1507 and 1508, in 1582, 1595–1599, 1616, and from 1648 to 1649. Towns were often quite utterly deserted, described again and again as "stinking necropoli." The plague was in Amsterdam throughout every year from 1622 to 1628: The count was 35,000 dead. Paris suffered in 1612, 1619, 1631, 1638, 1662, and 1668. In London, the plague struck 5 times between 1593 and 1664–1665, claiming, it is said, a total of 156,463 victims. The last spectacular appearance of this disease in Western Europe took place in Toulon and Marseilles in 1720; it was extremely virulent, and "a good half" of the population of Marseilles died. According to one historian, for nearly a year the streets were full of "putrid bodies, gnawed by dogs." Most critical for social-system operation, these 4 centuries of plague provoked massive derelictions of public duty. Municipal magistrates, officers, and prelates fled their offices and obligations; in France, whole *parlements* emigrated. The governing body of Grenoble absented itself wholly in 1467, in 1589, and in 1596; in Bordeaux, all governance was in abeyance in 1471 and again in 1585; this was also the state of affairs in Besançon in 1519 and in Rennes in 1563 and in 1564.

It is notable that Europe's economic revival in the seventeenth and eighteenth centuries coincided with the retreat of the plague and a burst of rapid population growth (Langer, 1964, p. 7; Gasquet, 1893, 1908). In Eastern Europe, however, the plague continued its deadly rounds: The "Pugachev" in Moscow in 1770 was said to have carried off as many men as the partition of Poland. Kherson was hit in 1783, Odessa in 1814, the Balkans generally in 1828–1829 and again in 1841 (Braudel, 1973, p. 47). The bubonic plague remained endemic in

South China, India, and North Africa, in which Oran's sufferings were vividly recorded by Camus as recently as 1942.

Compensatory Adjustment Processes of the Sociocultural System

Unlike the series of European plagues prior to the eighteenth century, malnutrition, even in the extreme form of periodic and severe famine, does not constitute a significant lack stress for the sociocultural system as a whole. As Miller has formally hypothesized and tentatively demonstrated (1953, 1965c, p. 401), although a certain system component may develop some measure of strain under stress, the system of which it is a part has numerous ways to compensate for such strain in order that general equilibrium be maintained. Internal matter-energy processes of the system seem clearly pertinent here; these adjustment processes reduce system strains by moving their components about, reallocating material and/or energetic items. Rates of flow of (in this case) energy can be controlled, increased, for example, to that part of the system with a deficit of the same. The adjustment of transmission rates from the distributor subsystem could readily arrange for energy flows to reach the affected system component faster and/or in greater amounts (Miller, 1965b, pp. 364–366). In other words, the "decider component," the administrative and coordinating unit of the system, could quite simply arrange to allocate more food to those suffering the malnutrition characteristic of the deprived sector. Famine aid could be sent rapidly to distressed regions.

However, it is almost universally the case that this sort of adjustment process, based on the reallocation of energy, is *not* in fact utilized to reduce the stress suffered by the energy-poor component of the social system. While it is theoretically possible for the system as a whole to respond in this fashion to distress in a component part, *empirically* such a response is highly exceptional.

While clearly (due to these available compensatory processes) what is significant stress for one system component may be only moderate stress for the total system, a further step, a corollary hypothesis, as it were, is required in tentative explanation of this empirical observation. It is proposed that localized "stress" can, in certain cases, enhance rather than disrupt the long-term maintenance of the generalized system equilibrium. In other words, the apparently relevant compensatory measures are not utilized because they are not in the best interests of the system as a whole; a more subtle but most efficient compensatory device is already built into the system, in the form of the localized stress itself, to adjust for a more significant preexisting system-wide strain—the strain of overpopulation. The quietly systematic pruning of the population represented by the higher morbidity and mortality rates of the poor obviates a wider and considerably more serious system strain. Those of the poor who have not adapted to a chronically low dietary intake generally die in sufficient numbers to ensure some moderation of an overburdened resource base. The poor, then, are ultimately the expendable, a relatively cheap price for the system to pay for self-regulation.

A brief consideration of certain aspects of recent and historical instances of famine should serve to illustrate this general thesis. True famine can be defined in statistical terms as a severe food shortage resulting in a significant increase in the death rate of the affected area (Mayer, 1975, p. 572). Darwin (1871, Vol. I, p. 130) called them "periodical dearths," noting that such dearths were probably the most important of all the checks on population growth. In terms of the end result for the affected portion of the population, the reaction of the system as a whole to famine has altered little since the sixteenth century. Into the French town of Troye, the famine of 1573 brought a veritable invasion, an "army of the poor." Described as starving, clothed in rags, and alive with fleas and vermin, the desperately hungry crowds were dealt with most expeditiously by the well-fed bourgeois of the town. Lured outside the gates of the town with the promise of a loaf of bread and a piece of silver, the poor were told over the now-securely impregnable walls that they must go to God for their livelihood, for the city walls of Troye would be closed against them until the next harvest. Matters grew only worse in the following century. As Braudel (1973, p. 40) has aptly noted, the problem was to ensure that the poor were in a position "where they could do no harm." In Paris, the sick and invalid were directed to the hospitals from which few emerged cured; the fit were chained together in pairs and made interminably to scour the drains and sewers of the city. In England, the Poor Laws, which were in fact laws *against* the poor, were enacted at the end of Elizabeth's reign. Increasingly, the poor were condemned to forced labor in the various workhouses (*Zuchthaüser* or *Maisons de Force*) that spread throughout the West. The seventeenth century was truly "relentless in its rationality"; but as Braudel further observes, it was perhaps an almost inevitable response to the increasing numbers of the poor in that hard century (1973, p. 41). And despite the fine and ringing phrases of humanitarian brotherhood so common today, the "improvisational," "ad hoc," and always inadequate measures that characterize the mid-twentieth-century response to famine (Mayer, 1975, p. 571) do tend to confirm that the cost of resolving the problem of the nutritional stress of the poor is not a cost the social system will—or can—pay. It is, after all, a cost apparently less severe for the system as a whole than any other that the rigorous and inescapable workings of the iron law of Malthus might exact were the death rates sharply lowered in the face of a generally unchecked growth rate. This terrible clarity of the logic of natural systems, a logic wholly impersonal and without regard for the passions and ethical notions of man, is the cause of a certain amount of alarm to many—to those, in fact, who in pre-Copernican fashion believe human-containing systems to be somehow exempt from the operation of the general regularities to which all other systems are clearly subject. Our failure to check the growth rate of world population at some point before the deleterious effects of overcrowding began to do it for us is a significant warning. We will continue to be ruthlessly subject to the most profound and unmoderated ramifications of such natural laws as that of Malthus only so long as we persist in denying their intimate relevance to man.

ACKNOWLEDGMENTS

The author wishes most particularly to thank Richard I. Ford and A. Roberto Frisancho for their generous assistance and invaluable critical advice on an earlier draft of this manuscript.

REFERENCES

Abelson, P. H. Food and nutrition. *Science,* 1975, *188,* 501.
Ackerknecht, E. H. *History and geography of the most important diseases.* New York: Hafner, 1965.
Allen, G. Genetic variation in mental development. In N. S. Scrimshaw & J. E. Gordon (Eds.), *Malnutrition, learning and behavior.* Cambridge, Massachusetts: MIT, 1968. Pp. 92–106. (a)
Allen, G. Short comments. In N. S. Scrimshaw & J. E. Gordon (Eds.), *Malnutrition, learning and behavior.* Cambridge, Massachusetts: MIT, 1968, P. 108. (b)
Angel, J. L. The bases of paleodemography, *American Journal of Physical Anthropology,* 1969, *30,* 427–438.
Angel, J. L. Ecology and population in the eastern Mediterranean. *World Archaeology,* 1972, *4,* 88–105.
Angel, J. L. Paleoecology, paleodemography and health. In S. Polgar (Ed.), *Population, ecology, and social evolution.* The Hague: Mouton, 1975. Pp. 167–190.
Ashby, W. R. *Design for a brain.* New York: Wiley, 1954.

Ashby, W. R. The set theory of mechanism and homeostasis. *General Systems*, 1964, *IX*, 83–97.
Ashby, W. R. Principles of the self-organizing system. In W. Buckley (Ed.), *Modern systems research for the behavioral scientist: A sourcebook.* Chicago: Aldine, 1968. Pp. 108–118.
Barnicot, N. A. Human nutrition: Evolutionary perspectives. In P. J. Ucko & G. W. Dimbleby (Eds.), *The domestication and exploitation of plants and animals.* New York: Aldine-Atherton, 1969. Pp. 525–529.
Barringer, B. Neolithic growth rates. *American Anthropologist*, 1966, *68*, 1253.
Barth, F. *Nomads of south Persia: The Basseri tribe of the Khamseh confederacy.* Boston: Little, Brown, 1961.
Béhar, M. Prevalence of malnutrition among preschool children of developing countries. In N. S. Scrimshaw & J. E. Gordon (Eds.), *Malnutrition, learning and behavior.* Cambridge, Massachusetts: MIT, 1968. Pp. 30–41.
Beisel, W. R. Synergistic effects of maternal malnutrition and infection on the infant: recommendation for prospective studies in man. *American Journal of Diseases of Children*, 1975, *129*, 571–574.
Bertalanffy, L. Von. General system theory—a critical review. *General Systems*, 1962, *VII*, 1–20.
Bickel, W. Bevölkerungsdynamik und gesellschaftsstruktur. *Schweizerische Zeitschrift für Volkswirtshaft und Statistik*, 1956, *92*, 317–328.
Birch, H. G. Field measurement in nutrition, learning and behavior. In N. S. Scrimshaw & J. E. Gordon (Eds.), *Malnutrition, learning and behavior.* Cambridge, Massachusetts: MIT, 1968. Pp. 497–508.
Birdsell, J. Some population problems involving Pleistocene man. *Cold Springs Harbor Symposia on Quantitative Biology*, 1957, *22*, 47–69.
Birdsell, J. Some predictions for the Pleistocene based on equilibrium systems among recent hunter-gatherers. In R. Lee & I. DeVore (Eds.), *Man the hunter.* Chicago: Aldine, 1968. Pp. 229–249.
Black, F. L. Infectious diseases in primitive societies. *Science*, 1975, *187*, 515–518.
Blau, P. M. A formal theory of differentiation in organizations. *American Sociological Review*, 1970, *35*, 201–218.
Boulding, K. E. *The organizational revolution.* New York: Harper, 1953.
Boulding, K. E. The Malthusian model as a general system. *Social and Economic Studies*, 1955, *4*, 195–205.
Boulding, K. E. General systems theory—the skeleton of science. In W. Buckley (Ed.), *Modern systems research for the behavioral scientist: A sourcebook.* Chicago: Aldine, 1968, Pp. 3–10.
Brace, C. L. & Livingstone, F. B. On creeping Jensenism. In D. E. Hunter & P. Whitten (Eds.), *Anthropology: Contemporary perspectives.* Boston: Little, Brown, 1975. Pp. 108–119.
Braudel, F. *Capitalism and material life 1400-1800.* New York: Harper & Row, 1973.
Brock, J. F. Dietary protein deficiency: Its influence on body structure and function. *Annals of Internal Medicine*, 1966, *65*, 877–899.
Brothwell, D. R. Teeth in earlier human populations. *Proceedings of the Nutrition Society of Great Britain*, 1959, *18*, 59–65.
Brothwell, D. R. Dietary variation and the biology of earlier human populations. In P. J. Ucko & G. W. Dimbleby, (Eds.), *The domestication and exploitation of plants and animals.* New York: Aldine-Atherton, 1969. Pp. 531–545.

Brothwell, D. R. Palaeodemography. In W. Brass (Ed.), *Biological aspects of demography*. London: Taylor and Francis, 1971. Pp. 111–130.

Brothwell, D. R. Palaeodemography and earlier British populations. *World Archaeology*, 1972, *4*, 75–87.

Brown, R. E., & Wray, J. D. Nutrition and population: Is it paradoxical that improved nutrition promotes interest in birth planning? *Medikon International*, 1974, *4*, 4–10.

Brues, A. The spearman and the archer—an essay on selection in body build. *American Anthropologist*, 1959, *61*, 457–461.

Bryant, V. M., Jr. Prehistoric diet in Southwest Texas: The coprolite evidence. *American Antiquity*, 1974, *39*, 407–420.

Cabak, V., & Najdanvic, R. Effects of undernutrition in early life on physical and mental development. *Archives of Diseases of Children*, 1965, *40*, 532–534.

Caillé, J. *La ville de Rabat jusqu'au Protectorat Français*. Vol. I. Paris: Vanoest, 1949.

Callen, E. O. Diet as revealed by coprolites. In D. Brothwell & E. Higgs (Eds.), *Science in archaeology: A survey of progress and research* (2nd ed., rev.). New York: Praeger, 1969. Pp. 234–243.

Cannon, W. B. *Wisdom of the body*. New York: Norton, 1939.

Canosa, C. A. Ecological approach to the problems of malnutrition, learning and behavior. In N.S. Scrimshaw & J. E. Gordon (Eds.), *Malnutrition, learning and behavior*. Cambridge, Massachusetts: MIT, 1968, Pp. 389–396.

Carneiro, R. L. Slash and burn cultivation among the Kuikuru and its implications for cultural development in the Amazon Basin. In J. Wilbert (Ed.), *The evolution of horticultural systems in native South America, causes and consequences*. Anthropologica Supplement publication 2. Caracas: Sociedad de Ciencias Naturales La Salle, 1961. Pp. 47–67.

Carneiro, R. L., & Hilse, D. F. On determining the probable rate of population growth during the Neolithic. *American Anthropologist*, 1966, *68*, 177–181.

Cipolla, C. *The economic history of world population*. Baltimore: Penguin, 1962.

Clement, A. J. Variations in the micro-stucture and biochemistry of human teeth. In D. R. Brothwell (Ed.), *Dental anthropology*. New York: Pergamon, 1963. Pp. 245–269.

Cravioto, J., & DeLicardie, E. R. Intersensory development of school-age children. In N. S. Scrimshaw & J. E. Gordon (Eds.), *Malnutrition, learning and behavior*. Cambridge, Massachusetts: MIT, 1968. Pp. 252–268.

Dairy Council Digest. Malnutrition, learning and behavior. *Dairy Council Digest: An interpretive review of recent nutrition research*, 1973, *44*, 31–34.

Dairy Council Digest. Nutritional needs during pregnancy. *Dairy Council Digest: An interpretive review of recent nutrition research*, 1974, *45*, 19–22.

Darwin, C. *The descent of man, and selection in relation to sex*. 2 vols. New York: Appleton, 1871.

Darwin, C. *Charles Darwin's natural selection: Being the second part of his big species book written from 1856 to 1858*. R. C. Stauffer (Ed.). London: Cambridge University Press, 1975.

Davies, C. T. M. Relationship of maximum aerobic power output to productivity and absenteeism of East African sugar cane workers. *British Journal of Industrial Medicine*, 1973, *30*, 146–154.

Deevey, E. S. The human population. *Scientific American*, 1960, *203*, 194–204.

Dumond, D. E. Population growth and culture change. *Southwestern Journal of Anthropology*, 1965, *21*, 302–324.

Dumond, D. E. The limitation of human population: A natural history. *Science*, 1975, *187*, 713–721.
Dunn, F. L. Epidemiological factors: Health and disease in hunter-gatherers. In R. B. Lee & I. DeVore (Eds.), *Man the Hunter*. Chicago: Aldine, 1968, Pp. 221–228.
Durkheim, E. *Les règles de la méthode sociologique*. Paris: Felix Alcan, 1895.
Durkheim, E. *The division of labor in society*. New York: Free Press, 1933.
Dwyer, J. T. & Mayer, J. Beyond economics and nutrition: The complex basis of food policy. *Science*, 1975, *188*, 566–570.
Echols, J. R. Population vs. the environment: A crisis of too many people. *American Scientist*, 1976, *64*, 165–173.
Eichenwald, H. F. Pre-natal and post-natal infectious diseases affecting the central nervous system. In N. S. Scrimshaw and J. E. Gordon (Eds.), *Malnutrition, learning and behavior*. Cambridge, Massachusetts: MIT, 1968. Pp. 426–437.
F.A.O. Assessment of the world food situation. UN, *World Food Conference*, Rome, 5–16 November, 1974.
Flannery, K. V. The origins of agriculture. *Annual Review of Anthropology*, 1973, *2*, 271–310.
Ford, R. I. Review of *Seed to civilization: The story of man's food* by C. B. Heiser. *American Anthropologist*, 1974, *76*, 887–889.
Frankova, S. Nutritional and psychological factors in the development of spontaneous behavior in the rat. In N. S. Scrimshaw & J. E. Gordon (Eds.), *Malnutrition, learning and behavior*. Cambridge, Massachusetts: MIT, 1968. Pp. 312–322.
Frisancho, A. R., Garn, S. M., & Ascoli, W. Childhood retardation resulting in reduction of adult body size due to lesser adolescent skeletal delay. *American Journal of Physical Anthropology*, 1970, *33*, 325–336.
Frisancho, A. R., Sanchez, J., Pallardel, D., & Yanez, L. Adaptive significance of small body size under poor socioeconomic conditions in southern Peru. *American Journal of Physical Anthropology*, 1973, *39*, 255–261.
Frisch, R. E. Critical weights, a critical body composition, menarche, and the maintenance of menstrual cycles. In E. Watts, F. E. Johnson, & G. W. Lasker (Eds.), *Biosocial interrelations in population adaptation*. The Hague: Mouton, 1975.
Frisch, R.E. & McArthur, J. Menstrual cycles: Fatness as a determinant of minimum weight for height necessary for their maintenance or onset. *Science*, 1974, *185*, 949–951.
Furetière, A. *Dictionnaire de Trévoux* (rev. ed). 1771.
Fussell, G. E. The change in farm labourer's diet during two centuries. *Economic History*, 1927, *1*, 268–274.
Garn, S. M., Nagy, J. M., Paznanski, A. K., & McCann, M. B. Size reduction associated with brachymesophalangia-5: A possible selective advantage. *American Journal of Physical Anthropology*, 1972, *37*, 267–270.
Garrow, J. S. & Pike, M. C. The long-term prognosis of severe infantile malnutrition. *Lancet*, 1967, *1*, 1–4.
Gasquet, F. A. *The great pestilence*. London: Simpkin, Marshall, 1893.
Gasquet, F. A. *The black death of 1348-1349* (2nd ed.). London: G. Bell, 1908.
Gavan, J. D., & Dixon, J. A. India: A perspective on the food situation. *Science*, 1975, *188*, 541–549.
Geertz, C. *Agricultural involution: The processes of ecological change in Indonesia*. Berkeley: University of California Press, 1963.
Goldsmith, G. A. More food for more people. *American Journal of Public Health*, 1969, *59*, 694–704.

Goldstein, M. S. The palaeopathology of human skeletal remains. In D. Brothwell & E. Higgs (Eds.), *Science in archaeology: A survey of progress and research.* New York: Praeger, 1969. Pp. 480–489.

Gopalan, C. Some recent studies in the nutrition research laboratories, Hyderabad. *American Journal of Clinical Nutrition,* 1970, *23,* 35–51.

Gordon, J. E. Epidemiological critique. In N. S. Scrimshaw & J. E. Gordon (Eds.), *Malnutrition, learning and behavior.* Cambridge, Massachusetts: MIT, 1968. Pp. 535–542.

Gorman, C. The Hoabinhian and after: Subsistence patterns in Southwest Asia during the late Pleistocene and early Recent periods. *World Archaeology,* 1971, *2,* 300–320.

Graham, G. G. Short comments. In N. S. Scrimshaw & J. E. Gordon (Eds.), *Malnutrition, learning and behavior.* Cambridge, Massachusetts: MIT, 1968. P. 84–87.

Graham, G. G., & Adrianzen, B. Growth, inheritance, and environment. *Pediatric Research,* 1971, *5,* 691–697.

Graham, G. G., & Morales, E. Studies in infantile malnutrition: Nature of the problem in Peru. *Journal of Nutrition,* 1963, *79,* 479–487.

Greenburg, B. Some relations between territory, social hierarchy, and leadership in the green sunfish (*Lepomis cyanellus*). *Physiological Zoology,* 1947, *20,* 267–299.

Greene, L. S. Physical growth and development, neurological maturation and behavioral functioning in two Ecuadorean Andean communities. *American Journal of Physical Anthropology,* 1973, *38,* 119–134.

Gruenwald, P. Short comments. In N. S. Scrimshaw & J. E. Gordon (Eds.), *Malnutrition, learning and behavior.* Cambridge, Massachusetts: MIT, 1968. P. 108.

Guzman, M. A. Impaired physical growth and maturation in malnourished populations, In N. S. Scrimshaw & J. E. Gordon (Eds.), *Malnutrition, learning and behavior.* Cambridge, Massachusetts: MIT, 1968. Pp. 42–54.

Hall, A. D., & Fagan, R. E. Definition of system. *General System,* 1956, *I,* 18–28.

Handley, J. E. *Scottish farming in the eighteenth century.* London: Faber, 1953.

Hansen, J. D. L., Wittmann, W., Moodie, A. D., & Fellingham, S. A. Evaluating the synergism of infection and nutrition in the field. In N. S. Scrimshaw & J. E. Gordon (Eds.), *Malnutrition, learning and behavior.* Cambridge, Massachusetts: MIT, 1968. Pp. 438–455.

Harner, M. J. Population pressure and the social evolution of agriculturalists. *Southwestern Journal of Anthropology,* 1970, *26,* 67–86.

Harner, M. J. Scarcity, the factors of production, and social evolution. In S. Polgar (Ed.), *Population, ecology, and social evolution.* The Hague: Mouton, 1975. Pp. 123–138.

Hassan, F. A. On mechanisms of population growth during the Neolithic. *Current Anthropology,* 1973, *14,* 535–542.

Hassan, F. A. Determination of the size, density, and growth rate of hunting-gathering populations. In S. Polgar (Ed.), *Population, ecology, and social evolution.* The Hague: Mouton, 1975. Pp. 28–52.

Hawley, A. H. *Human ecology.* New York: Ronald Press, 1950.

Heiser, C. B. Jr. *Seed to civilization: the story of man's food.* San Francisco: W. H. Freeman, 1973.

Heizer, R. F. The anthropology of prehistoric Great Basin human coprolites. In D. Brothwell & E. Higgs (Eds.), *Science in archaeology: A survey of progress and research.* (2nd ed., rev.) New York: Praeger, 1969. Pp. 244–250.

Herlihy, D. *Pisa in the early Renaissance.* New Haven, Connecticut: Yale University Press, 1958.

Higgins, B. *Economic development: Problems, principles and policies.* New York: Norton, 1968.

Ho, P-T. *Studies on the population of China, 1368–1953.* Cambridge, Massachusetts: Harvard University Press, 1959.

Holmberg, A. R., & Dobyns, H. F. The Cornell project in Vicos, Peru. In C. R. Wharton (Ed.), *Subsistence agriculture and economic development.* Chicago: Aldine, 1969. Pp. 392–414.

Issac, G. The diet of early man: Aspects of archaeological evidence from Lower and Middle Pleistocene sites in Africa. *World Archaeology,* 1971, *2,* 278–299.

Jarman, M. Culture and economy in the north Italian Neolithic. *World Archaeology,* 1971, *2,* 255–265.

Jelliffe, D. B. The assessment of the nutritional status of the community, with special reference to field surveys in developing regions of the world. *World Health Organization Monograph Series,* 1966, No. 53.

Jelliffe, D. B. *Infant nutrition in the subtropics and tropics.* Geneva: WHO, 1968.

Kempf, E. J. Basic biodynamics. *Annals of the New York Academy of Science,* 1958, 73, 869–910.

Keppel, F. Food for thought. In N. S. Scrimshaw & J. E. Gordon (Eds.), *Malnutrition, learning and behavior.* Cambridge, Massachusetts: MIT, 1968. Pp. 4–9.

King, J. C. *The biology of race.* New York: Harcourt, Brace and Jovanovich, 1971.

Krippendorff, K. Communications and the genesis of structure. *General Systems,* 1971, *XVI,* 171–185.

Kunitz, S. J., & Euler, R. C., Aspects of Southwestern paleo-epidemiology. *Prescott College Anthropological Reports,* 1972, No. 2.

Langer, W. L. Europe's initial population explosion. *American Historical Review,* 1963, 69, 1–17.

Langer, W. L. The black death. *Scientific American,* 1964, *210,* 114–121.

Langer, W. L. Checks on population growth: 1750–1850. *Scientific American,*1972,*226,* 92–99.

Lasky, R. E., Lechtig, A., Delgado, H., Klein, R. E., Engle, P., Yarbrough, C., & Martorell, R. Birth weight and psychomotor performance in rural Guatemala. *American Journal of the Diseases of Children,* 1975, *129,* 566–569.

Latham, M. C. Nutrition and infection in national development. *Science,* 1975, *188,* 561–565.

Le Chatelier, H. Recherches expérimentales et théoriques sur les équilibres chimiques. *Annales des Mines,* 1888, Mémoires XIII (huitième série).

Lechtig, A., Delgado, H., & Lasky, R. E., Maternal nutrition and fetal growth in developing societies. *American Journal of Diseases of Children,* 1975, *129,* 434–437. (a)

Lechtig, A., Delgado H., & Lasky, R. E., Maternal nutrition and fetal growth in developing countries. *American Journal of Diseases of Children,* 1975, *129,* 553–556. (b)

Lee, R. B., & DeVore, I. (Eds.) *Man the hunter.* Chicago: Aldine, 1968.

Mackenroth, G. *Bevölkerungslehre: theorie, soziologie und statistik der bevölkerung.* Berlin: Springer-Verlag, 1953.

Malcolm, L. A. Growth and development of the Kaiapit children of the Markham Valley, New Guinea. *American Journal of Physical Anthropology,* 1969, *31,* 39–51.

Malcolm, L. A. Growth and development of the Bundi child of the New Guinea highlands. *Human Biology,* 1970, *42,* 293–328.

Malthus, R. T. *An essay on the principle of population.* London: J. Johnson, 1798.

Malthus, R. T. *An essay on the principle of population and a summary view of the principle of population.* Baltimore: Penguin Books, 1970.

Marshall, C. L., Brown, R. E., & Goodrich, C. H., Improved nutrition vs. public health services as major determinants of world population growth. *Clinical Pediatrics,* 1971, *10,* 363–368.

Mayer, J. Management of famine relief. *Science,* 1975, *188,* 571–577.

Mahew, B. H. System size and ruling elites. *American Sociological Review,* 1973, 38, 468–475.

McDermott, W. Modern medicine and the demographic disease pattern of overly-traditional societies: A technological misfit. *Journal of Medical Education,* 1966, *41* (suppl.), 137–162.

McKeown, T. *Medicine in modern society.* London: Allen and Unwin, 1965.

McKeown, T., & Brown, R. G., Medical evidence related to English population changes in the eighteenth century. In D. M. Heer (Ed.), *Readings on population.* Englewood Cliffs, New Jersey: Prentice-Hall, 1968. Pp. 16–38.

Messenger, J. C. *Inis Beag: Isle of Ireland.* New York: Holt, Rinehart & Winston, 1969.

Michels, R. La democrazia e la legge ferrea dell' oligarchia. *Rassegna Contemporanea,* 1910, *3,* 259–283.

Miller, J. G. The development of experimental stress-sensitive tests for predicting performance. *Psychological Research Association,* 1953, Report 53–10.

Miller, J. G. Living systems: Basic concepts. *Behavioral Science,* 1965, *10,* 193–237. (a)

Miller, J. G. Living systems: Structure and process. *Behavioral Science,* 1965, *10,* 337–379. (b)

Miller, J. G. Living systems: Cross-level hypotheses. *Behavioral Science,* 1965, *10,* 380–411. (c)

Mols, R. *Introduction à la démographie historique des villes d'Europe du XIVe au XVIIIe siècle,* Tome II. Louvain: Université de Louvain, 1955.

Montesquieu, C. L. de S. *De l'esprit des loix.* Tome I. Genève: Barrillot et Fils, 1748.

Mosca, G. *Elementi di scienza politica.* Roma: Fratelli Bocca, 1896.

Newberne, P. M. Animal models for investigation of latent effects of malnutrition. *American Journal of Diseases of Children,* 1975, *129,* 574–577.

Odum, E. P. *Fundamentals of Ecology.* (3rd ed.) Philadelphia: Saunders, 1971.

Öttingen, A. K. von. *Die moralstatistik* (3rd ed.). Erlangen: A. Deichert, 1882.

Pareto, V. *Tratto di sociologia generale.* 2 vols. Firenze: Barbèra, 1916.

Pearson, P. B. Scientific and technical aims. In N. S. Scrimshaw & J. E. Gordon (Eds.), *Malnutrition, learning and behavior.* Cambridge, Massachusetts: MIT, 1968. Pp. 10–13.

Pfanner, D. E. A semisubsistence village economy in lower Burma. In C. R. Wharton (Ed.), *Subsistence agriculture and economic development.* Chicago: Aldine, 1969. Pp. 47–60.

Poirier, F. E. *Fossil man: An evolutionary journey.* St. Louis: C. V. Mosby, 1973.

Poleman, T. T. World food: A perspective. *Science,* 1975, *188,* 510–518.

Prigogine, I. *Introduction to the thermodynamics of irreversible processes.* Springfield, Illinois: C. C Thomas, 1955.

Rafalski, H., & Mackiewicz, M. An epidemiological study of physical growth of children in rural districts of Poland. In N. S. Scrimshaw & J. E. Gordon (Eds.), *Malnutrition, learning and behavior.* Cambridge, Massachusetts: MIT, 1968. Pp. 72–81.

Randsborg, K. Population and social variation in early Bronze Age Denmark: A systemic approach. In S. Polgar (Ed.), *Population, ecology and social evolution.* The Hague: Mouton, 1975. Pp. 139–166.

Renfrew, C. Patterns of population growth in the prehistoric Aegean. In P. J. Ucko, R.

Tringham, & G. W. Dimbleby (Eds.), *Man, settlement and urbanism*. London: G. Duckworth, 1972. Pp. 383–399.

Richardson, S. A. The influence of social-environmental and nutritional factors on mental ability. In N. S. Scrimshaw & J. E. Gordon (Eds.), *Malnutrition, learning and behavior*. Cambridge, Massachusetts: MIT, 1968. Pp. 346–361.

Riecken, H. W. Panel discussion, Part VIII. In N. S. Scrimshaw & J. E. Gordon (Eds.), *Malnutrition, learning and behavior*. Cambridge, Massachusetts: MIT, 1968. P. 528.

Robson, J. R. K. *Malnutrition: Its causation and control, with special reference to protein-calorie malnutrition*. 2 vols. New York: Gordon and Breach, 1972.

Rosenbleuth, A., Wiener, N., & Bigelow, J. Behavior, purpose and teleology. *Philosophy of Science*, 1943, *10*, 18–24.

Russell, J. C. That earlier plague. *Demography*, 1968, 5, 174–184.

Sahlins, M. *Stone age economics*. Chicago: Aldine, 1972.

Salusbury, G. T. *Street life in medieval England* (2nd ed.). Oxford: Pen-in-Hand, 1948.

Sanderson, F. N. The great food fumble. *Science*, 1975, *188*, 503–509.

Schaller, G. B., & Lowther, G. R. The relevance of carnivore behavior to the study of early hominids. *Southwestern Journal of Anthropology*, 1969, *25*, 307–341.

Schjelderup-Ebbe, T. *Beiträge zur sozial- und individualpsychologie bie* Gallus domesticus. Griefswald: Author, 1921.

Scrimshaw, N. S. The effect of infection on nutritional status. *Bibl. "Nutr. Dieta."*, 1973, No. 18.

Scrimshaw, N. S., & Béhar, M. Protein malnutrition in young children. *Science*, 1961, *133*, 2039–2047.

Scrimshaw, N. S., & Gordon, J. E. (Eds.) *Malnutrition, learning and behavior*. Cambridge, Massachusetts: MIT, 1968.

Scrimshaw, N. S., Taylor, C. E., & Gordon, J. E. Interactions of nutrition and infection. *World Health Organization Monograph Series*, 1968, No. 57.

Shêng-Han, S. On 'Fan Sheng-Chih Shu', an agriculturistic book of China written by Fan Sheng-Chih in the 1st century BC. Peking: n.p., 1965.

Simpson, G. G. Forces of evolution and their integration. In P. Dolhinow & V. Sarich (Eds.), *Background for man*. Boston: Little, Brown, 1971. Pp. 7–25.

Sjoberg, G. *The pre-industrial city: Past and present*. New York: Free Press, 1960.

Smith, C. A. The effect of wartime starvation in Holland upon pregnancy and its product. *American Journal of Obstetrics and Gynecology*, 1947, *53*, 599–606.

Smith, T. *Parasitism and disease*. Princeton, New Jersey: Princeton Univ. Press, 1934.

Spencer, H. A theory of population, deduced from the general law of animal fertility. *Westminster Review*, 1852, *57*, 468–501.

Spencer, H. *The evolution of society: selections from Herbert Spencer's Principles of sociology*. R. L. Carneiro (Ed.). Chicago: Aldine, 1967.

Spurr, G. B., Barac-Nieto, M., & Maksud, M. G., Energy expenditure cutting sugarcane. *Journal of Applied Physiology*, 1975, *39*, 990–996.

Stein, Z., Susser, M., Saenger, G., & Marolla, F. *Famine and human development: The Dutch hunger winter of 1944–45*. New York: Oxford University Press, 1975.

Stini, N. A. Evolutionary implications of changing nutritional patterns in human populations. *American Anthropologist*, 1971, *73*, 1019–1030.

Summer, W. G., & Keller, A. G. *The science of society*. Vol. 1. New Haven, Connecticut: Yale Univ. Press, 1927.

Tanner, J. M. Human growth and constitution. In G. A. Harrison, J. S. Weiner, J. M.

Tanner, & N. A. Barnicot (Eds.), *Human biology: An introduction to human evolution, variation, and growth*. New York: Oxford Univ. Press (Clarendon), 1964. Part IV, pp. 299–397.

Thompson, W. S. *Population and progress in the Far East*. Chicago: University of Chicago Press, 1959.

Thomson, A. M. Historical perspectives of nutrition, reproduction, and growth. In N. S. Scrimshaw & J. E. Gordon (Eds.), *Malnutrition, learning and behavior*. Cambridge, Massachusetts: MIT, 1968. Pp. 17–28.

Trotter, M., & Glaser, G. C. A re-evaluation of estimation of stature based on measurement of stature taken during life and of long bones after death. *American Journal of Physical Anthropology*, 1958, *16*, 79–124.

Tylor, E. B. On a method of investigating the development of institutions; applied to laws of marriage and descent. *Journal of the Royal Anthropological Institute*, 1889, *18*, 245–272.

Vernon, P. E. Measurements of learning. In N. S. Scrimshaw & J. E. Gordon (Eds.), *Malnutrition, learning and behavior*. Cambridge, Massachusetts: MIT, 1968. Pp. 486–496.

Walters, H. Difficult issues underlying food problems. *Science*, 1975, *188*, 524–530.

Weiss, P. Animal behavior as system reaction. *General Systems*, 1959, *IV*, 1–44.

White, L. A. *The evolution of culture: the development of civilization to the fall of Rome*. New York: McGraw-Hill, 1959.

Widdowson, E. M. The place of experimental animals in the study of human malnutrition. In R. A. McCance & E. M. Widdowson (Eds.), *Calorie deficiencies and protein deficiencies*. Cambridge, Massachusetts: MIT, 1968. Pp. 225–236.

Wills, V. G., & Waterlow, J. C. The death rate in the age-group 1–4 years as an index of malnutrition. *Journal of Tropical Pediatrics*, 1958, *3*, 167–170.

Wrigley, E. A. *Population and history*. New York: McGraw-Hill, 1969.

Yudkin, J. Archaeology and the nutritionist. In P. J. Ucko & G. W. Dimbleby (Eds.), *The domestication and exploitation of plants and animals*. New York: Aldine-Atherton, 1969. Pp. 547–552.

9

Nutrition, Behavior, and Culture

EDWARD FOULKS AND SOLOMON H. KATZ
University of Pennsylvania

INTRODUCTION

Over the last several decades, considerable effort has been directed toward developing an understanding of the biological effects of specific and general forms of malnutrition on human neurological and psychological development. Now, as we begin to refine our understanding of these consequences, we can start considering their relation to the overall functioning of the societies in which they occur. This paper will attempt to explore these implications at several levels in the context of traditional, rapidly changing, and modern societies. More specifically, this chapter will explore some ways in which diet and the physical environment interact to affect, and be affected by, human behavior and social processes. In this context, culture will be understood as a system that often serves as a socially and sometimes physiologically adaptive interface between humans and their environment. Rather than dwelling on the effects of diet on individual development per se, we will attempt to extend our understanding of malnutrition by demonstrating that the nature of social organization, interpersonal relationships, and culture are profoundly influenced by nutrition.

It is obvious that the behavioral consequences of malnutrition in human populations are manifold. Malnutrition affects human behavior directly by disturbing brain growth and function and indirectly by influencing the social institutional responses to this perturbation. In some circumstances, cultural patterns represent responses to potential malnutrition and may be considered biologically adaptive. We will cite examples of such cultural adaptations in protein-poor societies in Amazonia and in niacin-poor societies in Latin America. In other circumstances, cultural responses to malnutrition do not appear to be directly biologically adaptive but nevertheless have a powerful influence on social structure and psychology. Such cultural responses, like biological adaptations, have required centuries of modification and selection. In order to develop some of these interrelations further, we will discuss our research on disturbances in calcium metabolism and central nervous system functioning among the North Alaskan Eskimo and show how many psychological and social functions articulate with these disturbances. We will also evaluate the ties between recent social, dietary, and psychological changes among the North Alaskan Eskimo.

PROTEIN–CALORIE MALNUTRITION (PCM)

Turnbull (1972) has recently called attention to the psychosocial responses to severe malnutrition exhibited by a mountain people of northern Uganda, the Ik. These people had been, in the past, rather successful nomadic hunters and gatherers; however, with the advent of nationhood, territories became important, and a process of settlement occurred. Originally, relationships were close: "A child was brought up to regard an adult living in the same camp as a parent, and any age mate as a brother or sister. These were the real and effective relationships [Turnbull, 1972, p. 28]" With settlement, however, these people were pushed higher and higher into the mountains, which were relatively barren of flora or fauna. Food was scarce, and starvation became common. Turnbull points out that the once close-knit social structure disintegrated, and altruism, love, and social attachments vanished. Individuals used each other for their own ends; even adults used children. Individual concern and self-sufficiency became the new order. "They were, each one, simply alone, and seemingly content to be alone [Turnbull, 1972, p. 238]." People did hunt together and forage together for mutual protection or for necessary cooperation; however, such good will as might have been generated by this companionship was "quickly dispelled by the acrimony involved in the division of the spoils [Turnbull, 1972, p. 238]." In the case of the Ik, mental retardation, lassitude, and passivity were not as much the apparent effects of severe malnutrition as were acrimony, envy, suspicion, and a dispassionate callousness toward other human beings. Such interaction as there was within this system was one of mutual exploitation.

Here we can see how the effects of these states of malnutrition extend throughout the entire fabric of social organization. Of course, in this case, we do not have precise estimates of PCM. This example nevertheless poses important social questions that have highly significant implications for those populations that face this prospect.

At another level of psychosocial implication a series of studies by Whiting and others (Harrington & Whiting, 1972) have shown that PCM and kwashiorkor can be statistically correlated cross-culturally with a pattern of social institutions and ecological constants. Cross-culturally, kwashiorkor has been found to occur most frequently (1) in the tropics; (2) in societies that practice a prolonged postpartum sex taboo; (3) in societies in which exclusive child–mother residence is common; and (4) in societies in which women primarily work small garden plots, harvesting carbohydrate-rich foods. Such societies are most commonly patrilocal and patrilineal and practice polygamy. In addition, men often live together in a large communal dwelling. Initiates into the men's society are often subjected to severe initiation rites frequently involving genital mutilation.

These authors point to a complex web of overdetermined or multiple-determined behaviors. The cultural adaptations of societies existing over long periods of time in areas providing little protein foodstuff have evolved in response to these limitations. A developing child is assured of protein intake during the crucial years of his early life by prolonged breast-feeding. This in itself inhibits ovulation for some time. Also, such societies practice a prolonged postpartum sex taboo, which further limits fertility and ensures the present child a longer stay at the breast. Furthermore, the prolonged sexual unavailability of the female, as well as her economic value in farming, creates certain pressures on the male to accumulate more females—thus the practice of polygamy. In such a situation, it is more parsimonious to have a new bride live near her husband and trace the descent of all children through the male.

The prolonged exclusive child–mother residence is felt to create especially close bonds between the mother and the child that become problematical in later life. The female must ultimately leave her mother and move to the place of her husband. Likewise, the male child must leave his mother at a certain age and join the men's society.

These transitions create many anxieties and conflicts in identity formation that are felt to be partially solved through the harsh rites of passage. Circumcision and other genital mutilations are seen in this context as representing a counterphobic defense against a fantasied all-powerful father and his group. These ceremonies have given rise to many psychological speculations that lie beyond the scope of the present discussion. What should be apparent, however, is that the social adaptations that develop under long-term chronic PCM extend far beyond the framework we usually consider when we investigate mental retardation in rapidly changing societies. In light of the current problems of increasing population and decreasing food, we must expand our paradigms to include studies of the ways in which societies adapt to marginal nutritional circumstances by developing coherent patterns of psychological functioning involving dependency, interpersonal relationships, and gender identity. Moreover, these psychological variables are in turn enmeshed in and determined by a complex sociocultural system that includes patterns of residence, marriage, and descent and many aspects of ritual and economic life, all of which can be related to this primary limitation in protein–calorie nutrition.

In some cases, culture may express behavioral adaptations to low availability or protein, and as long as these mechanisms are in operation, overt PCM, as seen in marasmus or kwashiorkor, is not evident. Meggers (1971) notes the following adaptations in environments with a scarcity of animal foods: (1) Settlements are usually small and are characterized by certain cultural traits limiting population size. These include a lack of strong political leadership, disputes over women, accusations of witchcraft, seasonal dispersals, and other factors favoring the fission of settlements; (2) there is often warfare, which results in dispersion rather than clumping of settlements into a given area. Such dispersion prevents overlapping areas of exploitation; (3) warfare and raiding necessitate the existence of large land areas between settlements in which animal species may reproduce unhindered by human predation; (4) shifting agriculture, warfare, and group fission also encourage frequent movement of settlements, which in turn avoids overexploitation of animal species; and (5) direct population control through infanticide, particularly of female infants, lowers the number of reproducers. Also effective are abortion, contraception, and prolonged postpartum sex taboos. Chagnon (1968a, 1968b, 1973) has shown how many of these traits coexist among the Yanomamö, where polygamy and infanticide create a scarcity of women, which in turn promotes disputes leading to fission within the village and ultimately to warfare between villages. This in turn precipitates relocation to distant areas in order to escape attack.

Gross (1975) has recently presented an extensive discussion of the role played by animal protein in limiting population size in many native settlements in Amazonia. He argues that the size, form and permanence of settlements, social complexity, and warfare patterns in the Amazon basin may vary with differences in the availability of animal proteins in the diet. He points out that when indigenous methods of population control were prohibited by modern governments, local populations exceeded the carrying capacity of the land, which led to malnutrition, disease, and rapid population decline.

PCM is particularly difficult to describe quantitatively; however, an evaluation of the effects of more specific nutritional deficiencies can give us added insights into the overall social implications of malnutrition. Iodine malnutrition is one example of this kind of specific deficiency (Stanbury, this volume; Greene, this volume). Another example is calcium deficiency.

CALCIUM–VITAMIN D MALNUTRITION AND GRAND HYSTERIA IN THE INDUSTRIALIZED NATIONS

Calcium is an element essential to the functioning of the brain. Vitamin D, with its intimate metabolic link to calcium, is equally essential. Calcium is involved in bone formation, muscle contraction, and several steps of blood clotting. Two of its other functions have direct relevance to the adequate function of the nervous system. It is involved in membrane permeability to other ions both during the process of muscle contraction and in the conduction of the neural impulse. At the synapse, or nerve ending, calcium is involved in the regulation of the amount of synaptic transmitter agent, such as acetylcholine, released upon stimulation (Schmidt, Parvati, & Smith, 1976). The net effect of lowering calcium ion concentration is to increase neutral excitability. Clinically, we see this manifested as an increased neuromuscular irritability that results in increased reflex activity, the extreme case of which is tetany. A classic sign of tetany is carpopedal muscular spasm.

There are three factors that have an important effect on calcium homeostasis. First is parathormone (PTH), which is secreted by the parathyroid glands in response to hypocalcemia. Next calcitonin (TCT), which is a hormone secreted from the thyroid gland during hypercalcemia. And last is vitamin D, which is obtained from the diet and/or is synthesized by the action of ultraviolet light from the sun on chemical (sterol) precursors in the skin. This vitamin is fat soluble and may be stored in the liver for up to several months. Calcium is ingested as a normal constituent of most diets, but its richest sources are milk and dairy products. The factors affecting the absorption of calcium are outlined in Figure 9.1.

Abnormalities in calcium homeostasis are capable of simulating and potentiating epileptic seizures. In addition, certain emotional factors are capable of acutely altering calcium homeostasis. One that is frequently encountered in states of anxiety and stress is hyperventilation, or overbreathing. Overbreathing has the physiological effect of increasing the pH of the blood and binding the free calcium, which reduces its availability for neuronal functioning, increases synaptic transmission rates, and is known under conditions of surgical hypothyroidism to produce frank psychosis (Denko & Kaelbling, 1962).

Wallace (1972) has proposed that the growth of cities during the Industrial Revolution in Europe and the United States created a temporary problem in the distribution of perishable farm products in large cities, wherein many sectors of the population were ill supplied with dairy products containing calcium. In addition, the fashions of the day dictated that ladies cover most of their skin surface with elaborate clothing. The pale cheek protected by bonnet and parasol and unexposed to solar ultraviolet radiation, was considered the hallmark of femininity. Wallace argues that low dietary levels of calcium and the limit placed on the autosynthesis of vitamin D by such fashions may

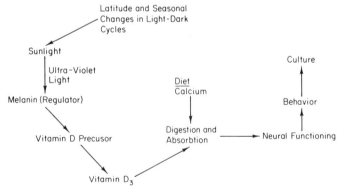

Figure 9.1. The relationship between dietary calcium, ultra-violet radiation levels and Vitamin D synthesis, blood calcium levels, neural functioning, behavior and culture among the North Alaskan Eskimo.

have been responsible for increasing the prevalence of rickets and osteoporosis at that time. In addition, European and American women of the time were commonly afflicted with a mental disorder that involved numerous somatic disturbances, altered states of consciousness, and convulsions. This disorder was called grand hysteria, and sufferers occupied over 50% of the beds at such famous hospitals as the Salpetrier in Paris, where Sigmund Freud, studying with Charcot, began to develop his famous theories about neurosis. Wallace points out that these grand hysterics, whatever their psychodynamics and connections to the unconscious, may have been suffering the behavioral symptoms of hypocalcemia. Noteworthy is the fact that as marketing in large cities improved, and as changing fashions allowed more exposure to sunlight, rickets decreased, as did grand hysteria, a disorder now considered rare in psychiatrists' offices.

ARCTIC HYSTERIA AMONG THE ESKIMO

Stefansson (1945, pp. 286–288) presented one of the first reports suggesting that the exclusively carnivorous diet of the Eskimo might be very low in calcium. The ketosis produced by the high protein diet also contributes to decalcification of bone and higher renal excretion of calcium. In addition, the cold climate of the Arctic requires heavy clothing, and sunlight is only available in the summer months. Thus, Eskimos, like Victorian Europeans, may have been candidates for disorders of calcium metabolism.

During his polar expeditions, Peary (1910) encountered a number of Eskimos who manifested hysterical attacks similar in form to the grand hysteria seen in Europe. He observed:

Aside from rheumatism and bronchial troubles, the Eskimos are fairly healthy; but the adults are subject to a peculiar affliction which they call piblokto, a form of hysteria. . . . The immediate cause of this affliction is hard to trace, so sometimes it seems to be the result of a brooding over absent or dead relatives or a fear of the future. The manifestations of this disorder are somewhat startling.

The patient . . . begins to scream and tear off and destroy clothing. If on a ship (he) will walk up and down the deck, screaming and gesticulating, and generally in a state of nudity, though the thermometer may be in the −40's. As the intensity of the attack increases, (he) will sometimes leap over the rail upon the ice, running perhaps ½ a mile. The attack may last several minutes, an hour or even more; and some sufferers become so wild that they would continue running about on the ice completely naked until they froze to death, if they were not forcibly brought back [pp. 166–67].

Explorers, scientists, missionaries, and more recently, social scientists have been frequently impressed by the high incidence of these dramatic behaviors exhibited by some inhabitants of arctic regions (Jochelson, 1908, Czaplica, 1914; Gussow, 1960; Wallace; 1972, and Parker, 1962). Gussow (1960) summarized the symptomatology of this syndrome from an extensive review of the literature. He described the following behaviors in decreasing order of frequency.

1. Tearing off clothing, achieving partial or complete nudity. This was frequently one of the first behavioral signs of the attack.
2. Glossolalia, muttering meaningless syllables, "speaking in tongues," making animal sounds.
3. Fleeing across the tundra, wandering into the hills, if indoors running outdoors in an agitated state.
4. Rolling in the snow, placing ice on oneself, jumping into water.
5. Bizarre acts such as attempting to walk on the ceiling.
6. Flinging things and thrashing about.
7. Mimetic acts.

Gussow felt that these behaviors represented a basic way Eskimos react to situations of intense stress. He emphasized the Eskimos' ability to regress and act out infantile needs for love and emotional support and pointed to the individual's desire to be pursued and to be attended to and held by family and friends.

Wallace (1972), on the other hand, argued that Piblokto-hysteria, like grand hysteria, may be a result of hypocalcemia that stems from an inability to physiologically adapt to a low level of calcium in the diet. They pointed out that the symptoms cited previously are often precipitated by hyperventilation, which results in a decrease in calcium ion concentration climaxed by a classic sign of hypocalcemic tetany, carpopedal spasms. They suggest that low levels of dietary calcium, in combination with these other factors, has probably influenced the functioning of the central nervous system, thus producing these dramatic behavioral changes.

It has been subsequently discovered that calcium intake among Eskimos is indeed low. A nutritional survey was conducted in Alaska by Heller and Scott (1961). They collected a total of 4840 diet records of about 7 days' duration on a seasonal basis for both sexes and all age levels from nine Eskimo and two Athabascan villages. The mean daily calcium intake levels among Eskimos and Athabascans were considerably below those recommended by the National Research Council for all age groups and genders. Three-fourths or more of the diets for each age and sex were deficient.

These authors estimated the probable intake level in aboriginal times by comparing the calcium content of adult female diets at Hooper Bay (southwestern Eskimo) and Pt. Hope (northern Eskimo). Hooper Bay women obtained more than three times as much calcium from local foods, chiefly from whole blackfish and needlefish. Calcium intake must have been still lower in the past in the Pt. Hope diet in which these particular fish are not available and other calcium sources are limited. Even at Hooper Bay, such fish sources are not continuously available throughout the year, nor are they so abundant that significant supplies can be dried or otherwise preserved for off-season use (Heller & Scott, 1961, p. 50). Levels for mean daily intake and availability of calcium from local foods and imported foods are consistently low for northwestern Alaskan Innuit villages.

In a recent study, Foulks (1972) has demonstrated the complex interactions between calcium malnutrition and Eskimo behavior and culture. He found that in North Alaskan Eskimos the mean blood levels of calcium were significantly lower (although still within the physiological range) than levels drawn from urban populations in Alaska. Furthermore, it was demonstrated that calcium was the only urinary electrolyte that exhibited dissynchronization of circadian variation. While hypocalcemia has been shown to be generally associated with emotional disorders, Foulks' study found that serum drawn from Eskimos with hysteria (during attack-free periods) did not differ from co-villagers in terms of calcium or phosphate levels.

However, certain emotional factors were found to be capable of acutely altering calcium homeostasis. One that was so frequently encountered among Eskimos as to be institutionalized was hyperventilation. (The ritualization of overbreathing was recently illustrated in James Houston's film *The White Dawn* in a ceremony during which two women breathed rapidly back and forth into each other's mouths.) Altered states of consciousness were traditionally induced by hyperventilation and were explained to be the soul exiting the subject through the mouth. Hyperventilation occurs naturally with anxiety and effectively raises serum pH, thereby binding free calcium ions to protein, thus rendering a temporary lowering of ionic calcium. Neural transmission is affected peripherally and centrally. Hyperventilation was found to precipitate epileptic seizures in some Eskimos.

In North Alaska, we have demonstrated a complex synergism between disturbances in the blood levels of calcium and their circadian variation and epilepsy, psychological states and culturally patterned hyperventilation resulting in arctic hysteria. These altered mental

states are temporary and characterized by culturally stereotyped behavior apparently modeled after behaviors of shamanistic trances.
These relationships are outlined in Figure 9.1.

The complex and subtle interaction of physiological state on
psychology and culture becomes manifest in the example of the Eskimo shaman. Through hyperventilation he is able to enter an altered
state of consciousness, "losing his soul" through his breath. The soul
travels to supernatural places and engages in struggles and negotia-
tions with other spirits and the souls of animals. Such soul trips
provide magical methods for solving many real problems of Eskimo
life such as finding food, curing illness, or solving interpersonal
conflicts. The behavior of the shaman during soul loss often includes
"walking into the sky," glossolalia, tearing off clothes, and finally
spasms and convulsions. Shamans are active, of course, in times of
group stress and in this way provide a model of "how Eskimos are to
behave in times of stress." The intricate psychology of this behavior is
reviewed in another paper (Foulks, Freeman, & Freeman, 1977).

We would like to reiterate and emphasize these interrelationships
between environment, behavior, and culture among the North Alaskan Eskimo. Malnutrition affecting the central nervous system must
affect behavior and psychology. The cultural system in turn is shaped
by, and shapes, psychology and behavior. In some cases, as pointed
out previously, these "superorganic" systems may represent adaptations to biological imbalances.

Shamans are now a thing of the past. Today, Eskimo societies are
moving into the modern world. Eskimo psychology is shifting, as has
the Eskimo diet. With modernization, the Eskimo probably no longer
experiences such extremes of calcium-vitamin D malnutrition, although Mazess and Mather (1975) have recently demonstrated there
are still important effects in older adults. Instead, recent shifts to a
cash economy and to dried and preserved "store foods" has resulted in
sharp increases in the amounts of refined carbohydrate in their diet.
This shift has in turn been accompanied by increasing rates of dental
problems, diabetes mellitus, and obesity. Further shifts to modernity
and affluence have led to decreased patterns of activity and changes in
the percentages of protein, carbohydrate, fat, and salt in the Eskimo
diet. The consequences of a high intake of these foodstuffs on the
functioning of the central nervous system is still a subject of some
debate. However, evidence seems clear that chronic high intake of
NaCl is associated with hypertension, which, in itself, is both a determinant and a result of certain psychological states commonly observed
among urban people. High animal fat intake and low activity patterns

are, of course, contributors to cholesterol hypernutrition. This substance has been implicated in the genesis of arteriosclerotic disease, which affects many organs of the body, including the heart and the brain. The psychological and social consequences of early death threat from myocardial infarction and of chronic brain syndrome associated with cerebral arteriosclerosis have an immediate and obvious relevance to modern life styles.

From this perspective progress to modernity seems to be not so much characterized by absolute improvement in quality of diet and lifeways as by the movement from a traditional set of ecological constraints to a modern set, perhaps equally as restricting to human life and functioning. In this chapter, we have attempted to demonstrate that the psychology of a people is affected by these constraints, the foremost of which is nutrition. More work is obviously needed in studies of malnutrition and central nervous system functioning, particularly in the area of cognitive growth and development. In addition, however, we feel increased attention might profitably be focused on the social–psychological sequellae of the various forms of malnutrition and on the exact mechanisms by which environmental stresses such as malnutrition influence attitudes, moods, and personality development. Attitudes, moods, and personality, of course, also affect school, work, and social performance, thus demanding a model capable of integrating nutritional, cognitive, and psychosocial factors.

Recently, Marc LaLonde (1974), Minister of Health of Canada, has proposed a new national strategy for dealing with the health problems associated with populations living in nations with high levels of affluence, health care, and access to nutritional requirements. His approach is similar to those advocated by Canosa (1968), Gordon (1968), Jellife (1966), and Robson (1972). These authors view health and disease in a total ecological context. Instead of linearly tracing diseases influencing health and well-being separately, they demonstrate a strong association among a whole series of cases of mortality and morbidity of which malnutrition is one.

CONCLUSIONS

This paper suggests some themes for future specific investigations. First, it is evident that over long periods most societies establish an equilibrium with regard to nutritional resources that allows living members to survive. Most sociocultural systems have elaborate mechanisms to deal with nutritional resources during periods of scarcity. However, there are limits to these adaptations, and they warrant further study.

Another important problem is related to specific excesses and/or deficiencies in diet. When malnutrition results in specific behavioral impairment (Thomson & Pollitt; Stanbury; Greene; Read; this volume), it becomes imperative to study the potentially dramatic consequences that corrective actions can have on social organization. It is possible that replacement of dietary deficiencies for which there have already been significant social organizational adaptations may produce some unplanned-for consequences due to the rapid rate of change in behavior and health status of the afflicted individuals.

The ultimate social and economic costs of malnutrition associated with overconsumption and misconsumption are particularly great in nations just achieving modernity. Health and nutritional planning must include ecosystem approaches capable of identifying the feedback relationships linking diet and social–psychological behaviors. The problems of malnutrition are obviously not only limited to developing nations but are important factors in the social-psychological structures of developed nations as well.

REFERENCES

Canosa, C. A. Ecological approach to the problem of malnutrition, learning and behavior. In N. S. Scrimshaw & J. E. Gordon (Eds.), *Malnutrition, learning and behavior.* Cambridge, Massachusetts: MIT Press, 1968. Pp. 389–396.

Chagnon, N. Yanomamö social organization and warfare. In M. Fried, R. Harris, & R. Murphy (Eds.), *War: The anthropology of armed combat and aggression.* Garden City, New York: Doubleday, Natural History Press, 1968. Pp. 109–159. (a)

Chagnon, N. *Yanomamö: The fierce people.* New York: Holt, Rinehart & Winston, 1968. (b)

Chagnon, N. The culture-ecology of shifting (pioneering) cultivation among the Yanomamö Indians. In D. R. Gross (Ed.), *Peoples and cultures of native South America.* Garden City, New York: Doubleday, Natural History Press, 1973. Pp. 126–144.

Czaplica, M. *Aboriginal Siberia: A study in anthropology.* New York: Oxford Univ. Press (Clarendon), 1914.

Denko, J., & Kaelbling, R. The psychiatric aspects of hypoparathyroidism. *Acta Psychiatria Scandanavia,* 1962, *164,* (38), 1–70.

Foulks, E. F. *The arctic hysterias of the north Alaska Eskimo.* In David Maybury-Lewis (Ed.), Anthropological Studies #10. Washington, D.C.: American Anthropological Association Press, 1972.

Foulks, E., Freeman, D. M. A., & Freeman, P. Preoedipal dynamics in a case of Eskimo arctic hysteria. In W. Muensterberger (Ed.), *Psychoanalytic study of society.* Vol. 8. New Haven, Connecticut: Yale University Press, 1977.

Gordon, J., Ascoli, W., Mata, L., Gusman, M., & Scrimshaw, N. Nutrition and infection field study in Guatemala villages 1959–1964 VI. *Archives of Environmental Health*, 1968, *16*, 424–437.

Gross, D. Protein capture and cultural development in the Amazon Basin. *American Anthropologist*, 1975, *77*, (3) 526–549.

Gussow, Z. Pibloktoq (hysteria) among the polar Eskimo: An ethno-psychiatric study. In W. Muensterberger & S. Axelrad (Eds.), *The psychoanalytic study of society*. New York: International University Press, 1960. Pp. 218–236.

Harrington, C., & Whiting, J. Socialization process and personality. In F. Hsu (Ed.), *Psychological anthropology*. Cambridge, Massachusetts: Shenkman, 1972.

Heller, C., & Scott, E. The Alaska dietary survey 1956–1961. *Public Health Service Publication* #999-AH-2. Washington, D.C.: U.S. Government Printing Office, 1961.

Jellife, D. The assessment of the nutritional status of the community. *World Health Organization*, Monograph Series No. 53, Geneva, 1966.

Jochelson, W. The Koryak in the Jessup north Pacific Expedition. In F. Boas (Ed.), *Memoirs, American Museum of Natural History*, New York, 1908. Pp. 416–417.

LaLond, M. *A new perspective on the health of Canadians. Public Health Publication* #H31-1374, Government Printing Office. Ottawa, 1974.

Mazess, R., & Mather, W. Bone mineral content in Canadian eskimos. *Human Biology*, 1975, *47*, (1), 45–63.

Meggers, B. *Amazonia: Man and culture in a counterfeit paradise*. Chicago: Aldine, 1971.

Parker, S. Eskimo psychopathology. *American Anthropologist*, 1962, *64*, 74–76.

Peary, R. *The north pole*. New York: Fredrich Stokes, 1910.

Robson, J. R. K. *Malnutrition: Its causation and control, with special reference to protein-calorie malnutrition*. New York: Gordon and Beach, 1972.

Schmitt, F. O., Parvati, D., & Smith, B. H. Electronic processing of information by brain cells. *Science*, 1976, *193*, 114–120.

Stefansson, W. *My life with the Eskimo*. New York: Collier, 1945.

Turnbull, C. *The mountain people*. New York: Simon & Shuster, 1972.

Wallace, A. F. C. Mental illness, biology and culture. In F. Hsu (Ed.), *Psychological anthropology*. Cambridge, Massachusetts: Shenkman, 1972. Pp. 363–403.

10

Malnutrition: Its Effect on Psychological Development and Cultural Evolution

EUGENE G. D'AQUILI AND GARY J. MIHALIK

University of Pennsylvania

INTRODUCTION

The purpose of this chapter is to consider the effects of malnutrition on both psychological development and cultural evolution via its effect on the genesis and transformation of cognitive structures. There are several steps that must be elucidated before we can understand the effect of malnutrition on psychological development and cultural evolution. First of all, we must understand the importance of cognitive structures in the psychological development of the individual and in the underlying mechanism generating cultural change. Next, we must understand the relationship of malnutrition to the development and function of the neocortex. Finally, we must understand the relationship of cognitive structures as classically understood (either by developmental psychologists, structural anthropologists, or linguists) to organic neurostructure (either macrostructure or microstructure) involving primarily anatomical relationships within the neocortex. Ultimately, the effects of malnutrition on neocortical development will be correlated with structure formation and transformation. Obviously, a detailed analysis of each of these steps would require much more space than is allotted. We must content ourselves, therefore, with a cursory examination of the major points in the hope that an understanding of the overall significance of malnutrition for the development and transformation of cognitive structures will compensate for the lack of detailed exposition at each individual step.

STRUCTURALISM

Vertical and Horizontal Structures

Before we can attempt to understand the devastating effect of malnutrition on psychological development and cultural evolution, we must first attempt to understand its effect on the development and transformation of structures, but this understanding itself depends on our awareness of the importance of structuralism to modern scientific thought. Perhaps Gunther Stent (1972) has most succinctly summarized the importance of structuralism. He states:

It is only in the past 20 years or so, more or less contemporaneously with the growth of molecular biology, that a resolution of the age-old epistemological conflict of materialism vs. idealism was found in the form of what has come to be known as structuralism.
. . . Both materialism and idealism take it for granted that all the information gathered by our senses actually reaches our mind; materialism envisions that thanks to this information reality is mirrored in the mind, whereas idealism envisions that thanks to this information reality is constructed by the mind. Structuralism, on the other hand, has provided the insight that knowledge about the world enters the mind not as raw data but in some already highly abstracted form, namely as structures. In the preconscious process of converting the primary data of our experience step by step into structure, information is necessarily lost, because the creation of structures, or the recognition of patterns, is nothing less than the selective destruction of information. Thus since the mind does not gain access to full set of data about the world, it can neither mirror nor construct reality. Instead for the mind reality is a set of structural transforms of primary data taken from the world. This transformation process is hierarchical, in that "stronger" structures are formed from "weaker" structures through selective destruction of information. Any set of primary data becomes meaningful only after a series of such operations has so transformed it that it has become congruent with a stronger structure preexisting in the mind. Neurophysiological studies carried out in recent years on the process of visual perception in higher mammals have not only shown directly that the brain operates according to the tenets of structuralism but also offer an easily understood illustration of those tenets [pp. 92–93].

For the most part, Stent is here advancing the understanding of structuralism that is most often propounded by biologists and that provides the most rational basis for an understanding of developmental psychology. Consequently, this "vertical" view of structures and structural transformation, that is, the more complex structures deriving from simpler structures, is very similar to the model propounded by Piaget (1948, 1971). There is another, "horizontal" view of structures that is most often presented within the social sciences and linguistics. This approach views a structure as a closed system in which transformation means the rearrangement of a given, and more or less unchangeable, number of elements. The confusion between the two approaches comes from the fact that social scientists and linguists appear to be primarily interested in a specific level of structural complexity, namely, cognitive structures, and in the rules of transformation that apply specifically to cognitive structures. A careful analysis of both approaches does not reveal that they are in any way disparate. Rather, *the social science model represents an intensive study of a specific level of structural complexity within the vertical scheme propounded by the biological model.* Perhaps some insight into this problem can be gained by viewing how each school regards transformations. Biologists and developmental psychologists generally deal with "open structures." The concept of transformation in this case often signifies the replacing of a set of elements (A) with another set of elements (B) with a one to one correspondence obtaining between a given element in set A and a given element in set B. Thus biologists will often speak of subjective perception as a transformation of incoming sensory stimuli. In a theoretical vein, psychoanalysis uses much the same meaning of transformation in the replacement of elements of cognition and affect with a totally different set of elements resulting in the symbology of dreams and fantasy material. The second, or social science, understanding of transformation and structure is best exemplified by the sense given to the word by Chomsky (1957) and Lévi-Strauss (1963 a, b). In this case, the elements of a structure are invariant, and the meaning of transformation is associated only with the rules of their recombination. Structures understood in this sense are closed systems, and the meaning of transformation is here the polar opposite of the sense just given for open system. This "social science" sense of the word transformation is more in keeping with the understanding of structure that we will consider in our subsequent analysis of psychological development and culture change. It is, however, important that we be able to integrate this sense of structure and transformation into the more general biological understanding.

A third and more comprehensive meaning of the words structure and transformation can be formulated that, we feel, can integrate both senses of the words that we have delineated above. In this third sense, more complex structures develop from simpler ones. More specifically, developmental psychology can be viewed as the progressive elaboration of a series of nesting structures of increasing complexity. At any given level of complexity, the elements that make up that level remain reasonably stable in number, and transformation within any given level of complexity involves rearrangement of elements only within that level. In this view, transformation can be understood as three processes:

1. Possible alteration or substitution of one element for another as in the case of full open structures
2. Addition of new elements of content that were not previously present in the simpler structures
3. Specific rules of reorganization of all the elements of content at a given level such as is typically understood in the Levi-Straussian or Chomskian understanding of transformation.

Such an overall view of structures and transformation allows for a classical Piagetian model of nesting structures, which has often been described as "the form of the simpler structure becoming the content of the more complex." This comprehensive understanding of structure may be called a "semiclosed" system. We choose to call it "semiclosed" because we feel that this term emphasizes the fact that structures are highly stable neural systems not easily changed but not absolutely and permanently fixed in either an ontogenic or in a phylogenetic sense. This approach also allows for the rules of synchronic reorganization of elements within a given level of complexity, usually the cognitive level, which is the sense of structure and transformation understood in the social sciences. There has been so much confusion recently about the various usages of the terms "structure" and "transformation" that we feel that the foregoing clarification is essential. To give some perspective of the level at which we are operating, we must state at this point that, for the purposes of this chapter, we are interested only in the level of complexity that comprises cognitive structures. From here on, therefore, *structure* will be used in the sense of a *"semiclosed" system* and *transformation* in the sense of a *rearrangement of more or less invariant elements within a given cognitive structure.*

Properties of Structures

The next point that we must take up is to consider what is meant by a cognitive structure per se and to attempt to demonstrate that such structures are related, in fact, to the function of specific areas of the neocortex that can be and are affected by malnutrition. The concept of cognitive structure is neither revolutionary nor novel. Beck (1963, 1964) has discussed the nature of depression in terms of cognitive models. He described a *cognitive model* as a relatively enduring component of cognitive organization in contrast to *cognitive process*, which can and does often change. A number of other cognitive psychologists and psychiatrists have proposed similar concepts to explain observed regularities of cognitive behavior. One can cite Piaget's "schemata" (1948), Postman's "categories" (1951), Rapaport's "conceptual tools" (1951), Kelly's "personal constructs" (1955), the "coding systems" of Bruner, Woodnow, and Austen (1956), the "modules" of Sarbin, Taft, and Bailey (1960), and the "concepts" of Harvey, Hunt, and Schroder (1961). These are all entities similar conceptually to a "cognitive structure" as we have been considering it. Thus, there is a great deal of evidence from both experimental and cognitive psychology that regularities of cognition exist and, furthermore, that they are inordinately stable configurations.

From an evolutionary point of view, one would almost expect, *a priori*, that some stable organizational aspect of cognition had to develop in order that human behavior might possess an acceptable degree of predictability and cohesion. Although cognitive structures are stable, they are by no means unchangeable since immutability would be highly maladaptive in a radically changing environment. Consequently, cognitive structures possess not only the property of stability but also the capacity for transformation or rearrangement of elements generating a new meaning complex from those same elements. Such rearrangement can be described by what have come to be known as rules of transformation. Lévi-Strauss and the school of French structuralism (Lévi-Strauss, 1963a, b, c, 1969) have presented compelling evidence that the "surface structures" of cultural institutions represent only transformations of a "deep structure" for any given cultural institution. Chomsky and his school arrive at similar conclusions with respect to the "deep" and "surface" structure of language. If one accepts the conclusions of these anthropologists and linguists, it becomes obvious that any given language or any given cultural institution represents but a transformation of a deep structure that itself is seen not so much as a social entity but as a property of a mental activity projected into the social domain. Lévi-Strauss himself maintains that cultural institutions can be explained primarily as a social projection of psychology or, more properly, as a social projection of cognitive structures and their rules of transformation.

We have alluded above to the property of structures that can best be termed stability. We must now turn to that other property, the ability for the rearrangement of their elements, which we have called transformations. It should be obvious that the ability of a given structure to undergo transformation when presented with external exigencies with which it is noncongruent is absolutely essential for survival. If an individual cannot generate alternate transformations of a given structure when challenged by changing environmental exigencies, then his coping mechanism is severely inhibited, and under primitive circumstances of adaptation, he will most probably perish. In an industrialized society, he will most probably be institutionalized with a label of some sort, either of mental illness or of decreased mental capacity, depending on how severely the transformation mechanism is impaired. All the evidence to date indicates that we organize our knowledge systematically and, furthermore, that its reorganization or change is itself systematic, representing system within a system. Not only sound mental health but actual physical survival is dependent on the ability of the individual to generate viable structural transformations.

What we have said about the individual is equally applicable to society and to the mechanism of cultural change. If indeed it is true that social structures are but a projection of cognitive structures, then the spectrum of variability on which selection acts to foster alternate societal forms under conditions of environmental change is quantitatively directly proportional to the number of individuals in the society who generate viable transformations of the cognitive structures underlying the cultural institutions. Put another way, if a large number of individuals in any society are capable of cognitive transformations of social institutions that are no longer adaptive, then the society presents a great number of alternatives on which selection can act. In such a case, the probability of the society's reshaping its institutions into more adaptive forms becomes markedly increased. If, on the other hand, for any reason (such as malnutrition, as we shall see presently), only a relatively small number of individuals are able to generate transformations of the cognitive structures underlying the societal institutions, then the number of alternative forms on which natural selection can operate becomes diminished. In such circumstances, the probability of the society's surviving under altered circumstances decreases. Of course, the mechanisms for an individual's coping with the environment and a society's adapting to the environment are identical because they are both based on the mechanism of transformation of cognitive structures. In the case of the individual, alternate transformations are tried and tested against input from the environment until the "best fit" is obtained. In the case of societal change, a number of viable alternatives must be presented by a number of individuals in the society. Thus, for example, if only 10 or 20 individuals cognitively generated an adaptive transformation, one still might not be selected for social implementation since there would probably not be enough people proposing the same alternative to allow it to be "heard" as a societal movement. Therefore, for adaptive culture change, the variety on which selection acts is composed not simply of a number of potentially viable cognitive transformations of the institution but of a number of clusters of individuals. Each cluster must be large enough to be perceived as a societal movement, and each cluster must represent one viable transformation of an existing cultural institution. In any case, the capacity for the great majority of the population of a given society to generate alternative transformations in times of stress and for members to cluster with other members proposing the same alternative (so that a number of clusters of individuals are present in the society, with each cluster proposing alternative plans) is essential for the survival of societies, especially under conditions of radical environmental change. Therefore, it appears that not only the adequate coping of the individual but also the potential for societal change rests squarely on the ability of individuals to organize their world into cognitive structures that are, to some degree, isomorphic with the external world, and which structures are capable of undergoing transformation in predictable ways under the stress of environmental change.

STRUCTURAL TRANSFORMATION

We now come to the most important part of this chapter, that is, the relationship of certain types of malfunctions of the structural-transformation system to malnutrition. First of all, it is our task to present at least a tentative model by which cognitive structures and their transformations can be seen to involve neural processes and, if possible, to delineate specific neural mechanisms underlying such processes. If, for example, we can demonstrate that it is highly probable that the generation and transformation of structures involve a certain localized area of the neocortex, then the extensive evidence indicating gross and microanatomical cortical abnormalities following severe protein-calorie malnutrition (PCM) would point to very specific and predictable consequences both in terms of psychological development of the individual and in terms of cultural evolution. This would be due to interference with these neural mechanisms and consequently with the structural-transformation system. One of the major problems heretofore has been that the concepts of cognitive structure, transformation, schemata, models, coding devices, etc., have been conceptual entities inferred by cognitive psychologists, anthropologists, or linguists from behavioral data. We feel strongly that until such constructs can be shown to have a basis in neuroanatomy and neurophysiology, they will be of heuristic value only. Conversely, if at least a tentative model, based on recent research in the neurosciences, can be presented relating cognitive structure to organic neurostructure, then important conclusions can be drawn as to the probable effects of physical agents on the neurostructure and consequently on the system of cognitive structures and transformation. We will now attempt to present a model for the biological basis of structures and transformations preparatory to considering the effect of severe malnutrition on them.

NEOCORTICAL FUNCTIONING AND THE "BIOLOGY" OF STRUCTURES

Localization of Structures

The very existence of cognitive structures presupposes the ability of an organism to abstract dimensions of meaning from the universe by which he can define the set of elements that are contained within a semantic field. We have elsewhere (d'Aquili, 1972; Laughlin & d'Aquili, 1974) described in detail the importance of the evolution of the inferior parietal lobule and its interrelationship with the anterior convexity of the frontal lobes (Luria, 1966) in the evolution of the capacity for abstraction and conceptualization. Suffice it to say here that it was most probably the evolutionary elaboration of these neural structures among the *Hominidae* that ultimately resulted in the capacity for abstract conceptualization characteristic of *Homo sapiens*. In short, the ability to generate the abstract dimensions that define a semantic field necessary to the generation of cognitive structures most probably resulted from the morphological development of these areas of the neocortex.

Thus far, we have attempted to relate the definition of a semantic field and its abstract cognitive contents (concepts) to the evolution and morphological interrelationship (via fiber tracts) of the anterior convexity of the frontal lobes and the area that Geschwind (1965) terms the inferior parietal lobule, that is, the area comprising the angular gyrus, supramarginal gyrus, and some immediately adjacent areas. This model only explains, as it were, the limits of the set and the neural origin of the cognitive structure *if* one considers a cognitive structure as analogous to a mathematical set. But cognitive structures have other properties (Piaget, 1970) that must be explained in terms of a biological model. Those properties include the circumstance that each element of the set is in fact related to each other element at a specific point in time and, furthermore, that the elements can be rearranged in terms of alternate relationships between the elements over time and under specific circumstances. It is this latter property that we term the transformation of structures and for which we are also attempting a biological model.

Let us now turn our attention to the possible basic relationships that can exist between elements of any cognitive structure. We maintain that on the simplest and most primitive level those relationships are essentially spatial, temporal, affective, or some combination of the preceding three. It has been known for a long time that the parietal lobe on the nondominant side is concerned with the perception of spatial relationships. Recent experiments with animals as well as observations of humans who have had their corpus callosum and anterior commissure sectioned to prevent the spread of epilepsy have strongly supported the early clinical observations of neurologists that the parietal lobe on the nondominant side is intimately involved in the perception of spatial relations. Indeed, most of the recent evidence indicates that this perception is of a holistic or gestalt nature (Bogen, 1969; Gazzaniga, 1970; Sperry, Gazzaniga, & Bogen, 1969; Gazzaniga & Hillyard, 1971; Levy-Agresti & Sperry, 1968; Nebes & Sperry, 1971; Trevarthen, 1969). It is of more than passing interest that specific areas on the opposite or dominant side are related to the performance of mathematical operations (specifically, the angular gyrus) and to the performance of certain basic logical–grammatical operations. These operations include the perception of opposites and the ability to set one object off against another to emphasize more fully its semantic properties, a quality that underlies the use of the comparative degree of adjectives in language (Luria, 1966). These and other basic logical–grammatical functions are related to areas of the parietal lobe adjacent to the angular gyrus and proximate to the anterior margin of the occipital lobe. Lesions of this area in man prevent the generation of antonyms as well as the use of the comparative degree of adjectives. In short, such lesions prevent the formation of *abstract dyadic oppositions* or polarities, which is a function basic to human cognition, and one that we have considered elsewhere in relation to the generation of myths (d'Aquili & Laughlin, 1975). The point of all this is that it is probably no coincidence that those neural structures that appear to generate gestalt spatial perception on the nondominant side are homologous to those structures that underlie mathematical, logical, and grammatical relationships. It is certainly no news that mathematics and mathematical operations appear to derive from the quantification of spatial properties. It is our contention that basic logical-grammatical operations are likewise so derived.

If one considers the holistic perception of spatial relationships as the more primitively evolved or more "basic" function of the parietal lobe, one could easily postulate that this has been preserved or even elaborated in man on the nondominant side. Modification on the contralateral, or dominant, side has been in the opposite direction, that is, breaking down the spatial gestalt into various composite units and relationships. This goes along with our contention that the evolution of the *Hominidae* is most characteristically marked by the evolution of analytical cognitive processes that permitted the evolution of abstract thought and problem solving. Such analytical processes most probably involved a modification and elaboration of the more primitive gestalt operations on what we now call the nondominant side into what we recognize as the analytical functions that we associate with the dominant hemisphere of the brain. Such elaboration of function, and probably also of microstructure, was just that, that is, a modification of more primitive functions.

The analytical functions of the dominant side do not arise out of nothing but are intimately related to the more primitive operations preserved, and probably further elaborated, on the non-dominant side. Thus, one can postulate that the parieto-occipital area on the dominant side developed not so much to perceive spatial relationships in their total configuration but developed the ability to perform the operation that we would now call the division of space into coordinate axes and, furthermore, the capability of cognitively defining axes in terms of the polar termini of each axis. In this second operation, one can begin to perceive the basis of conceptual dyadic opposition beginning to derive from the evolution of an analytical perception of space. Furthermore, there is considerable neurophysiological evidence (Luria, 1966; Pribram & Luria, 1973) that the ordering of events in time, or, more properly, into a temporal sequence, is a result of the reciprocal interrelationship between these parietal areas and the anterior convexities of the frontal lobes via evolved fiber tracts. Furthermore, we have elsewhere attempted to show (d'Aquili & Laughlin, 1974) that this basic temporal ordering of conceptual material underlies the faculty of abstract causal thinking, which in turn underlies both abstract problem solving and the development of "cultural tradition." In short, we propose that the most sophisticated mathematical, logical, or grammatical operation can ultimately be reduced to the simplest spatial and temporal analyses, which themselves can be understood as an evolutionary elaboration of the more gestalt operations of the primitive neocortex, more or less preserved in the nondominant hemisphere of the brain.

Consequently, we would argue that the apparent multiplicity of relationships between elements of a cognitive structure can be reduced to a relatively small list of ultimately basic analytical relationships, including (1) inside–outside, (2) above–below, (3) in front–behind, etc. These relatively few basic spatiotemporal relationships can be enriched by combining them with an affective or emotional valence. Thus, "inside" is usually identified with good and "outside" with bad, "above" with good and "below" with bad, etc. These affective valences are *not* absolute, and the reverse of any of them may appear. However, it is interesting to note how frequently the relationships just mentioned do in fact culturally receive the affective valence stated. We feel that there is a reason for this association, which involves issues of simple preservation, "above" usually being safer than "below" and therefore good, "inside" being usually safer than "outside" and therefore good, "in front" being usually safer than "behind" and therefore good, etc. Nevertheless, we must reiterate that the reverse of these associations *can* theoretically occur, and, in fact, occasionally does.

Instead of embarking on the nearly impossible task of listing all the possible complex relationships that can exist between elements of a cognitive structure, we have chosen rather to attempt to reduce them to a handful of simple spatiotemporal relationships. We feel that it can be practically demonstrated that all complex relationships, whether they be mathematical, logical, or grammatical, can be reduced to either one or a combination of the basic spatiotemporal relationships that we have just considered. This is true with respect to all relationships with the single exception of affective or emotional relationships. These latter represent feeling states and are of crucial importance since they, in one way or another, enter into moral and value judgments. On the most primitive level, they can be resolved into whether a stimulus is positive or aversive for an organism. Simply put, that which is good is that which provides either immediate or delayed gratification for the organism; that which is bad is that which the organism experiences as unpleasurable or not conducive to survival. As with the spatiotemporal relationships, the basic affective relationships can be elaborated into a number of subtle feeling states and can be related to perception and cognition in various ways. The neurophysiological substrate for such affective-cognitive perceptual linkages is undoubtedly the numerous connections known to exist between various limbic structures and either the secondary sensory association areas (in the case of perceptions) or the inferior parietal lobule (in the case of cognition).

Structural Transformation and the Neocortex

Thus far, we have attempted to delineate the basic classes of relationships that obtain between elements of a cognitive structure, that is, spatial, temporal, and affective. We have attempted to present a tentative neurophysiological model for the evolution of such relationships. All this brings us to the problem of transformations themselves, which represents, as we have noted above, the rearrangement of the relationships of elements of a cognitive structure.

The major question with which we are concerned here is, given the principal cognitive elements contained within a semantic field and given a number of possible relationships between each dyad of the cognitive elements (the possible relationships being generated by the neural structures that we have discussed above), why is it that any given set of relationships changes? Put in other words, this last question could be formulated: "Under what circumstances does the surface manifestation of a structure undergo a transformation?"

Considering the work of Lévi-Strauss and his school, as well as the findings, of a number of cognitive psychologists (Harvey et al., 1961; Lévi-Strauss, 1963 a,b; Piaget, 1970) it seems that structures are not only composed of relationships between dyads of cognitive elements, such relationships setting one element off against another for semantic clarity but that the relationships *themselves* can be grouped into dyads involving opposing the spatial, temporal, of affective relationships that we have considered above, such as, up–down, left–right, before–after, good–bad, etc. Thus, every pair of relationships involves three or four cognitive elements, four cognitive elements if each pole of the two relationships is separate or three cognitive elements if one cognitive element is common to two polar dyads. One of the few ways in which the work of cognitive psychologists and particularly of Lévi-Strauss (1963a, b, c, 1969) can be made to make sense is if we postulate that it is inherent within the machinery of the brain to relate the cognitive elements of a structure in such a way that, for every pair related by one aspect of a relationship such as "up" *at least* one other pair must be related by the opposite relationship, that is, "down." Furthermore, one must postulate that these relations obtain in such a way that if the elements related by "up" are changed so that they are now related by "down," those related by "down" must now become related by "up," otherwise the reciprocal change would result in nonsense. Unless one postulates some such system of reciprocal change attendant upon transformation, one simply cannot explain, for example, the almost algebraic neatness of Lévi-Strauss's famous solution of the problem of affective valence between son-father, nephew-mother's brother, etc. (Lévi-Strauss, 1963).

Note that we stated that the postulate of reciprocal change is operative only when the reciprocal change involves a new surface structure that has meaning. Certain combinations can obviously involve nonsense. It would appear at this point that we are invoking the subjective entity of meaning to be the constraint within which basic neurophysiological processes operate. If this were true, then the phenomenon would be dependent on the epiphenomenon, and we would be reduced to absolute idealism. On the contrary, we would state rather that those constellations of relationships between cognitive elements of a structure that we consider meaningful possess that quality of "meaningfulness" simply because they *are* the subjective manifestations of inherently stable relationships within the neural microstructure, the locus of which probably resides in various configurations of postsynaptic slow wave potentials. The very stability of the overall constellation of relationships and of the neural events that generate them is precisely what we mean when we state that a given surface manifestation of structure is meaningful. "Meaningfulness" therefore derives from the stability of neural connections, and this stability in turn derives from the selection of certain combinations of neural configurations as being adaptive and thus conducive to survival. It is only in this sense of the word "meaning" that we will say that meaning imposes constraints on the postulate of reciprocal change during a transformation. Thus, any given cognitive (and by extension social) structure is limited in the number of possible transformations not by the theoretical total of all the permutations generated by the postulate of reciprocal change but to a number that represents a subset of the total set, that is, those possible transformations that are also meaningful subjectively, which is to say those that have adaptive properties and represent a high degree of isomorphism with the external world.

The answer to why any given constellation of relationships between elements of a semantic field is stable at all at a given time is simply because it is the most adaptive psychologically for an individual or sociologically for a group. It is the environment, therefore, that ultimately imposes the constraints that define exactly which surface manifestation of a deep structure will obtain, either cognitively or socially, at any given time. It is change in the environment ultimately that causes a disconfirmation of a given surface structure as representing the external world and that forces a change in one or more relationships between cognitive elements. Once one change is forced, multiple relationships within the entire system become rearranged by the postulate of reciprocal change, generating a number of possible configurations, until that configuration that is most adaptive to the circumstances becomes fixed (either for the individual or for the group). It seems to us that when Wallace (1970) speaks of mazeway resynthesis, what he is essentially talking about is the rearrangement of relationships between multiple dyads (usually under the influence of intense limbic arousal) of a superordinate structure involving the relationship of the individual to the universe as a whole. Thus, mazeway resynthesis can be seen as a transformation of the most encompassing superordinate cognitive structure under conditions of intense stress. It is a testimony to the stability of cognitive structures that only the most severe stresses, the most intense states of limbic arousal, are able to facilitate the transformation of important superordinate structures.

As we have seen, it is the environment that is the principal determinant of both the content of cognitive elements that comprise structures and of the fixing of a given constellation of relationships of cognitive elements at any point in time. Furthermore, it is the environment that ultimately governs when either an individual cognitive structure (or a social structure) will undergo transformation. We hope we have emphasized the crucial quality of the *interrelationship* between the central nervous system and the environment in generating culture and cultural change in presenting a biological model for structures and transformations that rests heavily on environmental determinants to explain structural stability and the conditions generating structural change.

MALNUTRITION AND STRUCTURAL TRANSFORMATIONS

And so we come at last to the effect of severe PCM on the cognitive structural–transformation system. We have just seen that there is con-

siderable evidence implicating certain areas of the neocortex, specifically the parieto-occipital region and the anterior convexity of the
frontal lobes. If further investigation supports these initial findings,
and if the model presented in this paper for a biological basis of the
cognitive structural-transformation system is valid, then one must
postulate that whatever affects the development and functioning of
the neocortex, particularly of the regions mentioned, must necessarily
affect the cognitive structural–transformation system with all the implications that such a deficit would have for the psychological development of the individual and for the mechanism of cultural evolution.

Lester (1975) has demonstrated an attentional deficit in malnourished infants. If this malnutrition is early and severe enough, it
can permanently damage intellectual functioning (Cabak & Najdanvic, 1965; Monckenberg, 1968). Indeed, in a study of children rehabilitated from kwashiorkor (occurring from 6 months onward), most
were found to have significant decreases in IQ (Champakam, Srikantia,
& Gopalan, 1968; Birch, Pineiro, Alcade, Toca, & Cravioto, 1971).
Geber and Dean (1956) showed that early, severe kwashiorkor resulted in most impairment to language and locomotor skills.

A study done by Evans, Moodie, and Hansen (1971) of children
admitted to the hospital between the ages of 10–48 months for
kwashiorkor found few significant differences in mental functioning
between them and controls. It is most important to note, however, that
there were *no early admissions* (6 months or less) in this study.
Cravioto and Robles (1965) have suggested that if the onset of
kwashiorkor is late enough (significantly beyond 6 months), it may
leave no noticeable effects after rehabilitation.

There is also significant evidence that indicates that whatever effects do remain from a serious episode of either marasmus or
kwashiorkor, these effects tend to diminish with time. (Champakam *et
al.*, 1968; Brockman & Ricciuti, 1970).

It appears, then, that there is a critical period in neurological development before which malnutrition has a severe effect and after
which the effects are nearly totally reversible. Since the onset of
kwashiorkor is usually after this critical period, whereas marasmus
may begin from shortly after birth, the detrimental effects of
kwashiorkor may ameliorate with time. All of this is summed up in the
Waterlow-Rutishauser hypothesis (Waterlow & Rutishauser, 1974),
which relates the average onset times of these two forms of PCM with
their long-term effects on intellectual functioning.

In spite of all the evidence, which shows that in some instances the effects of PCM may diminish with increasing age, there are many instances in which they do *not* diminish significantly. These, then, are of much more importance to the subject of this chapter. DeLicardie and Cravioto (1974) examined the behavioral response style to cognitive demands in 5-year-old children who had suffered from severe PMC between the ages of 4 and 38 months. Their results showed that the previously malnourished group (M) made a significantly smaller proportion of work responses to cognitive demands than either of 2 sets of controls. In addition, of the total number of responses, a significantly smaller proportion were verbal for group M.

Klein, Lester, Yarbrough, and Habicht (1975) showed that previously malnourished but subsequently rehabilitated 14-month-old infants did not respond as quickly to either a novel stimulus or a change in stimulus as did well-nourished children.

From the above brief discussion, it is obvious that there are neurological correlates to PCM during and subsequent to the period of malnutrition. For a more complete discussion of this subject, see Thomson and Pollitt; Stanbury; Greene; and Read (this volume–Chapters 2, 3, 4, and 5). In addition, the work of Marcondes *et al.* (1973) and Winick and Rosso (1969), indicating general reduction of brain weight and definite cortical atrophy in both forms of PCM (kwashiorkor and marasmus) but most especially marked in the marasmic condition, is of particular significance. On the basis of the anatomical finding of severe cortical atrophy alone, one would postulate *a priori* a deficit in the cognitive structural-transformation system that we have been discussing, especially if such atrophy were general (as it is), and clearly included the parieto-occipital region and the anterior convexities of the frontal lobes.

> Research data have indicated that the severely malnourished child is characterized by apathy, withdrawal, low responsivity to environmental stimuli, and poor attention maintenance. This lethargic behavior ensures that the child fares poorly in competition for attention with others in the environment. As a result, learning experiences are curtailed because of reduced reciprocal mother-child interaction. Low-level functioning also limits the child's capacity to act on his own environment. According to the theories of Piaget, limitations in child–environment interactions interfere with intellectual development. In Piagetian terms, the child and the environment form an interlocking system whose interactions generate mental structures, which are the substrates of knowledge. The low level of interaction typical of the malnourished child thus leads to developmental retardation [Thomson & Pollitt, this volume].

With respect to this "developmental retardation," we think it is important to consider in particular the studies of Brockman and Ricciuti (1970) and of Cravioto and DeLicardie (1972, 1975). In commenting on them Thomson and Pollitt have stated that these "two studies . . . in which such tests (categorization and bipolar concepts) were used failed to provide evidence of construct validity. In both cases, the assumption behind the choice was that the process selected for analysis is central to overall cognitive development." Whether these two processes, that is, categorization and bipolar conceptualization, are in fact central to overall cognitive ability is a matter for dispute. But that these processes are indeed central to cognitive structure development and transformation should by this time be very clear in view of the evidence that we have presented above. Since these investigators have indeed implicated a fairly severe deficit of categorization and bipolar conceptualization as a result of severe PCM, we must assume that the processes of cognitive structure formation and transformation are severely impaired under such circumstances. One would postulate that, in the case of maximal impairment, stable structures are simply not produced. The expectation would be that meaningful, consistent behavior would thus be severely hampered and that individuals possessing such a deficit would perish without the specific agency of society providing institutions to care for them. However, if the impairment of these functions is not total, one would expect the imposition on the individual of rigid cognitive structures that, once established, would not undergo transformation even in the presence of overwhelming disconfirming evidence from the environment. Such a lack of plasticity of neural functioning is a direct corollary of the anatomical changes resulting in atrophy on the "macro" level and of the impoverishment of dendritic–synaptic connections on the "micro" level. In the face of this, there can be little doubt that severe malnutrition results in impairment of the cognitive structural–transformation system. Furthermore, at least with regard to the marasmic state during the first year of life, it is fairly clear that some degree of deficit in this system is permanent even after proper nutrition has been initiated.

The implications of such a situation are staggering in terms of the mechanisms both for personal survival and for culture change and societal survival that we have discussed above. As we have seen these mechanisms are intimately related to the proper functioning of the cognitive structural–transformation system. In short, severe malnutrition can prevent the individual from adapting to his environment by preventing the proper development and especially the appropriate transformations of structures or models of the world that ordinarily are formed as a result of the interaction between the individual and his environment. Furthermore, fairly severe PCM in large segments of a society is likely to decrease the number of individuals with variable options (transformations) of social institutions, as well as probably to decrease the number of options themselves. Without a sufficient number of individuals clustering around the principal alternatives to any given social structure, there simply will not exist enough viable variability on which selection can operate. Simply put, such a situation will spell death for a society.

CONCLUSION

The path that we have taken in this chapter has been perhaps too circuitous for many scholars' ideal of simplicity. To traverse this path in reverse, we have seen the effect of serious malnutrition on the neocortex and on the development and transformation of cognitive structures. We have seen the importance of cognitive structures and their transformations for the adaptation of an individual to his environment as well as for the mechanism of cultural change. The overall conclusion, although several steps removed from its logical beginning, is nevertheless of major importance. For the individual, the effect of serious malnutrition at this point is obvious in terms of cognitive maladaptation to a changing environment. For societies as a whole in which severe malnutrition is endemically present, the consequences are just as devastating under conditions of major environmental stress. Such societies simply become nonviable. In a word, they lose the basis of the variability that any healthy society needs to survive.

REFERENCES

Beck, A. T. Thinking and depression. I. Idiosyncratic content and cognitive distortions. *Archives of General Psychiatry*, 1963, 9, 324–333.
Beck, A. T. Thinking and depression. II. Theory and therapy. *Archives of General Psychiatry*, 1964, 10, 561–571.
Birch, H. E., Pineiro, C., Alcalde, E., Toca, T., & Cravioto, J. Relation of kwashiorkor in early childhood and intelligence at school age. *Pediatric Research*, 1971, 5, 579–585.
Bogen, J. E. The other side of the brain. II. An appositional mind. *Bulletin Of the Los Angeles Neurological Societies*, 1969, 34, 135–162.
Brockman, L., & Ricciuti, H. Severe protein-calorie malnutrition and cognitive de-

velopment in infancy and early childhood. *Developmental Psychology*, 1970, *4*, 312.

Bruner, J. S., Goodnow, J. J., & Auston, G. A. *A study of thinking*. New York: Wiley, 1956.

Cabak, V., & Najdanvic, R. Effect of undernutrition in early life on physical and mental development. *Archives of Disease in Childhood*, 1965, *40*, 532–534.

Champakam, S., Srikantia, S., & Gopalan, C. Kwashiorkor and mental development. *American Journal of Clinical Nutrition*, 1968, *21*, 844–852.

Chomsky, N. *Syntactic Structures*. The Hague: Mouton, 1957.

Cravioto, J., & DeLicardie, E. Environmental correlates of severe clinical malnutrition and language development in survivors from kwashiorkor or marasmus. In *Nutrition, the nervous system and behavior*. Pan American Health Organization, Scientific Publication No. 251, 1972, 73–94.

Cravioto, J., & DeLicardie, E. Longitudinal study of language development in severely malnourished children. In G. Serban (Ed.), *Nutrition and mental functions*. Vol. 14. *Advances in behavioral biology*. New York: Plenum Press, 1975. Pp. 143–191.

Cravioto, J., & Robles, B. Evolution of adaptive and motor behavior during rehabilitation from kwashiorkor. *American Journal of Orthopsychiatry*, 1965, *35*, 449–464.

d'Aquili, E. G. *The biopsychological determinants of culture*. Reading, Massachusetts: Addison-Wesley Modular Publications, 1972.

d'Aquili, E. G., & Laughlin, C. *Mythmaking: A biogenetic structural analysis*. Paper presented at the annual meeting of the American Anthropological Association, Mexico City, 1974.

d'Aquili, E. G., & Laughlin, C. The biopsychological determinants of religious ritual behavior. *Zygon*, 1975, *10* (1), 32–58.

DeLicardie, E. R., & Cravioto, J. Behavioral responsiveness of survivors of clinically severe malnutrition to cognitive demands. In J. Cravioto, L. Hambraeus, & B. Vahlquist (Eds.), *Early malnutrition and mental development*. Uppsala: Almquist and Wiksell, 1974.

Evans, D., Moodie, A., & Hansen, J. Kwashiorkor and intellectual development. *South African Medical Journal*, 1971, *45*, 1413–1426.

Gazzaniga, M. S. *The bisected brain*. New York: Appleton-Century-Crofts, 1970.

Gazzaniga, M. S., & Hillyard, S. A. Language and speech capacity of the right hemisphere. *Neuropsychologia*, 1971, *9*, 273–280.

Geber, M., & Dean, R. F. A. The psychological changes accompanying kwashiorkor. *Courrier*, 1956, *6*, 3–14.

Geschwind, N. Disconnexion syndromes in animals and man. *Brain*, 1965, *88*, 237–294, 585–644.

Harvey, O. J., Hunt, D. E., & Schroder, H. M. Conceptual systems and personality organization. New York: Wiley, 1961.

Kelly, G. A. *The psychology of personal constructs* (Vol. 1), New York: W. W. Norton, 1955.

Klein, R., Lester, B., Yarbrough, C., & Habicht, J. On malnutrition and mental development: Some preliminary findings. In A. Chaves (Ed.), *Ninth International Congress of Nutrition*. New York: S. Karger, 1975.

Laughlin, C. & d'Aquili, E. G. *Biogenetic structuralism*. New York: Columbia University Press, 1974.

Lester, B. M. Cardiac habituation of the orienting response to an auditory signal in infants of varying nutritional status. *Developmental Psychology*, 1975, *11*, 432–442.

Lévi-Strauss, C. *The savage mind*. Chicago: University of Chicago Press, 1963. (a)
Lévi-Strauss, C. *Structural anthropology*. New York: Doubleday, Anchor Books, 1963. (b)
Lévi-Strauss, C. *Totemism*. Boston: Beacon Press, 1963. (c)
Lévi-Strauss, C. *The elementary structures of kinship*. Boston: Beacon Press, 1969.
Levy-Agresti, J., & Sperry, R. W. Differential perceptual capacities in major and minor hemispheres. *Proceedings of the National Academy of Science*, 1968, *61*, 1151–1165.
Luria, A. R. *Higher cortical functions in man*. New York: Basic Books, 1966.
Marcondes, E., Lefevre, A., Machado, D., Garcia de Barros, N., Cavallo, A., Gazal, S., Quarentei, G., Setian, N., Valente, M., & Barbieri, D. Neuropsychomotor development and pneumoencephalograph changes in children with severe malnutrition. *Environmental Child Health*, 1973, *19*, 135–139.
Monckeberg, F. Effect of early marasmic malnutrition on subsequent physical and psychological development. In N. Scrimshaw & J. Gordon (Eds.) *Malnutrition, learning and behavior*. Cambridge, Massachusetts: MIT Press, 1968.
Nebes, R. D., & Sperry, R. W. Hemispheric disconnection syndrome with cerebral birth injury in the dominant arm area. *Neuropsychologia*, 1971, *9*, 247–259.
Piaget, J. *The moral judgment of the child*. (Trans. by M. Gabain) Glencoe, Illinois: Free Press, 1948.
Piaget, J. *Structuralism*. New York: Harper & Row, 1970.
Piaget, J. *Biology and knowledge*. Chicago: University of Chicago Press, 1971.
Postman, L. Toward a general theory of cognition. In J. H. Rohren & M. Sherif (Eds.), *Social psychology at the crossroads*. New York: Harper, 1951.
Pribram, K. H., & Luria, A. R. (Eds.) *Psychophysiology of the frontal lobes*. New York: Academic Press, 1973.
Rapaport, D. *Organization and pathology of thought*. New York: Columbia University Press, 1951.
Sarbin, T. R., Taft, R., & Bailey, D. E. *Clinical inference and cognitive theory*. New York: Holt, Rinehart & Winston, 1960.
Sperry, R. W., Gazzaniga, M. S., & Bogen, J. E. Interhemispheric relationships: The neocortical commissures; syndromes of hemisphere disconnection. In P. J. Vinken & G. W. Bruyn (Eds.), *Handbook of clinical neurology* (Vol 4). Amsterdam: North Holland Publishing Co., 1969. Pp. 273–290.
Stent, G. S. Prematurity and uniqueness in scientific discovery. *Scientific American*, 1972, *227*(6), 84–93.
Trevarthen, C. *Brain bisymmetry and the role of the corpus callosum in behavior and conscious experience*. Presented at The International Colloquium on Interhemispheric Relations, Czechoslovakia, June 10–13, 1969.
Wallace, A. F. C. *Culture and personality*. New York: Random House, 1970.
Waterlow, J. C., & Rutishauser, H. E. Malnutrition in man. In J. Cravioto, L. Hambraeus, & B. Vahlquist (Eds.), *Early malnutrition and mental development*. Uppsala: Almquist and Wiksell, 1974.
Winick, M., & Rosso, P. Head circumference and cellular growth of the brain in normal and marasmic children. *Journal of Pediatrics*, 1969, *74*, 774–778.

11

Toward a New Concept of
Nutrition

SOLOMON H. KATZ

University of Pennsylvania and the W. M. Krogman Center, Children's
Hospital of Philadelphia, and the Eastern Pennsylvania Psychiatric Institute,
Philadelphia.

In this the 201st year of our nation, it is relevant to add a sober
reminder to this discussion of malnutrition, behavior, and social organization. Suskind (this volume) has indicated that there are as many as
100 million malnourished children now living, mostly in less advantaged parts of the world. The science of understanding malnutrition
should *never* be disconnected from the reality facing these 100 million
children. When leaders of this nation begin to talk about "agropower"
in the same political and economic terms that other nations speak of
"petropower," we as scientists must begin to ensure that our scientific
findings become integrated into the policymaking process. Anything
less borders on irresponsibility. (For an unusually comprehensive
source of new technical and scientific advances on world food problems, see *Science, 188*, pp. 501–650, 1975.) This must be done at all
levels of decision making and must reflect a scientifically valid and
humane approach that optimizes the best we have to offer those
involved.

It is clear that there is an important, albeit implied, link between the
policy-making process and the content of this volume. On the one
hand, we are dealing with the effects of malnutrition on the neurological and related aspects of behavioral development of individuals and,
on the other hand, with the collective effect of these phenomena on

the entire social structure of a population. If malnutrition influences neural and behavioral development of individuals, is it ever possible for a malnourished population to follow the model of economic and political development found in other societies in which malnutrition is not a significant problem? And if not, what kind of adaptations are open to such a population? Ultimately, how will this knowledge influence the policies that an affluent and agriculturally productive nation such as ours should adopt on "agropower"?

Of course, my queries and comments are based on the assumption that the data and models we have are of sufficient quality to be applicable to these problems. In one sense, we are all aware that there is a continuous process of improving and updating our models and techniques of measurement. However, it is essential to recognize that there is a real need to balance the realities of nutritional decision making today with the potentials of having improved data and models tomorrow. Both processes must go on simultaneously, and optimized feedback between them needs to occur continuously. This kind of planning system requires formal development and should be one of the goals of future symposia.

While there is a considerable need for models to incorporate sufficient scientific data to optimize decision making on policies and programs affecting human nutrition, there is also a need to develop a solid data base from which to make generalizations. For example, there is a strong need for a better definition of a human developmental or life-cycle approach in interpreting the results of nutritional studies. It is important to recognize that there are sensitive periods in infancy, childhood, adolescence, and in early, middle, and late adulthood, as well as senescence, in which nutrition plays an important role. It may be necessary but not sufficient to understand the effects of protein–calorie malnutrition (PCM) occurring in adolescents and older adults. Read (this volume) has reviewed recent findings that demonstrate a significant interaction between nutrition, social deprivation, and nutritional deprivation of the parents. He suggests that even when malnutrition in the young child is corrected, the behavioral functioning of these children does not improve significantly until the nutrition of the parents improves. The parents provide the social stimulation that the developing child needs.

When assessing behavior cross-culturally, we are cautioned by a number of investigators, including Thomson and Pollitt, Stanbury and Greene (this volume). There is a tremendous need for valid cross-cultural tests. Additionally, such tests must have validity within the expected behavioral functions for each society. This, according to

Thomson and Pollitt, raises an interesting question. Are there any direct, permanent results of kwashiorkor, as distinguished from marasmus, on behavior that cannot be explained by sociocultural deprivation? Thomson and Pollitt suggest that there are none; however, such conclusions require *careful validation* before they are used as a basis for policies concerning nutritional supplementation.

Not only is there a need for more sensitive and specific psychological measures of malnutrition, but there is an equal need in the area of physical assessments. Suskind alluded to an interesting problem when he observed that in Southeast Asia many children who are normal in body proportions and behavior are stunted in overall size. Inherent in this observation is an important need for clarification of the question: "Is bigger really better?" Our society gears many of its attitudes toward the theme that bigger body size, so characteristic of the "secular growth trend," is better than the smaller sizes of previous generations. We are led to conclude that at least some of this increase in body size is a result of better nutrition and health care, but we rarely ask if "bigger" is more adaptive later in the human life cycle than "smaller" when all other variables are equal. Smaller individuals may be better adapted to withstand the stresses of malnutrition later in their lives. What is needed is a careful assessment of how to apply growth standards and how to interpret our findings.

Also striking are the remarkable statistics on the extent of both marasmus and kwashiorkor and their interaction with infant diseases. There has been a decline in breast-feeding in many of the same regions of the world in which marasmus and kwashiorkor are prevalent, and as Suskind has indicated, most of the diseases of nutrition and deprivation appear in the child between the ages of 6 months to approximately 2 years. This is precisely the time when most of the populations have entirely ceased breast-feeding. Of course, breast-feeding alone cannot support most infants after 6 months. However, if supplemented with iron and calories, breast milk is probably the best nutritional resource available to solve many of the problems described in this volume.

This discussion relates closely to another issue raised by Suskind's suggestions for a program to prevent malnutrition (Suskind, this volume). He lists five objectives for this preventive program to combat malnutrition:

1. Improvement in the nutritional status of women of child-bearing age, particularly through adolescence, pregnancy, and lactation;

2. Spacing of pregnancies at reasonable intervals;
3. Reduction in perinatal mortality and morbidity;
4. Reduction in the frequency and severity of infectious diseases;
5. Dedection of early signs of malnutrition in order to take remedial action.

Of these five objectives, the first four could be met by promoting and advocating a continuation and/or a return to breast-feeding. However, this recommendation carries with it questions about nutritional supplementation for the mother, its economic and social impact, and its long-term effect on the social organization of the various societies most in need.

In order to evaluate such recommendations and answer important questions about nutrition, we need more comprehensive models to account for the important variables. I would like to present a simple heuristic model that I have developed over the past several years (Figure 11.1). This model suggests that we must examine the interactions of four classes of variables at all levels. These include environmental, biological, demographic, and sociocultural factors. For example, if we are considering goiter and cretinism in highland Ecuador (Greene, this volume), we must ask questions not only about how the sociocultural and the biological systems interact through the changes in behavior produced by lowered thyroid activity but also about (1) the presence of goitrogens and other variables influencing iodine in the environment; (2) the effects of the deficiency on fertility, population size, and composition; and (3) the effects of thyroid compensation on the subsequent development of toxic goiter in later life and its subsequent effects on individual and group behavior. In order to complete an analysis of complex nutritional problems, we must continue to be inclusive in our models in order to be able to answer questions of such a broad scope.

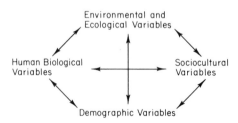

Figure 11.1. This figure shows the importance of the possible interaction of the principal variables involved in a consideration of various nutritional problems.

We have also applied such approaches to other problems, such as the nutritional significance of the methods used in preparing maize (Katz, Hediger, & Valleroy, 1974) and the nutritional problems related to calcium metabolism (Foulks & Katz, this volume). More recently, we have attempted to integrate this approach for breast-feeding (Katz & Young, 1976) and for the nutritional practices and patterns surrounding the consumption of fava beans (Katz, Adair, & Schall, 1976). The latter are particularly interesting because *Vicia fava* (fava beans) may contain antimalarial agents that help to balance the glucose-6-phosphate dehydrogenase polymorphism that seems to co-occur with their consumption. Many of these investigations have led us to expand our concept of "malnutrition" and how it should be controlled. For example, we have come to recognize that hypercaloric nutrition and the excessive intake of minerals may be as negative as the lack of calories, proteins, and minerals. Obesity for the population of the United States is a much more significant problem than is caloric insufficiency. Likewise, excessive sodium intake and alcohol consumption are also potentially debilitating.

There are numerous psychosomatic illnesses involving nutrition, and there are potential effects on central nervous system functioning of such flavor-intensifying additives as monosodium glutamate and serious threats of bladder cancer from cyclamates. We must begin to ask about the health-care cost in human and economic terms of the use of various additives to prolong the shipping and shelf life of foods. Similarly, with the example of milk supplementation of cereal grains and the inability of many populations to digest milk lactose after infancy, we must begin to ask about genetic differences and how they fit nutritional supplementation programs.

What we need in order to solve these problems is a new kind of agency. For want of a better term and a better analogy, we need a nutritional protection agency—one that, like the Environmental Protection Agency, can mandate a nutritional-impact statement for each food we store, process, and ship abroad. Domestically, the impact of preservatives, flavor and color additives, and nutritional *quality*, not just quantity, of food proteins must be evaluated. We must weigh seriously, in a much more holistic manner, our policies of agricultural support and nonsupport of food assistance and know and understand the complete impact of their effects. It is not sufficient, for example, to separate food policy from population policy. We must know the impact of a nutritional supplementation program on population growth if our ultimate aim is to stabilize population expansion. We must also investigate new food alternatives and integrate them into the customs and local cuisines of various peoples. This latter need is clearly an anthropological problem.

In conclusion, the papers in this volume prove beyond all doubt that highly significant effects of nutrition on behavior and social organization regularly occur. It is my hope that we can begin to take the steps toward understanding them better and integrating a scientifically valid and humane organizational framework to solve some of the universally tragic consequences of malnutrition now apparent throughout the world.

REFERENCES

Katz, S. H., Adair, L., & Schall, J. *Fava bean consumption in regions with endemic malaria and G-6-PD deficiency*. Paper presented at the meetings of the American Association of Physical Anthropologists, St. Louis, April 1976.
Katz, S. H., Hediger, M. L., & Valleroy, L. A. Traditional maize processing techniques in the New World. *Science*, 1974, *184*, 765–773.
Katz, S. H., & Young, M. V. *Biosocial aspects of breast-feeding*. Paper presented at the meetings of the American Association for the Advancement of Science, Boston, Massachusetts, February 1976.

12

Contemporary Implications of the State of the Art

MARGARET MEAD

The American Museum of Natural History

I would like to try to pull together these complex and contrasting chapters and consider their implications for the immediate future. Although Segraves (this volume) speaks in terms of system, I would suggest that the population of this planet—or the societies of this planet—are not yet a system. They are only partially a system; there-fore, any insistence that we think about the population of the planet in general system terms is premature. We are approaching the level of a system, and it is quite possible that within a reasonably short time the kind of analysis that we have used for smaller systems will be applica-ble. It is also quite possible that we have reached the state of a system in terms of the spread of disease.

The nature of things is not yet quite so inexorable. The degree of leeway that is present for individuals and for groups in making choices about what they are going to do about the population problem and about the food problem is still very wide, and the beliefs that people have—at least those beliefs in things they think have been demon-strated by science—are going to be extraordinarily important in directing their action.

Perhaps one of the most conspicuous examples of this is the position that the Soviet Union and eastern European countries have taken on

Malthusian theory and the effect that this has had on the deliberations of international conferences. Our belief or disbelief in Malthusian theory and the position that we take on the effects of early malnutrition (whether it produces reversible or irreversible damage) will determine whether intervention is attempted and what such programs will be like. Our beliefs will thus guide our actions.

Greene's work (this volume) has very clearly demonstrated the effect of severe iodine malnutrition and endemic goiter on human populations and the extent to which this can be altered by the inclusion in the diet of iodine from various sources. The reduced functioning of a large portion of the population and the lowered expectation of "normal" functioning in the whole population are, I think, very important points. Thus, the presence of these deaf-mute "cretins" in the population made everyone else look "normal," and the standard of normalcy went way, way down. The presence of such large numbers of grossly retarded individuals created a situation in which the social expectation of behavior was lower than it would have been if the more moderately deficient individuals were the lowest element in society. If this example can serve as a model, then we would expect to encounter similar situations, in varying degrees, in many parts of the world. There are different kinds of impairment as a result of different kinds of deficiency, which are affecting, in a variety of ways, the expectations and the functioning of different populations.

I would like to add a note to the discussion of endemic iodine deficiency. While in Bali, I chose to work in a particular village because it was the only village in which the walls of the courtyards were unfinished. The walls of the courtyard were simply made of a kind of rattan over which clay should have been applied, but parts of the walls were left undone. I decided that it would be an easy place to work because I would be able to see into the courtyards before entering. I selected the village on that basis without realizing that this village had a high prevalence of hypothyroidism. The people shrank the pattern of their cultural activities without entirely destroying that pattern. This is a point that Dr. Greene did not mention, but it appears to be characteristic of the behavior of hypothyroid individuals. Cultural patterning is preserved but with an enormous reduction in the complexity of the patterning. The villagers did not finish the walls in the same context that they left many other things unfinished. They knew how walls should be constructed, but they merely erected a skeleton of the original pattern and never finished it.

Now this sort of specific behavioral deficit, and that illustrated in the discussion of calcium deficiency among the Eskimos and in the behavior of the pale-faced fading ladies of the Victorian period (Foulks & Katz, this volume), are specific behavioral deficits subsequent to some particular type of malnutrition. At one level, it is easy to alter these conditions: You just take off some of the lady's clothes and give her a little better food, and there is no longer a problem, or you introduce iodine in the proper amounts, and the problem is similarly resolved.

This is encouraging. However, there is the second level on which a population adjusts, in a more or less permanent fashion, to a low plane of nourishment and a lower level of general efficiency. It was very striking that in this village in Bali, although we brought in iodine, we could not persuade anybody born in the village to take it. Women who married in from other villages and who were alarmed when their children began to show signs of hypothyroidism would use it, but the local population had become accustomed to goiter. The chief priestess had a goiter larger than her head, and she was the leader of the village. Goiter and its consequences were the norm rather than the extreme, and a goiter, or an extra finger, did not place an individual at a social disadvantage.

Another instance of this type of social inertia is reflected in the work of John Gwaltney (1970) in the villages of the blind in Oaxaca, Mexico, in which local inhabitants refused to move even though they would have benefited by leaving. They were afraid that they would later go blind, so they wanted to stay in a place in which they had previous visual experience and with which they were thus familiar.

Now, discussion at this second level may make us very pessimistic—the first level that I mentioned should make us very optimistic. It suggests the possibility of large populations adjusting to a level of misery that is physically destructive, characterized by malnutrition and by the consequences of malnutrition in different aspects of functioning. The contemporary population of the City of New York may fit this paradigm. It has slowly adjusted to a level of pollution and a level of misery that has numerous deleterious effects that can reduce the functional capacity of whole populations. What may happen is that people will neither move away nor do anything about the situation; conditions may just slowly grow worse and worse. This is not too encouraging.

The FAO calculates that there are 400 million severely malnourished people in the world. These individuals tend to be concentrated in particular geographical areas. If we accept the suggestion that malnutrition has some effect on the development of the brain and that the ability for high abstract thought is permanently and irreparably damaged by various sorts of malnutrition, then we face a complex ethical problem in attempting to devise a world system that will alter these circumstances. We encountered this problem in 1966 at the New York Academy of Sciences. Edward Hunt presented the proposition, not too well supported (but neither are the rest of these contentions), that if malnutrition produces impaired intellectual functioning, and if it had been demonstrated that Black children in this country were severely undernourished, then this might account for their poor achievement in school (Hunt, 1966). The New York anthropological community blew up in response to this suggestion, regarding it as racist. This emotional overreaction delayed our recognition of the fact that even the effects of many of the extreme forms of malnutrition are reversible with adequate nutrition and changes in the home environment. The result of an ideological inflexibility in dealing with such problems may be an inability to do anything to ameliorate the situation. In actuality, a good deal of the data that have been presented indicate that many of these behavioral effects are reversible (Thomson & Pollitt, this volume).

In populations that have experienced long-term malnutrition (Buchbinder, Greene, this volume), it is likely that many adults may be severely affected. Should we label these populations as being "inferior" as the result of this situation? Such circumstances obviously present us with difficult ethical questions, as on ideological grounds we must treat all human beings as people who should be fed and cared for. Thus, I think that all of these implications must be considered with a tremendous degree of caution.

It is quite plausible to conclude that a community needs a certain number of flexible individuals in order to foster change (d'Aquili & Mihalik, this volume) and that a better nourished population is more likely to manifest this flexibility. On the basis of my experience in New Guinea, I found that coastal populations were likely to be well supplied with protein, and we know that they are flexible people. Forty-seven years ago, we observed, in the Admiralty Islands, that the coastal people had far and away the best diets, showed the greatest degree of enterprise, and had the greatest capacity for social change. On the other hand, the people in the interior of the Great Admiralty Islands had a much poorer diet and showed all of the characteristic behavior of people under nutritional stress. They were extremely passive; pregnant women simply sat and waited for their babies to come out. If they did not, well, that was just too bad. It seemed likely that this degree of apathy and passivity was a consequence of prolonged malnutrition, of living on the very poor soil of the interior with limited access to animal protein.

Twenty-five years later, the south-coast lagoon-dwelling Manus had developed an imaginative response to modern society, and many of them had gone on to higher education (Mead, 1956). In contrast, many of the poor miserable "country bumpkins" in the interior were living exactly as they always had. The general improvement in education pioneered by the sea people benefited the land people also. I have followed these people for 47 years, and the idea that students of distinction would catch up so soon with the coastal people was unbelievable. However, the situation has changed markedly. In 1975, one of them from one of the most backward villages was a postdoctoral student in an American university. Thus, despite the well-documented poor quality of the local diet and the backward state of the village, some individuals were able to emerge intact and overcome the local low expectation for performance when they met higher expectations when they went away to school (Mead, 1976a).

My point is that although we have good data showing the damaging effects of marasmus and kwarshiorkor early in life in some individuals, these individuals comprise only a small segment of the population. We are not yet able to describe precisely the conditions that permit other individuals to survive these same nutritional stresses. This seems to be one of the very serious difficulties with which we are faced in understanding the effect of malnutrition on behavioral capacity.

It is also important that we examine the suggestion that social stratification results in a certain proportion of the population being ill fed, functioning on a lower level of competence, and ultimately being eliminated from the population (Greene, Segraves, this volume). Historically, this is undoubtedly true. No one questions European history where there were bishops who prayed that the Lord would send a plague to kill off the lower orders because they were too many of them. However, ideology has changed with the course of time, and at present most societies, at least those of Europe and North America, have some form of ideological commitment to caring for the dietary needs of all their citizens. I wish to stress the point that man is now in a position to intervene in the system, and that presents, I think, a very serious caveat for that line of reasoning. As we recognize the extent to which the present system of industrialized agriculture is responsible for hunger, new kinds of intervention are possible (Mead, 1976b; Lappé, 1977).

There are enormous social implications to these studies demonstrating behavioral defects subsequent to persistent malnutrition early in life. What if the idea of triage were to be accepted? If there are 400 million malnourished people in the world, and if, as suggested, many of them are impaired (they cannot think abstractly, they are not very flexible), then are these the people who would be sacrificed in a society employing an ideological "lifeboat psychology"? On the other hand, if you assume that we are now dealing with a world system in which our knowledge and expectations are very important in guiding our actions, and our ethical system and our scientific system are interrelated, then we have quite a different approach to things. Triage thinking would advise us, if we accepted it, to let the 400 million people starve to death because they would never be successful, anyway, and they would not be able to change their society. This would also change us into a different kind of people; in the end, we might turn out to be similar to the Iks (Turnbull, 1972), as was suggested by a recent *New York Times* editorial.

It is well documented that in most cases impairment of the neocortex produces behavioral limitations. But we do not yet know anything about an individual's ability to transcend such situations. We do not know whether there are some individuals who are *vulnerable* to these stresses and others who are not. In overcoming such nutritional stresses and harsh life circumstances, some individuals may even be stimulated to greater strength. We must consider the possibility that we are dealing with significant individual differences in response to these environmental circumstances.

If many of these effects are truly irreversible, then we are going to have to treat some people as handicapped and accept them and care for them exactly as we would care for the deaf or the blind or any other handicapped group in society. However, it is extremely dangerous to impute such deficits to large numbers of individuals in populations living in areas in which protein-calorie malnutrition (PCM) is prevalent. Although the papers presented in this volume are fascinating and rich in data, I have not seen any discussion of the possibility that there are individuals in these populations who do not succumb to these unfortunate life circumstances.

The Gluecks' early and follow up studies (Glueck & Glueck, 1962) in Boston are quite relevant here. These studies of white boys from slum environments attempted to determine why some became delinquents while their siblings and neighbors did not. The Gluecks concluded that extreme physical immaturity was one of the best predictors of delinquency. Yet, these findings were regarded as unacceptable by American behavioral scientists. They were considered to be virtually racist in character because whenever you present anything to Americans that they cannot change, they say it is racist. The Gluecks were very severely criticized for this study, but 35 years later they went back and studied that same set of people and found that many of them had matured and were no longer social problems.

The Gluecks had identified the vulnerable. Now, I suggest that much of what has been discussed in these chapters may in actuality apply to only a *vulnerable* segment of total populations and that we should be extremely careful of how far we generalize it to the rest of the population. The adverse response of Americans to the idea of irreversibility recalls Tanner's statement (Tanner, 1953): "Americans would like somatotypes when they find out how to alter them." Irreversibility is a concept fraught with both ethical and ideological danger and should be treated cautiously.

I think that the next step is to take a population in which malnutrition is severe and to study the bright people in it. Who are they? We are always hearing about the poor, depressed people from Appalachia. Yet many people who grew up under these impoverished conditions leave that setting and are quite successful elsewhere. There are many intelligent and superior people who have survived such hardships.

I think that we must do the same thing in the study of infectious diseases. Suskind (this volume) has clearly outlined the interrelationships between disease and malnutrition, yet it would be extremely profitable to study not only those babies who are most prone to illness and who die, but also the biological characteristics and social environments of those who are successful. I think it is unfortunate that many of these studies have focused so heavily on those individuals who are most vulnerable to these environmental stresses.

REFERENCES

Glueck, S., & Glueck, E. *Family environment and delinquency.* Boston: Houghton Mifflin, 1972.

Gwaltney, J. *The thrice shy.* New York: Columbia University Press, 1970.

Hunt, E. *Some new evidence on intelligence and race.* Paper presented at the New York Academy of Sciences, October, 1966.

Lappé, F. M. *Food first!* Hastings on Hudson, New York: Institute for Food and Development Policy, 1977.

Mead, M. *New lives for old.* New York: Morrow, 1956.

Mead, M. Return to Manus. *Natural History,* 1976, 85(6), 60–69. (a)

Mead, M. A comment on the role of women in agriculture. In I. Tinker & M. Bo Bramsen (Eds.), *Women and world development.* Washington, D.C.: American Association for the Advancement of Science, Overseas Development Council, 1976. Pp. 9–11. (b)

Tanner, J. M., S. Tax, L. Eiseley, I. Rouse, & C. F. Vogelin (Eds.), *An appraisal of anthropology today.* Chicago: University of Chicago Press, 1953.

Turnbull, C. *The mountain people.* New York: Simon & Schuster, 1972.

13

Toward an Appreciation of the Biological Bases of Behavioral Variation and Its Influence on Social Organization

LAWRENCE S. GREENE

University of Massachusetts/Boston

The contributors to this volume have shown how different forms of malnutrition may affect nervous system development and behavior in human populations. They have also discussed how the behavioral variation that is produced as a consequence of these conditions may, or may not, have a significant influence on the sociocultural characteristics of human communities. The following pages will comment on these findings, supplement them with additional data, and indicate why they are of particular theoretical and practical importance for an appreciation of human biological and sociocultural variation.

THE SYNERGISTIC EFFECT OF MALNUTRITION, INTERCURRENT DISEASE, AND ENVIRONMENTAL IMPROVERISHMENT ON BEHAVIORAL DEVELOPMENT

Although the American Association for the Advancement of Science symposium from which this volume is derived primarily focused on the effect of frank malnutrition on behavioral development, it soon became apparent that disease and experiential factors are equally important in accounting for the high prevalence of behavioral deficits in some human populations. A growing body of experimental and clinical data suggests that:

1. Exposure to "improverished" or "enriched" physical and social environments both have a measurable and significant effect on brain growth and behavioral development in experimental animals.
2. Many of the behavioral effects attributed to different types of malnutrition in human populations may be a consequence of inadequate mental stimulation due to an impoverished physical–social environment and/or a decrease in the child's interaction with his physical and social environment due to the metabolic effects of the nutritional stress.
3. Many of the apparently irreversible behavioral effects attributed to severe malnutrition, and other more concrete forms of brain damage, may be significantly ameliorated by exposure to "therapeutic" environments not only early in life but throughout much of the life cycle.

The first section of this chapter will review these findings.

Intercurrent Disease Factors

Suskind (this volume) has clearly outlined how protein–calorie malnutrition (PCM) affects the immune response in children, thus increasing the prevalence of respiratory and diarrheal diseases. The onset of the disease episode then acts to exacerbate preexisting marasmus or precipitate acute episodes of kwashiorkor. (Scrimshaw, 1973, 1975).

It has become apparent that in addition to being under increased metabolic stress, the malnourished and chronically ill child has an altered relationship with his surroundings. Because of these conditions, the child is irritable and has a decreased capacity for positive interaction with his physical and social environment. The most important aspect of this situation is that the maternal–infant relationship is markedly altered when the child is chronically ill. Instead of being a positive stimulus, the irritable and demanding child is perceived in a negative fashion and thus is less likely to elicit positive maternal behavior. This is particularly true among uneducated or poorly educated women having large families with closely spaced births, who may themselves be malnourished.

Thus, in addition to compounding the nutritional stress (in purely physiological terms), the increased disease experience of these children further alters their ability to successfully interact with their environment. This form of *experiential deprivation* may be of equal importance to the malnutrition in affecting nervous system maturation and behavioral development. The growing body of provocative literature on this subject will now be reviewed.

Environmental Experience, Nervous System Development, and Behavior

Effects on the Brain

During the past 20 years, a number of experimental studies on laboratory animals have indicated that experience within "enriched" (complex) sensory environments has a measurable and significant effect on many aspects of brain development (Rosenzweig, Krech, Bennett, & Zolman, 1962; Rosenzweig, Bennett, & Diamond, 1967, 1972; Walsh, Budtz-Olsen, Torok, & Cummins, 1971; Walsh, Cummins, Budtz-Olsen, O'Rourke, Brown, & Cameron, 1971; Walsh & Cummins, 1975, 1976). Normal rats reared in enriched environments have cerebral cortices that are heavier and wider than controls; there is an increased number of glial cells; and their neurons have larger cell bodies and nuclei.

The brains of these animals also show an increased arborization of the dendritic tree (Greenough & Volkmar, 1973; Walsh & Cummins, 1976), an increase in the number of dendritic spines, and an increase in the size of synaptic junctions (Rosenzweig *et al.*, 1972). Such changes increase neural interconnectivity, a factor that may be important in accounting for the behavioral effects produced by these environments. The brains of the "enriched" animals also show increased amounts of the enzymes acetylcholinesterase, cholinesterase, and choline acetyl transferase. These morphological and neurochemical differences are especially pronounced in the occipital cortex.

The effect of environmental enrichment on the brains of experimental animals is *not* confined to early "critical" phases of development. Mature animals exposed to "enriched" conditions show the same types of responses but may require somewhat longer periods of exposure to produce comparable results (Rosenzweig *et al.*, 1972; Walsh &

Cummins, 1976). Rearing under "impoverished" physical–social conditions produces opposite effects, with animals exposed to such environments showing lower values for the brain measures listed above. In experiments with rats that were placed in different combinations of enriched and isolated environments for 2 consecutive 30-day periods (4 groups: enriched-enriched; enriched-isolated; isolated-enriched; isolated-isolated), it was found that brain weight was highest in the E–E group and lowest in the I–I group. Results in the switchover groups were conflicting but seem to suggest that the final environmental condition was the major determinant of brain weight (Rosenzweig et al., 1967; Walsh & Cummins, 1976).

Comparable results have been reported in studies of rats subjected to experimental brain damage at birth and then reared in either isolated or complex environments. Lesioning led to a reduction in cerebral length and breadth that was ameliorated somewhat by rearing in complex environments (Walsh, Cummins, & Budtz-Olsen, 1973).

Behavioral Effects

Normal animals raised under different environmental conditions. A number of experiments with laboratory animals indicate that differential experience has an effect on behavioral development (Hebb, 1949; Bingham and Griffiths, 1952; Forgays & Forgays, 1952; Krech, Rosenzweig, & Bennett, 1962; Bennett, Rosenzweig, & Diamond, 1970; Greenough, Madden, & Fleischmann, 1972). In these studies, rats raised in "enriched" environments scored significantly better on various measures of problem-solving ability than rats reared under "isolated" conditions. However, in a careful comparison of behavioral data on rats raised in "enriched," "standard," and "isolated" conditions, Bennett et al. (1970) concluded that the problem-solving ability of the "enriched" and "standard" groups was approximately equal and that both were significantly superior to that of the "isolated group." Thus, the behavioral differences between "normal" animals raised under "enriched" and "isolated" conditions appear to be more a function of the effects of isolation than of enrichment. In contrast to the studies on rodent species, investigations carried out on rhesus monkeys *(M. mulatta)* raised in social isolation show a variety of personal and social abnormalities but not learning deficits when compared to colony-born and wild-raised controls (Harlow, Schlitz, & Harlow, 1968; Gluck & Harlow, 1971: Sackett & Rupenthal, 1973).

The interaction of malnutrition and environmental improverishment in affecting behavioral development Some of the most provocative and germane studies are those evaluating the relative effects

of, or interactions between, malnutrition and environmental deprivation on behavioral development. Animal studies by Fraňková (1968,
1970, 1972), Levitsky and Barnes (1972), and Wells, Geist, and Zim-
merman (1972) demonstrated that environmental isolation produces
behavioral deficits similar to those produced by PCM and that rearing
in an "enriched" environment alleviates, to a considerable degree, the
behavioral deficits of previously malnourished animals. Animals that
were *both* malnourished and raised in "inpoverished" environments
early in life showed by far the greatest behavioral deficits as adults.

Perhaps the most comprehensive and compelling studies are those
of Davenport on the role of "superenriched" environments in
ameliorating the effects of early hypothyroidism on behavioral development (Davenport, 1976; Davenport, Gonzalez, Carey, Bishop, &
Hagquist, 1976). In these experiments, normal-born rats and rats made
"cretinous" as a consequence of prenatal and neonatal exposure to
antithyroid drugs were reared either in an isolated environment or in a
"superenriched" environment similar to that employed by
Rosenzweig and his co-workers (Rosenzweig *et al.*, 1972). These experiments showed that the "cretin" rats reared in the "superenriched"
environment achieved scores comparable to the normal rats on a
number of behavioral tasks. Davenport (1976, p. 91) concluded that
"superenrichment" reduced the behavioral deficits of the cretinous
rats to a substantial degree in maze acquisition, almost entirely in
maze retention and bar pressing extinction, but not at all in passive
avoidance performance.

A recent study by Winick, Meyer, and Harris (1975) is the only
human investigation that really purports to evaluate the therpeutic
effect of home environment in ameliorating the behavioral consequences of early malnutrition. In this study of Korean children adopted
into American homes during the first 3 years of life, it was found that
those who were below the third percentile for height and weight for
age on Korean standards ("malnourished" group) upon admission to
the adoption service scored significantly lower on standard IQ tests at
6–14 years of age than similar adopted children who had been above
the 25th percentile for height and weight at that time ("well-
nourished" group). However, the "malnourished" children received
IQ and achievement scores that were comparable to those of average
American children. The authors suggest that the beneficial effects of
the American home environment compensated for whatever neurological effect may have been produced by early "malnutrition," thus
allowing the previously "malnourished" children to function within
the normal range of behavior.

Summary and implications for human population. The animal studies cited have demonstrated that complex physical and social environments have a beneficial effect on a number of morphological, histological, and neuro-chemical characteristics of the brain in laboratory animals at all ages and that social isolation in physically unstimulating settings has an opposite effect of decreasing these brain measures. Isolated rearing conditions produce behavioral deficits in laboratory animals as do PCM and hypothyroidism early in life. The effects on behavioral development produced by these nutritional and metabolic stresses are alleviated, to a significant degree, by rearing in "superenriched" environments.

Studies by Skeels and Dye (1939) and Skeels (1966) of children raised in orphanages have shown the powerful influence of environmental factors in affecting behavioral development in humans. The work of Winick *et al.* (1975) provides *preliminary* data suggesting an ameliorating effect of environmental enrichment on behavioral development in previously "malnourished" children.

These findings in laboratory animals, and the limited quasi-experimental observations on human subjects (Yarrow, 1961; Ainsworth, 1962) suggest that the high prevalence of behavioral deficits in some human populations may be accounted for by an interaction between malnutrition (with intercurrent diarrheal and respiratory disease) and environmental improverishment. I would expect many of these behavioral deficits to have a definite neurological basis, as both severe malnutrition and environmental–social deprivation have been shown to produce significant changes in the morphology and chemistry of the brain. Other investigators, however, are more hesitant to link the observed neurological changes to subsequent behavioral deficits, although they do admit that the two may be causally related (Thomson & Pollitt, personal communication).

We are rapidly becoming aware that socioeconomic differences and intrafamilial factors may make it extremely difficult to isolate the influence of malnutrition on behavioral capacity in human studies (Thomson & Pollitt, this volume; Cravioto & DeLicardie, 1975; Richardson, 1976). However, the animal studies cited above indicate that experiential factors (especially in extreme physical–social environments) have an enduring effect on brain development. Thus, the significant behavioral deficits manifested by many malnourished children from impoverished environments are likely to have a neurological basis. Whether such deficits are due to nutritional or experiential factors becomes somewhat problematic, at least at the level of description. The major point that we must consider is the probability that there are significant numbers of individuals in these populations who have neurologically based behavioral deficits, of varying degrees, irrespective of causation. If we can entertain or accept this prospect, then it is likely that we will be able to appreciate the effects that it may have on the sociocultural characteristics of these populations.

It was stated above that the causal factors producing these deficits are problematical. Our main concern is to describe the phenomenon (the high percentage of neurologically deficient and behaviorally limited individuals) as convincingly as possible. However, once description is accomplished, it is particularly important that we be able to delineate the causal factors producing this variation if we are to intervene and attempt to alter these circumstances. It has been our sad experience that food-supplementation programs produce, except under extreme conditions, limited results without changes in the home environment, while environmental enrichment without adequate nutrition is equally futile in affecting significant behavioral changes (Hunt, 1976).

COMMENTS ON STUDIES EVALUATING THE EFFECT OF MALNUTRITION ON BEHAVIORAL DEVELOPMENT IN HUMAN POPULATIONS

Thomson and Pollitt, Stanbury, Greene, and Read (this volume), have discussed the effect of several types and degrees of malnutrition on behavior in human populations. At this juncture, it might be useful to briefly comment on some of the issues raised by their provocative papers. I would first, however, like to reiterate a point that was made in the preceding section.

The major conceptual issue raised by this volume is whether there are significant numbers of individuals with neurological deficits and behavioral limitations living in human populations in which various types of malnutrition are prevalent. As was noted above, the causal factors producing this behavioral variation are important, and we certainly are suggesting that early malnutrition per se is a significant etiologic component. However, we should not lose sight of the primary phenomenon (the suggested high percentage of behaviorally limited individuals) in our attempt to assess the relative contributions of the various etiologic elements producing this variation.

Iodine Malnutrition

Stanbury (this volume) indicates that there is a high percentage of individuals with severe neurological and behavioral deficits ("cretins") in a number of populations experiencing extreme iodine malnutrition due to insufficient dietary iodine, possibly compounded by the ingestion of water and food crops that contain naturally occurring antithyroid compounds. Stanbury suggests that the "cretins" who at present comprise from 1 to 10% of these populations are likely to represent only the most severely affected end of a spectrum of neurological and behavioral deficit, and Greene (this volume) has presented evidence from a community in highland Ecuador that suggests that in addition to the 5.7% of the inhabitants who are deaf-mute "cretins," there are an additional 17.4% of the population who show significant but more moderate neurological deficits and behavioral limitation.

In 1960, it was estimated that approximately 200 million people throughout the world were subject to endemic goiter (Kelly & Snedden, 1960). These figures were undoubtedly much higher prior to the widespread introduction of iodized salt in the 1920s (Langer, 1960). It is thus almost certain that in the not too distant past there was a high percentage of individuals with severe and moderate neurological and behavioral deficits living in many populations in several different parts of the world in which iodine malnutrition was common (Querido, 1972). As demonstrated by Greene, this phenomenon undoubtedly has had some effect on the sociocultural characteristics of these human populations.

Protein–Calorie Malnutrition (PCM)

Both Suskind and Thomson and Pollitt (this volume) cite data from Bengoa (1974) indicating that the prevalence of *severe* forms of PCM varies between 0 and 20% among children less than 5 years of age in a number of communities surveyed in Latin America, Africa, and Asia. The median point prevalences for these *severe* forms of PCM are 1.6% in Latin America, 4.4% in Africa, and 3.2% in Asia. Based on these figures, Bengoa (1974) has estimated that over 9 million children in the 0–4-year age range suffer from severe forms of PCM in these geographical areas, while approximately 89 million experience more moderate forms (Table 13.1). However, Bengoa (1974, p. 5) states that "since the estimate is based on point prevalence studies the true prevalence of both severe and moderate protein calorie malnutrition

TABLE 13.1

Estimated Number of Children 0–4 Years of Age Suffering from Severe or Moderate Protein–Calorie Malnutrition (PCM) in Three Regions of the World[a]

Region	Severe PCM	Moderate PCM	Total
Latin America	700,000	9,000,000	9,700,000
Africa	2,700,000	16,000,000	18,700,000
Asia (excluding China and Japan)	6,000,000	64,000,000	70,000,000
Total	9,400,000	89,000,000	98,400,000

[a] After Bengoa (1974).

may be very much higher." Thus, if the nutritional status of children in these communities could be constantly evaluated throughout the year rather than at a single point in time, it is certain that many more children would be found to have experienced both severe and moderate forms of PCM, and the prevalence figures in Table 13.1 would be considerably higher.

Marasmus

Bengoa (1974, p. 6) notes that in studies that distinguished between marasmus and kwashiorkor, the prevalence of marasmus was greater in 77% of the cases. This suggests an estimate of over 5 million children, mostly younger than 1 year of age, in Latin America, Africa, and Asia suffering from marasmus at any one point in time.

In their review of the literature on the behavioral effects of severe PCM, Thomson & Pollitt (this volume) have concluded that marasmus throughout much of the first year of life frequently results in enduring behavioral deficits. It is thus possible that at least 5 million individuals with significant behavioral deficits are added to the populations of Latin America, Africa, and Asia each year. Using Bengoa's point prevalence data (Bengoa, 1974, Table 2, p. 6), these individuals would conservatively account for about 1.5–2% of the population of these communities, and possibly a much higher percentage. Many of these children are probably also living under conditions of extreme physical and social impoverishment. As was noted above, the combination of malnutrition and environmental deprivation has a particularly depressing effect on neurological development and behavioral capacity in experimental animals and is likely to have a similar impact in humans. It seems reasonable to expect fairly high *actual* prevalences of behavioral retardation (perhaps 2–3% or more among surviving adults) in many parts of the less developed world, solely on the basis of the synergism between marasmus and environmental deprivation.

Kwashiorkor

Again referring to Bengoa (1974), we would expect that perhaps 2–3% of children in many communities in Latin America, Africa, and Asia have experienced kwashiorkor during the first 5 years of life. As Bengoa points out, the point prevalence of this type of nutritional disease greatly underestimates its actual prevalence due to the acute nature of the condition. Bengoa (1974) reports a median prevalence of 18.9% for moderate forms of PCM in these parts of the world. The impact of these conditions on behavioral development is not entirely clear.

In their careful review of the behavioral consequences of severe PCM, Thomson and Pollitt minimize the effect on behavioral development of severe acute PCM (kwashiorkor) after the first year of life and also conclude that there is insufficient data to determine whether severe but acute episodes of PCM *during* the first year of life or severe and chronic PCM occurring after the first year of life result in any impairment of intellectual functioning. I agree that the most compelling documentation for an enduring behavioral effect is that pertaining to infantile marasmus. However, I believe that a number of studies provide evidence that both kwashiorkor (which is usually an acute exacerbation precipitated by intercurrent infectious disease and superimposed onto chronic malnutrition) and prolonged moderate forms of PCM (with possible intermittent acute episodes precipitated by intercurrent disease factors) combined with "impoverished" physical and social environments are likely to produce enduring behavioral deficits in the children so affected.

Again, I must reiterate an important point. The main conceptual issue with which I am concerned is whether it is likely that there are significant numbers of individuals with neurological deficits and behavioral limitations in human living populations in areas in which PCM is prevalent. The studies cited by Thomson and Pollitt are those that, due to certain methodological considerations, are most likely to provide data on the behavioral effects of *known* episodes of marasmus or kwashiorkor and are not likely to be confounded by covarying environmental variables. They thus attempt to evaluate the independent effect of malnutrition. Given the quasi-experimental nature (at best) of most human studies, the rigor and caution of their review is well founded. However, their methodological rigor allows inclusion of only clinical case studies, eliminating a consideration of retrospective community studies. I suggest that these latter studies, though less well documented and controlled, are likely to provide a more complete picture of the combined effects of malnutrition and environmental deprivation on behavioral development on a *population basis*.

Three entirely retrospective investigations are particularly pertinent (Cravioto, DeLicardie, & Birch, 1966; Mönckeberg, Tisler, Toro, Gattas, & Vega, 1972; Edwards & Craddock, 1973). These studies indicate that among children living in areas in which PCM is prevalent, those whose physical growth for age (height—Cravioto *et al.*, 1966; weight—Monckeberg *et al.*, 1972; head circumference, height, and weight—Edwards & Craddock, 1973) is at the lower end of their population-distribution score significantly more poorly on behavioral measures when compared to peers whose physical growth is adequate. This relationship between physical growth and behavioral development did not exist among middle (Monckeberg *et al.*, 1972) or upper class (Cravioto *et al.*, 1966) comparisons.

These data suggest that chronic malnutrition (not necessarily leading to hospitalization) has a significant effect on behavioral differences (Cravioto & DeLicardie, 1975). That there are significant differences between children so grouped does not *necessarily* mean that there are large numbers of individuals with significant behavioral limitations in these populations. However, an examination of the distribution of these scores suggests, at least to me, that many individuals are functioning at very low levels even when compared to members of their own population. Although the questions of construct validity raised by Thomson and Pollitt are legitimate, I think that the covariation of physical and behavioral test measures is, in itself, an indication of a considerable degree of concurrent validity.

I would also add in passing that my reading of studies by Stoch and Smythe (1963, 1967), Champakam, Srikantia, and Gopalan (1968) and Botha-Antoun, Babayan, and Harfouche (1968) suggests a significant effect of severe PCM (apparently mostly kwashiorkor) even when it occurs in the second year of life. The intercurrent effect of "environmental deprivation" is certainly a factor in producing these deficits (Cravioto & DeLicardie, 1975). However, I disagree with Richardson (1976, p. 265) who concludes, on the basis of multiple regression analyses, that nutritional experiences (history of hospitalization and height for age) have less of an effect on behavioral development than a measure of "family background." Problems with the reversibility of physical, as opposed to neurological, deficits and the likelihood that the comparison cases had also been malnourished but not hospitalized weaken the predictive strength of the nutritional variables. The family background variable is simultaneously overloaded since it is probable that unhospitalized malnutrition covaries with low socioeconomic status.

As noted above, the study by Winick *et al.* (1975) suggests that "enriched" home environments may have a significant ameliorating effect on the behavioral development of previously "malnourished" children. However, due to the manner in which the children were sampled, it is difficult to determine whether they were ever actually malnourished or were even from areas in which malnutrition was prevalent. Such data, although in the direction that we would expect from animal studies, should thus be considered quite preliminary and interpreted with extreme caution.

Small Body Size and Adaptation to Nutritional Stress

Segraves (this volume, pp. 199–203 cites work by Frisancho and others that indicates that reduced body size within a human population constitutes an adaptation to limited food resources by lowering the nutritional requirements for physical growth and body maintenance. She then states: "If, in fact, a physiological tolerance (such as that possibly conferred by reduced body size) for relatively more limited nourishment can reasonably be assumed to have developed over time in some proportion of the human population, then impairment of this population should not be anticipated" (Segraves, this volume, p. 202). I think that this statement requires some elaboration and comment.

I am in complete accord with findings by Frisancho, Sanchez, Pallardel, and Yanez (1973) and Stini (1972), among others, that there probably has been cross-generational genetic adaptation for smaller body size, and certainly ontologenical (developmental) adaptation limiting body size, among human populations living in areas in which malnutrition is prevalent. The smaller body is adaptive in that it has lower nutritional requirements and is thus able to survive and maintain a higher level of function at a lower nutritional plane. However, that populations adapt to nutritional stress through a decrease in body size does not mean that the nutritional stress has been overcome. It merely means that the population can effectively cope with a somewhat greater nutritional stress without pathological consequences. A more severe nutritional stress *exceeding* these new *limits* of adaptation will certainly have a detrimental effect on the physical and neurological growth and development and ultimately the survival of individual members of the population.

Summary

Severe malnutrition and "environmental impoverishment" both can have an effect on neurological development and behavioral capacity in studies with experimental animals. The simultaneous existence of both conditions leads to the most profound behavioral deficits, while "enriched" environments appear to ameliorate some portion of the behavioral deficits sustained by previously malnourished animals. These findings probably hold in humans; however, the relative impact of the deprivation stresses and the therapeutic benefit of enrichment has not been, and perhaps cannot be, precisely evaluated in human studies.

A growing number of investigations have described behavioral deficits in children who experienced some form of severe malnutrition for a prolonged period of time. Environmental impoverishment always co-varies with these nutritional stresses and probably has an influence on neurological and behavioral development equal to that of the malnutrition. It has been suggested (Pollitt, 1969; Latham, 1971) that the major impact of the nutritional stress is in the way it interferes with the child's interaction with its environment (maternal–infant, child–peer, child–physical), thus producing a form of environmental deprivation that itself leads to the neurological and behavioral deficits observed in these children.

The discussion in this chapter and in Thomson and Pollitt's paper indicates that there is obviously some controversy as to the impact of various types of PCM on behavioral development. The evidence is strongest for infantile marasmus. I have suggested that a reasonable case can be made for other types and degrees of PCM, especially when they coexist with "environmental impoverishment." We should also remember that specific deficiencies (lack of vitamins, minerals, especially iron) often coexist with PCM (Bengoa, 1974) and may also contribute to the pattern of behavioral retardation (Read, Stanbury, this volume).

Taking both nutritional and experiential factors into account, I have suggested that individuals with significant behavioral deficits *conservatively* account for 2–5% of the populations of many communities in Latin America, Africa, and Asia, in which PCM is prevalent. These figures may be considerably higher in areas in which iodine malnutrition is severe and goiter is hyperendemic.

MALNUTRITION AND SOCIAL ORGANIZATION

Malnutrition and Social Stratification

In her provocative chapter, Segraves (this volume) notes that malnutrition may be a consequence of differential access to strategic resources and is a function of the stratified nature of social systems. She argues that social stratification is a function of the size and complexity of social systems and maintains that a high percentage of individuals with behavioral limitations may be a *consequence* of this stratification but not a *cause*.

I concur with the position that malnutrition is a consequence rather than a cause of social stratification, and I agree with Segraves (pp. 193–195) that social stratification is generally a function of social size and complexity and, in some form and level of intensity, is a necessary prerequisite for social integration and stability. However, I do think that both of these points deserve some comment.

Widespread malnutrition in the lower strata of highly stratified social systems, due to the uneven distribution of essential resources, functions to preserve and potentiate the stratification in a very important way. The combined effects of malnutrition and "environmental impoverishment," both of which are a function of low social position, work synergistically to *create* a relatively large group of behaviorally limited individuals within the lower social strata. The high frequency of individuals with biologically based behavioral limitations of varying degrees in this group is, in a sense, the ultimate form of social control. It guarantees the self-perpetuation of the lower strata by assuring that there will be a group of individuals who are not capable of social mobility, irrespective of the existence of other forms of social restraint. The existence of significant numbers of these retarded individuals in the lower social strata reduces system strain by obviating the need for a heavy investment in other forms of social control. Thus, we can conceive of endemic malnutrition in this context not only as a consequence of intense social stratification that merely eliminates excessive population expansion but also as an important form of social control within highly stratified socieities that may be independent, to some degree, of population growth.

I believe that it is generally true that the prevalence of malnutrition within societies varies as a function of their degree of internal stratification and the relative power position of the society in the hierarchy of nation-states. As noted previously, the differential effects of malnutrition and environmental improverishment function to maintain the internal social hierarchy. The further pervasiveness of such behavioral retardation on a national level may reflect the environmentally determined poverty of a nation or, quite frequently, be a manifestation of extreme exploitation by external politico-economic interests. A foreign mercantile or colonial power usually desires a docile "native" population that will provide inexpensive labor for the production of primary products. The *unconscious* creation, or maintenance, of a broad stratum of behaviorally limited "natives" through an inequitable distribution of essential resources leading to chronic malnutrition is one way in which external forces (whether they be distant industrialized nations or a neighboring dominant ethnic group) maintain social control over subservient nation-states or societies.

   In summary, I still agree that malnutrition and a high prevalence of behavioral retardation are a consequence rather than a cause of social stratification. However, I suggest that these are not passive consequences that filter out of the system but are dynamic factors that feed back to serve important functions in the maintenance and potentiation of already existing highly stratified social systems.

Malnutrition and Overpopulation

   Segraves (p. 204) concludes that while malnutrition may produce a stress on certain subdivisions of biological populations, it does not constitute a lack stress for the sociocultural system as a whole (p. 205). In her view, one way in which populations adjust to the more important system-wide strain of overpopulation is through a higher rate of mortality and morbidity among their lower strata. Malnutrition among the poor, as a consequence of limited access to strategic resources, is one factor contributing to this differential mortality and morbidity (Segraves, p. 208). She suggests that a dispassionate view of the subject would lead us to conclude that, at the system level, malnutrition, although a local stress, serves the necessary function of limiting population expansion and thus alleviates a greater system-wide strain on sociocultural stability. Several of these points warrant further discussion.

   Historically, it certainly is true that malnutrition among lower social strata led to higher rates of morbidity and mortality in these groups and that this had some effect in adjusting to the strain of overpopulation. The ideologies that have supported most highly stratified social systems placed little value on the welfare of the lower strata. And there has been little or no awareness, until recent times, of the influence of environmental factors such as nutrition on human development.

However, ideologies have changed, as Mead (this volume, p. 263) has noted. The past 200 years—and on a worldwide basis, the last 30 years—have seen significant changes in the ideological underpinnings of many, or most, societies. The intensity of internal stratification has generally decreased, and most parts of the previously colonized world now possess governments that, at least nominally, represent the interests of their citizens. Governments are now involved in social welfare programs, whereas previously the poor rotted in the streets, or "outside the gates of Troye" (Segraves, this volume, p. 209).

At this point in time, malnutrition is not *so much* of a pruner of excess population as it has been in the past (though it certainly still operates in that fashion); instead, it has become a producer of relatively large numbers of individuals with some degree of behavioral limitation. Under the emergent humanistic democratic ideology, governments have greater obligations to these individuals than they did in the past.

These behaviorally limited individuals used to constitute part of a large pool of cheap labor within highly stratified societies that operated at low technological levels and were labor intensive; or these people were part of the lowest strata in certain more technologically advanced countries. Under the then-existing conditions, they were economically useful, and as noted above, most such societies owed them a low level of obligation. They thus contributed to system maintenance and created little or no strain.

In contrast, at the present level of technological intensification, the unskilled labor needs of societies have diminished enormously, and the basic level of competence required of workers (even tightening bolts on an assembly line) has increased significantly. Under the new ideology, wages, even at the minimum level, have increased markedly. The result of these factors is that individuals with behavioral limitations are incapable of many types of labor, or employers are unwilling to hire them at their level of competency for current wages. They thus remain unemployed. Whereas these behaviorally limited poor people were allowed to starve in the streets under the old order (thus reducing system strain), contemporary governments are ideologically committed to caring for them. However, the growing cost of such special maintenance and educational and medical programs can often lead to an *increase* in system strain.

Malnutrition may have had the consequence of limiting overpopula-

tion and reducing system
technological conditions. P
conditions, it has a much ˙
and through the creatior
some behavioral limit˙
sociocultural systems.
perative to eliminate
cost of widespread ˙
porary societies wi˙
tary terms, it is prc˙
with its social consequ˙

284

This is based on m˙
speculate that the ˙
not universal but ˙
Within the co˙
society in high˙
extremely do˙
severely re˙
ever, I su˙
als migh˙
less tr˙
grow˙
tim˙

I should add that I woulu
limit significantly population gru
very low technological levels. I thi˙
(Buchbinder, this volume) of regional pop˙
orous pioneering populations→ overpopulation→ ˙
radation→ endemic malnutrition, increased infection, iu˙
bidity, and increased mortality rates→ population declinu
vironmental recovery) aptly describes the sequence of events unu
these conditions. However, I doubt that under contemporary conditions, even among the less developed nations, that this effect in reliev-
ing system strain outbalances the strain caused by the behavioral
sequelae of endemic malnutrition.

The Influence of Cultural Context of the Personality Characteristics of Behaviorally Limited Individuals

Foulks (1972) and Foulks and Katz (this volume, p. 228) have discussed how certain types of hysterical behavior associated with hypocalcemia among North Alaskan Eskimos have become institutionalized
in shamanistic behavior. The high frequency of this aberrant behavior
has been fit into Eskimo culture so as to serve important social (group)
and psychological (individual) needs. Foulks and Katz have also
commented on Turnbull's study of personality change in response to
altered ecological conditions among the Ik (Turnbull, 1972) and
suggest further studies in this direction. I would like to offer some
brief *speculations* in relation to the personality characteristics of individuals who have behavioral limitations as a consequence of chronic
malnutrition and environmental deprivation.

In the discussion of my work in Ecuador and at several points
throughout this chapter, I have referred to individuals with severe and
moderate behavioral deficits as being docile and easily manipulable.

experience in Ecuador. I would now like to
ersonality characteristics of such individuals are
e greatly influenced by particular cultural contexts.
text of a traditional community in a highly stratified
and Ecuador, virtually all of these individuals were
cile. I believe that this would be the case for the most
rded individuals under almost any circumstances. How-
pect that the large numbers of *moderately* limited individu-
have been much less docile if they had spent their lives in a
ditional setting, such as in Quito. If such individuals were to
up in a poor urban ghetto in the United States at this point in
e, I would predict that rather than being docile they would proba-
y be extremely hostile.

A point by d'Aquili and Mihalik is extremely pertinent. These
authors suggest that the processes of cognitive structure formation and
transformation are severely impaired by early malnutrition (probably
in conjunction with early environmental deprivation) and that such
impairment of these functions would lead to "the imposition upon the
individual of rigid cognitive structures, which, once established,
would not undergo transformation even in the presence of overwhelming disconfirming evidence from the environment" (d'Aquili &
Mihalik, this volume).

I think that the extreme docility that I have described among these
individuals in Ecuador reflects an inflexible clinging to characteristics
of the modal personality (subservience) of the indigenous segment of
the community. I *wonder* whether individuals with similar behavioral
limitations, who may have been living in poor urban environments in
the United States in the late 1960s and early 1970s, might not have
manifested exaggeratedly hostile personalities that were a somewhat
inflexible rendition of the modal personal hostility that was characteristic of their environment at that point in time.

Behavioral Limitations and Social Flexibility

In their discussion of the effect of severe early malnutrition on the
cognitive structural transformation system, d'Aquili and Mihalik
(p. 250) note that

> furthermore, fairly severe PCM in large segments of a society is likely to
> decrease the number of individuals with variable options (transformations) of
> social institutions, as well as probably to decrease the number of options
> themselves. Without a sufficient number of individuals clustering around the
> principal alternatives to any given social structure, there simply will not exist
> enough viable variability on which selection can operate.

This is an extremely important point that goes to the core of the issues under discussion. Extinction through high rates of mortality directly associated with the combined effects of malnutrition and infectious disease is not the only threat to the survival of human breeding populations. A population surviving the ravages of severe malnutrition is likely to contain significant numbers of individuals with some degree of behavioral limitation. If the proportion of individuals with severe and moderate behavioral deficits is *extremely high* (Gajdusek, 1962; Greene, this volume; Stanbury, this volume), then we would expect the population to show a low degree of social flexibility as has been suggested by d'Aquili and Mihalik.

There would thus be a decrease in the total informational content of the sociocultural system, with relatively fewer individuals capable of expressing the full behavioral repertoire of the culture. The richness of the cultural tradition would decrease due to the fact that there are fewer "actors" capable of playing the requisite roles. Some social institutions, being meaningless to a large portion of the population, would be likely to diminish in elaboration or fall into decline. In sum, as d'Aquili and Mihalik have noted, there would be a decrease in sociocultural variability that would leave the population less responsive to change and thus at a selective disadvantage. Therefore, rather than resulting in the physical extinction of populations, endemic malnutrition is more often likely to lead to sociocultural rigidity and the dissolution of social units.

The model described above is applicable to the case in which fairly severe malnutrition affects virtually an entire population. In highly stratified societies, we would expect that endemic malnutrition and intercurrent infectious disease (along with "environmental deprivation") would produce some degree of social dissolution among the lower social strata, but that this dissolution would be molded and manipulated by the behaviorally and socioculturally intact upper strata. Further, we would expect that the elimination of the effects of endemic malnutrition, intercurrent infectious disease, and environmental deprivation among the lower strata would ultimately result in an increase in sociocultural cohesion among these strata and consequently an increased ability to effect social change.

I should add in passing that much of what has just been presented runs counter to Segraves' argument that biological and sociocultural systems are analytically separate entities (Segraves, pp. 205–206). In my view, sociocultural systems are systems of information that have been accumulated over time and that aid in adapting human populations to their environments. This accumulated information is collectively carried and transmitted by individual members of a society, each of whom carries a somewhat partial and discordant version of the totality of cultural data. Some people carry less (retarded individuals, people from all strata with limited experiences), and others carry more. The sociocultural system of a population is the aggregate of all the information carried by all members of the population. For the population, this information does not exist independently of its carriers. It must be carried and transmitted by people; thus, any factor (i.e., malnutrition) affecting the information-carrying capacity of a biological system (a human population) will ultimately have an effect on the sociocultural system.

Malnutrition: The Vulnerable and the Survivors

An important point that may need reiteration is that malnutrition is not and was not totally pervasive even in extremely poor isolated communities in which it is and was endemic or among the urban poor in industrialized societies. Even in these settings, the combined point prevalence of severe and moderate forms of PCM among children under 4 years of age is rarely over 30%. The exception, of course, is the case of famine. The reasons why some children become malnourished while others do not, and why the incidence of malnutrition is higher in some families than others, is uncertain and is presently the object of considerable inquiry (Richardson, 1976; Cravioto & DeLicardie, 1975). Constitutional factors, socioeconomic differences between families, family size, birth order, birth spacing, educational level, and personal hygiene of the parents (especially the mother) are all factors that contribute to the production of this variation (Richardson, 1976; Cravioto & DeLicardie, 1975; Greene, 1976; Montgomery, this volume).

As Mead (pp. 263, 264) has noted, many individuals emerge intact (physically, neurologically, psychologically) from developmental experiences under rather extreme conditions. I hope it is quite clear to the reader that despite our emphasis on people with behavioral deficits we expect the large majority of individuals in populations living under nutritional stress to be normal even if the stress is extreme and 25% of the population manifests moderate to severe neurological deficits (Greene, this volume). The remaining individuals in such populations have either avoided or survived these stresses. There is no question that most of these people do proceed to become useful members of their communities, or if they leave their place of birth, of society as a whole. This volume merely attempts to show how endemic malnutrition in combination with other factors (infectious disease, environmental impoverishment) may produce a broad spectrum of behavioral deficit in human populations and to indicate how this phenomenon may have a significant effect on the organization of human social units.

Ethical Implications

Mead (pp. 262–264) has raised many questions about the ethical implications of some of the issues that we have discussed. Perhaps the most poignant question revolves around the analysis of the relationship between malnutrition and overpopulation and the somewhat contrary positions taken by several of the contributors.

Segraves appears to view endemic malnutrition and high rates of mortality and morbidity among the poor as necessary consequences of overpopulation that have the positive effect of reducing system strain. Both Mead and Greene agree that this has certainly been a result of endemic malnutrition in the past but find it a morally unacceptable solution to the problem of overpopulation in the future. It certainly will be an inevitable consequence if present worldwide population trends do not moderate; however, a growing and more efficient technological ability to feed people and service human needs and to limit human births, coupled with a more equitable distribution of resources, both within and between nations, may provide a morally acceptable solution to present pressures on system stability. More likely than not, the *actual* if not the desired resolution of this complex problem on a worldwide basis will contain elements that are morally acceptable and other elements that are morally repulsive but probably less visible.

CONCLUSIONS

Data presented throughout this volume indicate that the simultaneous occurrence of early moderate-to-severe malnutrition, intercurrent infection, and environmental deprivation has a deleterious effect on neurological development and behavioral capacity in animal models and in humans. The exact nature of the interaction between different types and degrees of malnutrition and physical-social deprivation is unclear, yet environmental enrichment does appear to have an important effect in ameliorating the neurological and behavioral consequences of both PCM and iodine malnutrition.

288 Lawrence S. Greene

From 1 to 10% of the adults had severe neurological and behavioral deficits in several severely malnourished populations that have recently been studied, and there is some indication that another 15–20% of the adult members of these populations have more moderate neurological deficits and behavioral limitations. A variety of other data on the behavioral effects of PCM and its point prevalence in Latin America, Africa, and Asia suggests that anywhere from 2 to 20% of the people in many communities in these areas may have slight to moderate behavioral limitations. Few community studies of behavioral capacity, especially among adults, have been carried out. Existing studies among children have invariably sampled from among those attending schools; thus, the most behaviorally limited individuals have been selected out of these investigations. Community studies similar to that reported by Greene are needed in order to clarify the question of the degree and prevalence of such deficits in populations in which protein–calorie and other forms of malnutrition are endemic.

It appears that the past occurrence of endemic malnutrition, intercurrent infection, and environmental deprivation were likely to have been equal or greater in intensity and prevalence than present conditions among the lower social strata of many societies at different points in time. It seems reasonable to assume that under those conditions the prevalence of neurological deficits and behavioral limitations was particularly high in some populations.

The presence of relatively large numbers of individuals with behavioral limitations has a wide variety of influences on the sociocultural systems of human populations. There are ideational effects, structural effects, and effects on the culture-carrying capacity of social units. Under extreme conditions, these consequences may lead to the effective dissolution of social units.

Finally, we would be most pleased if this volume would stimulate social scientists to begin a more systematic analysis of sociocultural dynamics and change in terms of the effect of the differential division of environmental resources on the biologically based behavioral characteristics of human subpopulations.

REFERENCES

Ainsworth, M. D. S. The effects of maternal deprivation: A review of findings and controversy in the context of research strategy. In *Deprivation of maternal care: A reassessment of its effects*. World Health Organization Public Health Paper No. 14, Geneva: World Health Organization, 1962. Pp. 97–165.

Bengoa, J. M. The problem of malnutrition. *World Health Organization Chronicle,* 1974, *28,* 3–7.

Bennett, E. L., Rosenzweig, M. R., & Diamond, M. C. Time courses of effects of differential experience on brain measures and behavior of rats. In W. L. Bryne (Ed.), *Molecular approaches to learning and memory.* New York: Academic Press, 1970. Pp. 55–89.

Bingham, W. E., & Griffiths, W. J. The effect of differential environments during infancy on adult behavior in the rat. *Journal of Comparative and Physiological Psychology,* 1952, *45,* 307–312.

Botha-Antoun, E., Babayan, S., & Harfouche, J. K. Intellectual development related to nutritional status. *Journal of Tropical Pediatrics,* 1968, *14,* 112–115.

Champakam, S., Srikantia, S. G., & Gopalan, C. Kwashiorkor and mental development. *American Journal of Clinical Nutrition,* 1968, *21,* 844–850.

Cravioto, J., & DeLicardie, E. Longitudinal study of language development in severely malnourished children. In G. Serban (Ed.), *Nutrition and mental functions.* New York: Plenum, 1975. Pp. 143–191.

Cravioto, J., DeLicardie, E., & Birch, H. G. Nutrition, growth and neurointegrative development: An experimental and ecological study. *Pediatrics,* 1966, *38,* 319–372.

Davenport, J. W. Environmental therapy in hypothyroid and other disadvantaged animal populations. In R. N. Walsh & W. T. Greenough (Eds.), *Environments as therapy for brain dysfunction.* New York: Plenum, 1976. Pp. 71–114.

Davenport, J. W., Gonzalez, L. M., Carey, J. C., Bishop, S. B., & Hagquist, W. W. Environmental stimulation reduces learning deficits in experimental cretinism. *Science,* 1976, *191,* 578–579.

Edwards, L. D., & Craddock, L. J. Malnutrition and intellectual development. A study of school-age aboriginal children at Walgett, N.S.W. *Medical Journal of Australia,* 1973, *1,* 880–884.

Forgays, D. G., & Forgays, J. W. The nature of the effect of free-environmental experience in the rat. *Journal of Comparative and Physiological Psychology,* 1952, *45,* 322–328.

Foulks, E. *The arctic hysterias of the north Alaskan Eskimo.* Anthropological studies No. 10, David Maybury-Lewis (Ed.), Washington, D. C.: American Anthropological Association Press, 1972.

Fraňková, S. Nutritional and psychological factors in the development of spontaneous behavior in the rat. In N. S. Scrimshaw & J. E. Gordon (Eds.), *Malnutrition, learning, and behavior.* Cambridge, Massachusetts: MIT Press, 1968. Pp. 312–325.

Fraňková, S. Late consequences of early nutritional and sensoric deprivation in rats. *Activitas Nervosa Superior,* 1970, *12,* 155–156.

Fraňková, S. Influence of nutrition and early experience on behavior of rats. *Bibliotheca Nutritio e Dieta,* 1972, *17,* 96–110.

Frisancho, A. R., Sanchez, J., Pallardel, D., & Yanez, L. Adaptive significance of small body size under poor socio-economic conditions in southern Peru. *American Journal of Physical Anthropology,* 1973, *39,* 255–261.

Gajdusek, C. Congenital defects of the central nervous system associated with hyperendemic goiter in a Neolithic highland society of Netherlands New Guinea. I. Epidemiology. *Pediatrics,* 1962, *29,* 345–363.

Gluck, J. P., & Harlow, H. F. The effects of deprived and enriched rearing conditions on later learning: A review. In L. E. Jarrard (Ed.), *Cognitive processes of non human primates*. New York: Academic Press, 1971. Pp. 103–119.

Greene, L. S. Nutrition and behavior in highland Ecuador (Doctoral dissertation, University of Pennsylvania, 1976). (University Microfilms, 1976, 76–695).

Greenough, W. T., & Volkmar, F. R. Pattern of dendritic branching in rat occipital cortex after rearing in complex environments. *Experimental Neurology*, 1973, *40*, 491–504.

Greenough, W. T., Madden, T. C., & Fleischmann, T. B. Effects of isolation, daily handling, and enriched rearing on maze learning. *Psychonomic Science*, 1972, *27*, 279–280.

Harlow, H. F., Schlitz, K. A., & Harlow, M. K. Effects of social isolation on the learning performance of rhesus monkeys. In C. R. Carpenter (Ed.), *Proceedings of the Second International Congress of Primatology* (Vol. 1). New York: Karger, 1968. Pp. 178–185.

Hebb, D. O. *The organization of behavior*. New York: Wiley, 1949.

Hunt, J. McVicker. Environmental programming to foster competence and prevent mental retardation in infancy. In R. N. Walsh & W. T. Greenough (Eds.), *Environments as therapy for brain dysfunction*. New York: Plenum, 1976. Pp. 201–255.

Kelly, F. C., & Snedden, W. W. Prevalence and geographical distribution of endemic goitre. In *Endemic goitre*. World Health Organization Monograph Series, No. 44, Geneva: World Health Organization, 1960. Pp. 27–233.

Krech, D., Rosenzweig, M. R., & Bennett, E. L. Relations between brain chemistry and problem solving among rats raised in enriched and impoverished environments. *Journal of Comparative and Physiological Psychology*, 1962, *55*, 801–807.

Langer, P. History of goitre. In *Endemic goitre*. World Health Organization Monograph Series, No. 44, Geneva: World Health Organization, 1960. Pp. 9–25.

Latham, M. C. The effects of malnutrition on intellectual development and learning. *American Journal of Public Health*, 1971, *61*, 1307–1324.

Levitsky, D. A., & Barnes, R. H. Nutritional and environmental interactions in the behavioral development of the rat: Long term effects. *Science*, 1972, *176*, 68–71.

Mönckeberg, F., Tisler, S., Toro, S., Gattás, V., & Vega, L. Malnutrition and mental development. *American Journal of Clinical Nutrition*, 1972, *25*, 766–772.

Pollitt, E. Ecology, malnutrition, and mental development. *Psychosomatic medicine*, 1969, *31*, 193–200.

Querido, A. History of iodine prophylaxis with regard to cretinism and deaf-mutism. In J. B. Stanbury & R. L. Kroc (Eds.), *Human development and the thyroid gland. Relation to endemic cretinism*. New York: Plenum, 1972. Pp. 191–199.

Richardson, S. A. The influence of severe malnutrition in infancy on the intelligence of children at school age: An ecological perspective. In R. N. Walsh & W. T. Greenough (Eds.), *Environments as therapy for brain dysfunction*. New York: Plenum, 1976. Pp. 256–275.

Rosenzweig, M., Krech, D., Bennett, E., & Zolman, J. Variation in environmental complexity and brain measures. *Journal of Comparative and Physiological Psychology*, 1962, *55*, 1092–1095.

Rosenzweig, M. R., Bennett, E. L., & Diamond, M. C. Effects of differential environments on brain anatomy and brain chemistry. *Proceedings of the American Psychopathological Association*, 1967, *56*, 45–56.

Rosenzweig, M. R., Bennett, E. L., & Diamond, M. C. Brain changes in response to experience. *Scientific American*, 1972, *226*, 22–29.

Sackett, G. P., & Rupenthal, G. C. Development of monkeys after varied experiences during infancy. In S. A. Barnett (Ed.), *Ethology and Development*. Philadelphia: Lippincott, 1973. Pp. 52–87.

Scrimshaw, N. S. The effect of infection on nutritional status. *Bibliotheca Nutritio e Dieta*, 1973, *18*, 153–164.

Scrimshaw, N. S. Interactions of malnutrition and infection: Advances in understanding. In R. E. Olson (Ed.), *Protein calorie malnutrition*. New York: Academic Press, 1975.

Skeels, H. M. Adult status of children with contrasting early life experiences. *Monograph of the Society for Research in Child Development*, 1966, *31*, 1–56.

Skeels, H. M., & Dye, H. B. A study of the effects of differential stimulation of mentally retarded children. *Proceedings of the American Association for Mental Deficiency*, 1939, *44*, 114–136.

Stini, W. A. Reduced sexual dimorphism in upper arm muscle circumference associated with protein-deficient diet in a South American population. *American Journal of Physical Anthropology*, 1972, *36*, 341–351.

Stoch, M. B., & Smythe, P. M. Does undernutrition during infancy inhibit brain growth and subsequent intellectual development? *Archives of Disease in Childhood*, 1963, *38*, 546–552.

Stoch, M. B., & Smythe, P. M. The effect of undernutrition during infancy on subsequent brain growth and intellectual development. *South African Medical Journal*, 1967, *41*, 1027–1030.

Turnbull, C. *The mountain people*. New York: Simon & Schuster, 1972.

Walsh, R. N., & Cummins, R. A. Mechanisms mediating the production of environmentally induced brain changes. *Psychological Bulletin*, 1975, *82*, 986–1000.

Walsh, R.N., & Cummins, R.A. Neural responses to therapeutic environments. In R. Walsh & W. T. Greenough (Eds.), *Environments as therapy for brain dysfunction*. New York: Plenum, 1976. P. 171–200.

Walsh, R. N., Budtz-Olsen, O. E., Torok, A., & Cummins, R. A. Environmentally induced changes in the dimensions of the rat cerebrum. *Developmental Psychobiology*, 1971, *4*, 115–122.

Walsh, R. N., Cummins, R. A., Budtz-Olsen, O. E., O'Rourke, G., Brown, H., & Cameron, J. Effects of environmental enrichment and deprivation on cerebral histology and composition. *Proceedings of the Australian Society for Medical Research*, 1971, *2*, 478.

Walsh, R. N., Cummins, R. A., & Budtz-Olsen, O. E. Environmentally induced changes in the dimensions of the rat cerebrum: A replication and extension. *Developmental Psychobiology*, 1973, *6*, 3–8.

Wells, A. M., Geist, C. R., & Zimmermann, R. R. Influence of environmental and nutritional factors on problem solving in the rat. *Perceptual and Motor Skills*, 1972, *35*, 235–244.

Winick, M., Meyer, K. K., & Harris, R. C. Malnutrition and environmental enrichment by early adoption. *Science*, 1975, *190*, 1173–1175.

Yarrow, L. J. Maternal deprivation: Toward an empirical and conceptual reevaluation. *Psychological Bulletin*, 1961, *58*, 459–490.

Index